£50.00

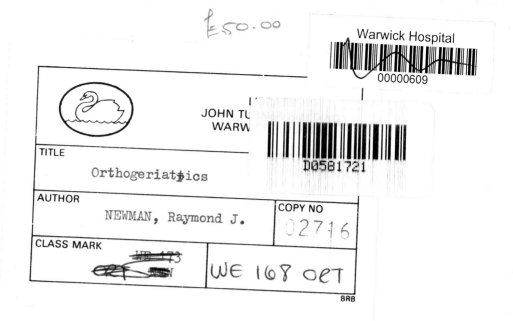

Orthogeriatrics

This volume is dedicated to my children
Esther Penelope Anne
and
Jonathan Philip Simeon
with the sincere hope that by the time they reach their old age
advances yet to be made in preventive medicine render the techniques
described in this book of historical interest only

ORTHOGERIATRICS
Comprehensive Orthopaedic Care for the Elderly Patient

Edited by

Raymond J. Newman BSc, MB ChB, DPhil, FRCS, FRCS (Ed), FRSH
Senior Lecturer in Orthopaedic Surgery, University of Leeds
Hunterian Professor and Member Court of Examiners, Royal College of Surgeons of England
Honorary Consultant Orthopaedic Surgeon, St James's University Hospital, Leeds

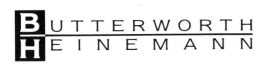

Butterworth–Heinemann Ltd
Linacre House, Jordan Hill, Oxford OX2 8DP

 PART OF REED INTERNATIONAL BOOKS

OXFORD   LONDON   BOSTON
MUNICH   NEW DELHI   SINGAPORE   SYDNEY
TOKYO   TORONTO   WELLINGTON

First published 1992

© Butterworth–Heinemann Ltd 1992

British Library Cataloguing in Publication Data
Orthogeriatrics.
  I. Newman, Raymond J.
  616.70084
ISBN 0 7506 1371 8

Typeset by Latimer Trend & Company Ltd, Plymouth, Devon
Printed in Great Britain at the University Press, Cambridge

Contents

Contributors

Dr **Jeffrey K. Aronson**, MA, MB, DPhil, FRCP
Clinical Reader in Clinical Pharmacology
   (Wellcome Lecturer),
MRC Unit and
University Department of Clinical
   Pharmacology,
Radcliffe Infirmary,
Oxford, UK

Dr **William E. Bagnall**, BSc, FRCP
Consultant Physician and Clinical Director –
   Medicine,
Department of Medicine for the Elderly,
St James's University Hospital,
Leeds, UK

Mrs **Diana Brahams**,
Barrister at Law,
15 Old Square,
Lincoln's Inn,
London, UK

Mr **Joseph J. Dias**, MD, FRCS (Ed)
Consultant Orthopaedic Surgeon,
Leicester Royal Infirmary and
Glenfield General Hospital,
Leicester, UK

Professor **Robert A. Dickson**, MA, ChM,
   FRCS, FRCS (Ed)
Professor of Orthopaedic Surgery,
St James's University Hospital,
Leeds, UK

Mr **David L. Douglas**, MD, FRCS (Ed)
Consultant Orthopaedic Surgeon,
Royal Hallamshire Hospital,
Sheffield, UK

Professor **Ian F. Goldie**, MD, PhD
Professor of Orthopaedic Surgery,
Karolinska Institute,
Karolinska Hospital,
Stockholm, Sweden

Mr **Richard J. Fordham**, BA, MA
Senior Lecturer in Health Economics and
   Management,
Centre for Advanced Studies,
Division of Health Sciences,
Curtin University of Technology,
Perth, Australia

Mr **Amar S. Jain**, MB, FRCS (Ed)
Consultant Orthopaedic Surgeon,
Royal Infirmary, Dundee
and Consultant in Charge,
Dundee Limb Fitting Centre,
Dundee, Scotland

Professor **Leslie Klenerman**, ChM, FRCS,
   FRCS (Ed)
Professor of Orthopaedic Surgery,
University Department of Orthopaedic and
   Accident Surgery,
Royal Liverpool University Hospital,
Liverpool, UK

Mr **Peter A. Millner**, BSc, FRCS
Orthopaedic Surgeon,
St James's University Hospital,
Leeds, UK

Professor **Graham P. Mulley**, DM, FRCP
Developmental Professor of Medicine for the
   Elderly,
St James's University Hospital,
Leeds, UK

Mr **Raymond J. Newman**, BSc, DPhil, FRCS,
   FRCS (Ed), FRSH
Senior Lecturer in Orthopaedic Surgery,
St James's University Hospital,
Leeds, UK

PD Dr **Dietmar Pennig**, MD
Director, Department of Trauma and
   Reconstructive Surgery,
St Vinzenz Hospital,
Köln, Germany

Professor **David I. Rowley**, B Med Biol, MD,
   FRCS (Ed)
Professor of Orthopaedic and Trauma
   Surgery,
Royal Infirmary,
Dundee, Scotland

Dr **Richard Sainsbury**, MB, ChB, FRACP
Senior Lecturer/Physician,
Department of Health Care of the Elderly,
The Princess Margaret Hospital,
Christchurch, New Zealand

Mr **Paul G. Stableforth**, MB, FRCS
Consultant Orthopaedic and Trauma Surgeon,
Bristol Royal Infirmary,
Bristol, UK

Professor **Jack Stevens**, MD, FRCS, FACS
Emeritus Professor of Orthopaedic and
   Traumatic Surgery,
University of Newcastle-upon-Tyne,
Newcastle-upon-Tyne, UK

Dr **Stephen R. Swindells**, BSc, FFARCS
Consultant Anaesthetist,
St James's University Hospital,
Leeds, UK

Professor **Anthony M. Warnes**, BA, PhD
Age Concern Institute of Gerontology,
King's College,
University of London,
London, UK

Foreword

It is becoming more popular in medical writing to combine derivatives from the ancient Greek language to find a descriptive term to cover a new field of clinical activity. The author has culled a hybrid, *Orthogeriatrics*, rather than using two words, *Geriatric orthopaedics*, but often the hybrid variety grows stronger than the single strain and this may well occur here.

It is excellent to see the result of combining surgical and medical disciplines in one book and covering such an important age group. In the 1981 Report of the Working Party on Orthopaedic Services to the Secretary of State for Social Services which I chaired, observations were made on the critical state of orthopaedic care for elderly patients. Because of this a recommendation was made that geriatric orthopaedic units should be formed since the perceived benefits of this method of rehabilitation would reduce the period that elderly patients remain in hospital, and in so doing, would shorten waiting times for elective orthopaedic procedures. St James's University Hospital in Leeds was one of the first to take up this recommendation. It is therefore most appropriate that a group of combined specialists from Leeds should provide the stage for this important publication. Michael Devas in Hastings has shown how many problems in geriatric orthopaedics can be solved by special units providing the basis for inter-disciplinary cooperation among staff. New knowledge and techniques subsequently spread from such a unit throughout the hospital and then into the wider community.

This textbook consists of a series of well written essays by many experts ranging from the demography of ageing, health resources, the special anaesthetic requirements of the elderly, appropriate medicines and drugs, the medico-legal aspects of ageing, to descriptions of many orthopaedic conditions and injuries as well as their treatment. It provides a thoroughly good read and should interest not only geriatricians and orthopaedic surgeons at all levels but also managers and administrators who must now appreciate the magnitude of the problems in this group of people. This book should provide the lever to obtain adequate resources and initiatives for caring for the aged, and should go far towards balancing the countless publications about hips, knees, spines and hands etc., each one concerned only with anatomical areas and not the whole person.

Robert B. Duthie
Nuffield Professor of
Orthopaedic Surgery
University of Oxford

Preface

Cast me not away in the time of age:
Forsake me not when my strength faileth me.
Prayer Book, 1662

The elderly are an important but often neglected group of patients who currently form approximately 15% of our population. However, over the course of the next 30 years this proportion will rise to at least 20%. Despite our growing awareness of their needs they are still not expected by many to enjoy painfree physical activity in the twilight of their life or qualify for elective surgery. I consider that the aged members of our population are at least entitled to this but when caring for them one must realize that the presentation of disease in this age group is unusual and often misleading. Furthermore, the ageing process confers a higher risk for surgery.

It is facile for an orthopaedic surgeon to consider himself not only to be a technical wizard but also to be sufficiently trained to deal with the many and varied medical, social and rehabilitative problems of the aged. Individuals in their 70s and 80s require a level of expertise comparable in many ways to that provided for a neonate. In the same way that mismanagement of the young can be disastrous so mismanagement of the elderly can be fatal. The only way that aged patients can be safely taken through their acute and elective orthopaedic surgery is by a collaborative approach with colleagues in different specialties and I hope that the wide choice of contributors chosen for this book emphasizes this point to the reader.

The neologism 'orthogeriatrics' has been coined to describe this collaborative approach but its etymological derivation is somewhat obscure. It is clearly a hybrid of two other words,

orthopaedics and geriatric. 'Orthos' is derived from Greek; *ortho* means straight, normal or correct whilst *pais* means child (*Dorland's Illustrated Medical Dictionary*). The word 'geriatric' was coined by Nascher in 1942. Once more its derivation is from the Greek with *geras* meaning old age and *iatrike* indicating medical involvement (*Dorland's Illustrated Medical Dictionary*). More comprehensively the British Geriatric Society defines geriatric medicine 'as that part of general medicine concerned with the preventative, social, diagnostic and remedial aspects of disease in old age'. Etymologically therefore, orthogeriatric literally means 'the medical straightening out or correction of old age!' However, it is currently applied to that collaborative rehabilitation process of elderly patients with orthopaedic conditions that is performed jointly by orthopaedic surgeons and geriatricians.

My interest in the field of orthogeriatrics was kindled during a period as lecturer in the University Department of Orthopaedic Surgery in Glasgow. There I was responsible for the day-to-day administration of patients on the so-called 'OGU' (orthogeriatric unit) at Gartnaval General Hospital. The remarkable rehabilitative achievements of that unit fascinated me and I continued my interest after moving to Leeds.

Here I decided to write a book on the subject with the aim of interesting not only surgeons and their trainees but also geriatric and general physicians. I also hope that general practitioners, nurses, physiotherapists and occupational therapists will find time to read it since it is essential that they also know how and when orthopaedic surgery can help an aged patient. Only in this way will orthopaedic procedures be made freely available to the elderly and not denied from those for whom it can impart significant benefit.

I would like to thank the medical illustration department in this hospital for preparing many of the figures, Dr Paul Butt for providing appropriate advice on radiology, Pamela Edmonson, Wendy Buswell and Denise Stirling of the physiotherapy and occupational therapy departments for their suggestions regarding the physical aspects of rehabilitation and Mrs Helen Radcliffe for typing so many drafts of the manuscript. Mr Peter Millner kindly undertook the daunting task of proofreading, for which I am grateful.

Finally, I should like to thank my wife Sandra Irene for her patience and skill in assisting in the editorship of this volume and for ungrudgingly spending many hours checking over manuscripts and figures – an ageing process in itself!

Raymond J. Newman
Leeds

References

Dorlands Illustrated Medical Dictionary, 24th edition. Saunders, London, 1965

Fletcher, P. J., MacMahon, D. G. (1989) The orthogeriatric unit – a suitable case for audit. *Care of the Elderly*, **1**, 170–174

Nascher, I. R. (1914) *Geriatrics: the Diseases of Old Age and Their Treatment*, Blakistons, Philadelphia.

A Crabbit Old Woman wrote this:

What do you see, nurses, what do you?
Are you thinking when you are looking at me—
A crabbit old women, not very wise,
Uncertain of habit, with far-away eyes,
Who dribbles her food and makes no reply
When you say in a loud voice 'I do wish you'd try.'
Who seems not to notice the things that you do,
And forever is losing a stocking or shoe.
Who unresisting or not, lets you do as you will,
With bathing and feeding, the long day to fill.
Is that what you are thinking, is that what you see?
Then open your eyes, nurse, you're not looking at me.
I'll tell you who I am as I sit here, so still;
As I do at your bidding, as I eat at your will,
I'm a small child of ten with a father and mother,
Brothers and sisters, who love one another.
A young girl of sixteen with wings on her feet,
Dreaming that soon a lover she'll meet;
A bride soon at twenty—my heart gives a leap,
Remembering the vows that I promised to keep;
At twenty-five now I have young of my own,
A woman of thirty, my young now grow fast,
Bound to each other with ties that should last;
At forty, my young sons have grown and are gone,
And my man's beside me to see I don't mourn;
At fifty once more babies play round my knee,
Again we know children, my loved one and me.
Dark days are upon me, my husband is dead,
I look at the future, I shudder with dread,
For my young are all rearing young of their own,
And I think of the years and the love that I've known.
I'm an old woman now and nature is cruel—
'Tis her jest to make old age look like a fool.
The body it crumbles, grace and vigour depart,
There is now a stone where I once had a heart;
But inside this old carcass a young girl still dwells,
And now and again my battered heart swells.
I remember the joys, I remember the pain,
And I'm loving and living life over again.
I think of the years all too few—gone too fast,
And accept the stark fact that nothing can last.
So open your eyes, nurses, open and see
Not a crabbit old woman, look closer—see ME.

*This poem was found among the possessions of an old lady
after her death in a Dundee hospital. A copy was given to every
nurse and it has since been reproduced in several journals.*

1

Demographic processes and health forecasts

Anthony M. Warnes

The process of demographic ageing

The ageing of the population and its attendant sociodemographic changes have a prominent place in current public debates and political concerns in Britain, the United States and other affluent countries. A sound understanding of the long-term trends and underlying processes is unfortunately rarer and alarmist interpretations abound of the implications of the progression of ageing. This chapter provides brief digests of the key definitions and processes of age structure change and of recent demographic trends and forecasts for Britain (with a glance at the situation elsewhere). It concludes with an examination of the demographic component of current trends in the prevalence of specific disorders.

Under the most favourable genetic and environmental conditions humans may display impressive longevity. However, survival beyond 110 years is extremely rare (Hayflick, 1987; Kannisto, 1988). The mean age of death even in the most privileged societies and social groups barely exceeds 80 years. For most practical purposes the age structure of a national population may be understood through its dynamics over the previous century, i.e. the present and past levels of fertility, mortality and migration transfers. If for example marriages and births were relatively low during a period of economic recession, as was the case in Europe during the 1920s and 1930s, then 60 years later the number of people entering the conventionally-defined elderly age groups will fall temporarily, as has been the case during the 1980s and 1990s.

The prime determinant of the age structure and mean age of a large national population is fertility. This is best demonstrated by mathematical models of the stable population structure achieved after many generations with different combinations of fertility and mortality schedules. A population with a crude birth rate (CBR) close to the highest in modern human populations, e.g. 40 per 1000 per annum, sees large numbers of children added each year to its base. Within 20 years these augmented age groups themselves begin to reproduce at the high rate. However low the level of mortality and however high the average life expectancy, old people never exceed 1 in 10 of the population. The converse situation is when fertility is exceptionally low with CBRs below 10. Even without exceptional longevity in the population, those that survive beyond 60 years form a much greater share of the total population. The reason why populations in modern, developed countries have unprecedentedly high representations of elderly people is that for the first time (at least in many centuries) exceptionally low fertility and unprecedentedly low mortality have been achieved (Myers, 1985).

Different countries are at different stages of the process of demographic ageing. European populations have been ageing since the beginning of the century and the momentum is receding. In North America and Australasia the growth in numbers is presently high but will shortly decline. It is in other world regions which have recently experienced significant fertility decline (notably Latin America and south-east Asia) that the most rapid increases in the elderly population will occur in the near future (Warnes, 1989b).

People of 60 years and over form one-fifth of the population in the United Kingdom and Scandinavian nations, and projections suggest

Table 1.1 The population aged 60 years and over and 80 years and over during 1980–2000 (millions)

Country	Age 60–79 years				Age 80+ years			
	1980 (No.)	(%)	2000 (No.)	(%)	1980 (No.)	(%)	2000 (No.)	(%)
France	7.6	14.3	9.3	16.6	1.4	2.7	1.5	2.7
West Germany	9.9	16.3	11.6	19.8	1.5	2.4	1.6	2.8
Sweden	1.6	18.9	1.4	17.8	0.2	2.9	0.3	4.1
United States	29.6	13.2	34.2	13.0	4.3	1.9	5.8	2.2
United Kingdom	9.7	17.4	9.5	17.1	1.4	2.5	1.8	3.3

Source: United Nations Organization (1985) Tables 37 and 38

that their share will exceed one-quarter by 2025 in Austria, Belgium, Denmark, Finland, France, Germany, Italy, the Netherlands, Norway, Sweden, Switzerland and the United Kingdom (United Nations Organization, 1985). The younger elderly population, aged 60–79 years, is decreasing absolutely and relatively in Sweden and the UK during the period 1980–2000, alongside substantial increases in the population of 80 years and over (Table 1.1). France and Germany are presently witnessing rapid growth of their elderly populations as the post-First World War birth cohorts move into old age.

The marked change in the British age structure during this century which has taken the over 60s share from around 6% at its beginning to 20% today, is not therefore a new phenomenon. It has been in train since the earliest years of this century in most European countries (it began earlier in France). Arguably it is now largely spent. We have accommodated the main weight of the likely age-structure change, without, it appears, great damage to the general social welfare or prosperity. Certainly on a global scale it is the less developed countries that will have the fastest elderly population growth and the most challenging problems of service provision. In 1980 25% of the world's elderly people were European, but by 2025 it is expected that 71% will be in the less developed countries and only 12% in Europe (Torrey, Kinsella and Taeuber, 1987; Kinsella, 1988; Martin, 1988).

Migration and the distribution of elderly people

National statistics and forecasts are invaluable in the monitoring of aggregate population structures and for formulating national policies and budgets but a poor guide to regional and local trends. The age structure of small geographical

areas, such as hospital or general medical practice catchments, is more variable and temporally unstable than in larger areas such as health regions and they, in turn, have greater variability than national territories. The principal mechanism producing local variations is the age and social selectivity of migrations although regional variations in mortality are still significant. For example, new housing estates attract disproportionate numbers of young families and lead to a sharp rise in the demand for maternity services.

Local assessments of the likely treatment load from elderly people must examine the migrations into and from the district by older people. Since the 1950s they have shown an increasing propensity to migrate relatively long distances for and during retirement. Approximately 10% of the cohorts reaching retirement since the late 1950s have undertaken these 'total displacement' migrations in Britain. They are most common among owner-occupiers, married couples, middle and upper income groups, people in good health, and the population of the largest cities (Table 1.2) During the 1970s and early 1980s, approximately one-quarter of new retirees resident in Greater London and several surrounding Home Counties districts left the metropolitan region. These moves, unlike the migrations undertaken by people of working age, are focused on favoured destination regions and not usually balanced by reverse flows. They therefore lead to exceptional concentrations of elderly people, particularly in rural and coastal areas which do not attract large numbers of working-age migrants, e.g. north Norfolk and central Wales (Warnes, 1987). Recently, data from the National Health Service Central Register (NHSCR) of patients have provided a near-continuous record of inter-county and inter-Health Authority migration and can be used for detailed projections (Stillwell, Boden and Rees,

Table 1.2 Migration rates by distance—sex, age and marital status, Britain 1980–81

Age group	Rates of migration within Britain over 1 year per 100 persons					
	All moves		Inter-county		Intra-county district	
	M	F	M	F	M	F
Single persons						
50–54	5.16	4.67	1.04	1.03	3.42	3.03
55–59	4.85	4.24	0.88	1.03	3.39	2.74
60–64	4.64	4.51	0.85	1.21	3.27	2.84
65–69	4.83	3.86	0.87	0.82	3.47	2.66
70–74	4.19	3.80	0.62	0.69	3.15	2.75
75+	4.45	5.10	0.70	0.80	3.19	3.64
Married persons						
50–54	4.03	3.72	0.97	0.89	2.55	2.38
55–59	3.55	3.58	0.84	0.94	2.29	2.23
60–64	3.67	3.88	1.02	1.12	2.26	2.38
65–69	4.15	3.75	1.21	0.97	2.54	2.42
70–74	3.46	3.27	0.79	0.73	2.33	2.23
75+	3.35	3.38	0.69	0.68	2.33	2.35
Widowed persons						
50–54	5.28	5.54	1.09	1.04	3.60	3.94
55–59	4.70	5.32	0.88	1.08	3.28	3.71
60–64	4.83	5.50	0.97	1.15	3.36	3.81
65–69	5.27	5.08	1.09	1.01	3.64	3.58
70–74	4.97	4.89	0.99	0.94	3.45	3.47
75+	5.95	5.85	1.18	1.09	4.00	4.04

Source: Office of Population Censuses and Surveys (1983)

1990). An increasing rate of migration after the age of 75 years has also been detected from national register data in Belgium and The Netherlands and from the Office of Population Censuses and Surveys (OPCS) Longitudinal Study and NHSCR data (Grundy, 1987). These moves are mainly short-distance and, apart from migrations away from poorly serviced and remote rural areas, tend to be counterbalanced by reverse flows and not to change the distribution of areas of under- and over-representation.

At the regional level in Britain, the share of the pensionable population ranged in 1980 from 16.1% in the West Midlands to 20.7% in the South West. The range for the over 75 year population was 4.9 to 7.0% in the same regions. Among local authority districts, the pensionable population ranged from more than one-third in Eastbourne, Worthing and Rother (Bexhill) in Sussex, to less than 10% in Tamworth and Cumbernauld and Kilsyth. The fastest growth of the pensionable population between 1971 and 1981 was, however, in new towns and growing suburbs like Stevenage (72%) and Crawley, Cumbernauld, Harlow, Corby and Bracknell

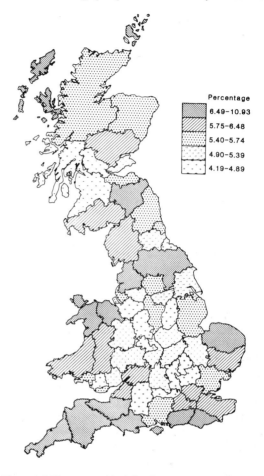

Figure 1.1 The geographical distribution of the population aged 75 years or over in Great Britain in 1981

(all over 50%). Losses of more than 5% were sustained in a dozen London boroughs and in Brighton, Worthing and Bournemouth (Law and Warnes, 1984). Areas with over-representations of the elderly population have a clear peripheral distribution in England and Wales and include all non-industrial coastal areas (Figure 1.1). Absolute numbers are concentrated in the urban-industrial core of the country, from West Yorkshire and Lancashire through the Midlands to South Wales and the Home Counties.

Trends in late age mortality and morbidity

Short-term forecasts of the change in an area's elderly population can assume a continuation of

Table 1.3 Age-specific death rates per 1000 per year, England and Wales 1961–87

Year	Males				Females			
	55–64	*65–74*	*75–84*	*85 +*	*55–64*	*65–74*	*75–84*	*85 +*
1961	21.9	54.7	124.4	256.9	10.8	30.9	87.8	214.1
1966	21.3	53.5	119.2	259.2	10.2	28.5	80.0	203.3
1971	20.1	50.5	113.0	231.8	10.0	26.1	73.6	185.7
1976	19.6	50.3	116.4	243.5	10.1	26.0	74.6	196.6
1981	17.7	45.6	105.2	226.5	9.5	24.1	66.2	178.2
1986	16.6	42.9	101.1	214.7	9.2	23.4	62.5	171.0
1987	16.0	41.2	96.3	191.6	9.1	20.8	60.1	158.6
Ratios of change over time								
1987:1961	0.73	0.75	0.77	0.75	0.84	0.67	0.68	0.74
1987:1976	0.82	0.82	0.83	0.79	0.90	0.80	0.81	0.81

Age-specific death rates, male:female ratios

		55–64	*65–74*	*75–84*	*85 +*
	1961	2.02	1.77	1.42	1.20
	1987	1.76	1.98	1.60	1.21

Sources: Office of Population Censuses and Surveys (1985) Table 20, and Office of Population Censuses and Surveys (1989b) Tables 1 and 3, HMSO, London

present mortality and migration rates and trends. Extrapolation is however an unsatisfactory technique for prediction beyond a decade. Given both the irrelevance of fertility to the number of elderly people up to 60 years ahead and the virtual impossibility of predicting birth rates so far into the future, the main opportunity for improving elderly population forecasts is to refine the mortality component. The greater our understanding of recent improvements in late-age mortality, the more reliable our forward projections.

During this century, child and working-age mortality has fallen more than that in old age. Deaths are now heavily concentrated in old age. In both the United States and Britain since the 1960s, there have been unexpected improvements in late age mortality. Official projections have repeatedly underestimated the growth of the over 70s and over 80s populations. Between 1961 and 1987 in England and Wales, mortality after the age of 65 years declined by around 24% for males and 30% for females (Table 1.3). The improvement has been greatest at ages 65–74 years for both sexes. The considerable male mortality disadvantage among those aged 55–64 years has moderated since 1961 but it continues to widen among those aged 65–84 years. As very low death rates are attained by successively older quinquennial age groups, it may be expected that their rates of improvement will slow, with the turndown first being evident for

females. The peak male to female ratio will shift to higher ages.

Substantial differentials in age-specific mortality rates by income, social group and region are still found within rich countries: there is considerable room for further improvement (Hunter, Kalache and Warnes, 1988). Age-specific death rates for those aged 50–74 years in Japan are at least 30% lower than in the United Kingdom and they are also substantially lower in Sweden. Mean life expectancy at birth improved considerably during 1960–87 in the richest 25 countries of the world, but the 5% gain in the United Kingdom was among the lowest and compares unfavourably with a 16% gain in Japan. The comparison for old-age mortality is more chastening: mean life expectancy at age 60 years improved since 1960 by 10% in the UK compared with 33% improvement in Japan (Table 1.4). Among octogenarians, the United States appears to have made most progress recently, including significant reductions in racial and geographical differences (Wing *et al.*, 1990).

Controversy over the causes of improving health continues, even for the nineteenth century decline in infectious morbidity and mortality, and is acute with respect to recent gains among the elderly population, not least because of the prevalence of multiple and degenerative disorders. Other problems are that good quality morbidity data are scarce and mortality data are

Table 1.4 International comparisons of average life expectancy at 0 and 60 years, 1960–87

Country	Life expectancy at birth						Life expectancy at 60 years					
	1960		1987		1987:1960		1960		1987		1987:1960	
	M	F	M	F	M	F	M	F	M	F	M	F
United States	66.7	73.3	71.5	78.3	1.07	1.07	15.9	19.6	18.2	22.5	1.14	1.15
France	67.0	73.6	72.0	80.3	1.07	1.09	15.6	19.5	18.4	23.7	1.18	1.22
Sweden	71.2	74.9	74.2	80.2	1.04	1.07	17.3	19.3	18.7	23.1	1.08	1.20
Japan	65.4	70.3	75.6	81.4	1.16	1.16	14.9	17.9	19.9	24.0	1.34	1.34
United Kingdom	68.3	74.2	71.9	77.6	1.05	1.05	15.3	19.3	16.8	21.2	1.10	1.10
Ratio UK:Japan	1.04	1.06	0.95	0.95	0.91	0.91	1.02	1.07	0.84	0.88	0.82	0.82
Ratio UK:France	1.02	1.01	1.00	0.97	0.98	0.96	0.98	1.08	0.91	0.89	0.94	0.90

Source: Organization for Economic Cooperation and Development (1990) Tables 50–55

often aggregated for open-ended large spans of the older age groups.

It is clear that during the twentieth century the survival curve has shifted upwards and to the right (Figure 1.2). By the first years of this century infant mortality had improved sufficiently in the United States for a notable benchmark in human welfare to be crossed: 50% of those born could expect to live for more than one-half of the maximum recorded human life span, i.e. 57 years. Nothing comparable had

been achieved before, even in privileged or aristocratic populations (Hendricks and Hendricks, 1986). Further substantial improvements have been achieved taking average life expectancy to the high 70s in many Western populations.

While the life-expectancy advance can be described, our understanding of the reasons and determinants is no more than propositional. Consequently, there is no attested model for the projection of mortality rates or life expectancy over the next 50 years and opposing theses

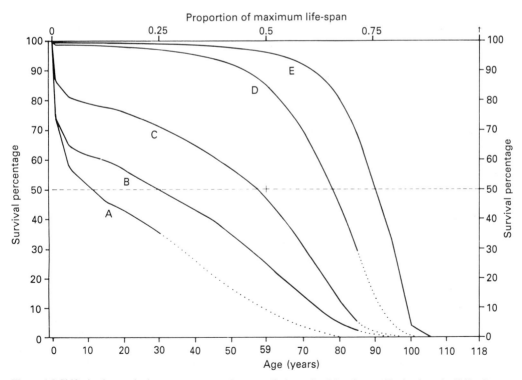

Figure 1.2 Shifts in the survival curve among modern populations: A—Manchester, England, early 1840s; B—United States, non-white males, 1900–2; C—United States, white males, 1900–2; D—United States, all males, 1982; E—hypothetical Western population with minimum disorders (Source: Warnes, 1989b, Fig. 5.1)

circulate and clash. One view (Fries, 1980, 1989) is that the maximum possible mean life expectancy had been approached in the 1970s, that further improvements would decelerate and the male to female mortality disadvantage narrow. Fries argues that the survival curve will become increasingly rectangular: it will advance to the right a little further, but mortality in middle age and early old age will continue to decline. He also believes that age-specific incidence rates for chronic illnesses will decrease faster than age-specific mortality rates, on the grounds that the United States population has been engaged in a 'national health habit experiment', which has reduced its exposure to widely-recognized risk factors such as tobacco smoking, the consumption of saturated fats and traffic accidents, e.g. through wearing seat belts.

This thesis underpins Fries's prediction that the variability in ages of death will fall. He expects higher proportions of the population to survive until near the modal age of death, following which the survival curve will descend more steeply than at present. The projected reduction of the duration of chronic illness implies a per capita reduction in health care costs, a forecast which caught the attention of government financial planners. If Fries is right the increase in the number of elderly people, and their heightened health expectations and demands, will be partly offset by delays in disease incidence and decreases in prevalence.

The opposing view is that further significant gains in average life expectancy can occur. Its proponents argue that there is no evidence yet that a 'ceiling' has been reached as data reported below for Japan confirm. Many also dispute the suggestion that age-specific mortality is falling faster than morbidity and argue the converse – that as the lethality of some of the most common disorders in later life is reduced, the duration of illness is increasing. In the absence of radical breakthroughs in our understanding of human ageing, an upper limit to mean life expectancy must exist. Its value will only be calculable when the distribution is specified of potential life spans in a supremely privileged population, i.e. in the (virtual) absence of environmental insults including disease. While attempts have been made to differentiate pre-senile (anticipated or avoidable) deaths from those attributable to senescence, the allocation is not yet supported by sufficient empirical evidence (Benjamin, 1989).

Forecasts of the elderly population

Projections of the size and the age and sex structure of the population of Britain are produced every 2 years by the Government Actuary in collaboration with the Office of Population Censuses and Surveys. Careful explanations of the assumptions about future fertility, mortality and external migration are given. The latest 1987-based projections to 2027 (with extrapolations to 2057) use the substantially revised assumptions introduced 2 years before, which significantly lowered the anticipated mortality rates (Warnes, 1989a).

The foundation for these changes is a detailed analysis of recent trends in the most common causes of death, ischaemic heart disease, lung cancer, bronchitis, asthma and emphysema, and other neoplasms (Alderson and Ashwood, 1985; Alderson, 1988). A substantial decrease in lung cancer mortality is predicted for males and an increase for females aged over 75 years. The new assumptions concerning overall late-age mortality rates are that they decline until 1991–92 at the same rates as recent years and then as assumed for the final 35 years of the 1985–2025 projections. The rate of improvement declines geometrically, halving every 10 years, and the rates fall over 40 years by about one-quarter for males and one-fifth for females (OPCS, 1987). Two minor adjustments in the 1987-based series are that for the first time there are projections of deaths from AIDS and methodological changes have reduced the projected numbers aged over 90 years.

Under these assumptions male life expectancy at birth rises from 72.4 years on 1987–88 mortality rates to 75.7 years in 2027, and female life expectancy from 78.0 to 80.5 years (OPCS, 1989a). The population aged 60–74 years will decrease during the 1990s by around 400,000 (Table 1.5). The total pensionable population will remain at about 10.5 million for the rest of the century and increase thereafter at about 1% per annum until a peak of 14.5 million around 2034. This surge reflects the relatively high birth rates experienced in the UK from the end of the Second World War until the mid-1960s. The subsequent period of low birth rates is likely to be reflected in a decline of the pensionable population after 2034 to 13.4 million by 2057 despite the assumed low mortality. Of particular interest for several hospital specialities including orthopaedics and geriatrics are the trends in the

Table 1.5 Projections of the elderly population of Great Britain 1987–2057

Age group	1991 M	1991 F	1996 M	1996 F	2001 M	2001 F	2011 M	2011 F	2021 M	2021 F	2041 M	2041 F	2057 M	2057 F
Standard projection assumptions (× 10⁵)														
60–64	14	15	13	14	13	14	18	19	18	19	15	15	18	18
65–74	22	27	22	27	22	25	24	27	27	32	29	32	28	31
75–84	11	19	12	19	12	19	13	18	14	20	19	27	15	21
85+	2	7	3	8	3	8	4	9	4	9	6	11	7	13
60+	49	67	49	67	51	67	58	73	64	79	69	85	68	82
All ages	273	287	279	290	283	293	288	296	293	300	291	298	286	289
											Percentage of total population			
60–64	5.1	5.2	4.7	4.8	4.6	4.8	6.2	6.4	6.1	6.3	5.2	5.0	6.3	6.2
65–74	8.1	9.4	7.9	9.3	7.8	8.5	8.3	9.1	9.2	10.7	10.0	10.7	9.8	10.7
75–84	4.0	6.6	4.3	6.6	4.2	6.5	4.5	6.1	4.8	6.7	6.5	9.1	5.2	7.3
85+	0.7	2.4	1.1	2.8	1.1	2.7	1.4	3.0	1.4	3.0	2.1	3.7	2.4	4.5
60+	17.9	23.3	17.6	23.1	18.0	22.9	20.1	24.7	21.8	26.3	23.7	28.5	23.8	28.4

Source: Office of Population Censuses and Surveys (1989a)

number of very old people. There are about 900 000 people aged over 85 years at present: this age group is projected to increase to about 1.1 million by the late 1990s. The increase is expected to continue at a declining rate to approximately 2 million by 2057.

The British 1985 and 1987 projections have followed their United States and United Nations counterparts in supplementing the 'standard' projections with alternatives generated under different assumptions. The two mortality variants are essentially that late age death rates improve either 50% faster or 50% slower. These changes have a substantial impact on the numbers of very old people expected in the future, e.g. the variant 1985-based projections for the over 75 year population in 2041 ranged from 4.1 to 5.3 million.

Age-structure change and health service demands

Declining late age mortality has increased survival into advanced old ages. As several of the most common physical and mental disorders have a prevalence that rises with age, it is usual to reason that demographic ageing leads to a rising quantum of disease and disability (Rosenwaike, 1985). Not least important is the increasing prevalence of multiple disorders and the complications of diagnosis, treatment and rehabilitation that they entail. However, age-specific incidence and prevalence rates are not constant. Successive cohorts have different exposures to risk factors: the decline in rates of tobacco

smoking among males is now firmly linked to the decreasing incidence of cardiovascular disease, and changes in occupations, conditions of work, domestic amenities, diet and exercise may all have impacts on mortality and morbidity. Changed treatment practices and technologies alter not only the lethality of diseases but also their duration. Long-term series morbidity data do not exist, making impossible models other than exploratory models of the relation between changing aggregate mortality and morbidity. Good progress has been made, however, in the detailed examination of the changing prevalence of specific conditions (Alderson and Ashwood, 1985; Manton, 1986; Wing *et al.*, 1990).

Considerable advances in projection models of health status were made during the 1980s. These use modified life-table techniques and require detailed and representative data on levels of health and disability. Early in the decade the World Health Organization promoted discussion of a common framework of definitions and models for the representation and forecasting of aggregate age-specific health status (Manton and Soldo, 1985). American and Japanese research opened up the field: Koizumi (1982) decribed the health status of the Japanese population using the categories: very healthy, almost healthy, not so healthy, ill, and receiving medical treatment. His age-specific schedules were compiled from life tables, patient surveys, a national health survey to determine disease prevalence and a population survey of health consciousness. Manton has specified for quinquennial age groups from 65–69 years upwards in the United States the fraction of survivors in six

Table 1.6 Distribution of functional disability by age and sex among non-institutional patients of the Norton Medical Centre, Teesside, 1985–86

Age group (years)	Males				Females			
	Fit and active (%)	Partially disabled (%)	House-bound (%)	Total (No.)	Fit and active (%)	Partially disabled (%)	House-bound (%)	Total (No.)
75–79	41	51	8	143	32	54	14	268
80–84	31	58	10	77	20	58	22	149
85+	25	53	22	32	11	44	44	106

Source: Hall and Channing (1990), Table I

health categories: those in nursing homes, those reporting 5–6, 3–4, or 1–2 limitations in 'activities of daily living' (ADL), and those reporting only one limitation in an 'instrumental activity of daily living' (IADL) (Manton and Soldo, 1985). These show a strong age relationship with institutional living among females, positive relationships between age and disability, and that both the prevalence of disability at all levels and the rates of institutionalization are lower at most ages for males than for females. From these data, projections of disability among the total and the non-institutionalized population are produced.

The new contractual requirement upon United Kingdom general practitioners to provide comprehensive medical care for elderly people and annually to screen those aged 75 years and over has prompted an urgent search for functional, cost-effective, unobtrusive and ethically sound approaches. Methods of forecasting consultation loads and of identifying from medical records individuals with a high probability of severe disability are sought (Freer, 1990). One thorough study has surveyed the elderly patients of a large general practice in north-east England (Hall and Channing, 1990). Health status life tables and logistic predictive models of the disabled patient population have been constructed, separating the institutional population and using the King's Fund Centre's categories of functional disability in the community population: fit and active, lifestyle appreciably disturbed by disability but not housebound, lifestyle severely modified by disability (housebound) and bedfast. The survey revealed significantly more prevalent and severe age-specific disability among women than men (replicating the Japanese and American aggregate population findings). The positive age relationship was also stronger for females than

males (Table 1.6). Although the rates of partial and severe disability increase markedly with age, the population at risk is concentrated in the younger age groups, and more than 33% of the 75 years and over population were 'fit and active' and only 11% housebound.

Incidence and prevalence of specific disorders

A major characteristic of the expression of disease in late life is its great variability: the older people are the less like each other they become. There are however several disorders with strong age-specific incidence and prevalence relationships in old age. Epidemiological research into these age relationships in populations living at different times and in different areas has generated many useful hypotheses concerning the aetiology and avoidable risk factors of disease. Its results also provide a basis for projections of treatment requirements. There have been many methodological and data problems. Until recently, few representative series were available either because of inadequate attention to the at-risk population or through small sample size. Inappropriately long open-ended upper age categories, such as 75 years and over, have been another handicap.

Recent research on several of the more common, lethal and costly age-related disorders has been most productive. A common characteristic of conditions as diverse as cardiovascular disease, diabetes, Alzheimer's disease and femoral neck fractures is a complex aetiology involving prolonged development through the adult ages, a significant role for lifestyle and environmental variables, and poorly understood interactions between the contributory factors.

Table 1.7 Selected age-prevalence series for organic brain syndrome

Age	Mean age for age group	Organic disorder Clackmannan Scotland[a] Mild	Severe	Both	Mild + severe dementia New-castle[b]	Tokyo[c]	New Zealand[d]	Organic brain syndrome Pooled[e]
65–69	67.5 ⎫ 69.8 ⎧	1.5	0.4	1.9	2.3	0.7 ⎫	3.8 ⎧	2.1
70–74	72.4 ⎭ ⎩	2.0	2.3	4.3	2.8	1.5 ⎭	⎩	3.3
75–79	77.3	3.7	5.1	8.8	5.5	2.2	6.4	8.0
80–84	82.2	7.8	10.4	18.2 ⎫		7.7 ⎧	11.0	⎫
85–89	87.1 ⎫ 88.8 ⎧ 84.7 ⎫	10.4	18.9	29.3 ⎭	22.0	17.7 ⎫⎭	23.6 ⎧	⎬ 17.7
90+	92.9 ⎭ ⎩ ⎭						40.4 ⎭	⎭

[a] Bond (1987) Table 4
[b] Kay *et al.* (1970), as presented in Jorm (1987), Table 2.1
[c] Karasawa *et al.* (1982), as presented in Jorm (1987), Table 2.1
[d] Campbell *et al.* (1983), as presented in Jorm (1987), Table 2.1
[e] Bergmann (1985) Table 1

Recent reviews of the age-specific prevalence of organic brain syndrome and studies of community populations rather than hospital admissions have enabled improved specifications of the exponential relationship between age and dementia (Bergmann, 1985; Bond, 1987; Jorm, 1987; Katzman, 1988). The apparent inconsistency between a 40% prevalence for mild and severe dementia among those aged 90 years and over in a New Zealand study, and a 22% rate for the 80 years and over in Newcastle-upon-Tyne is partly resolved if the mean ages of the open-ended age categories are estimated (Table 1.7). Logarithmic plots of apparently divergent series which use different age categories suggest that there is an underlying age-prevalence relationship in large populations (Warnes, 1989c, Figure 1).

Fracture of the femoral neck is another age-related condition with severe implications for the sufferers and the health services. These fractures have a strong exponential relationship with age, particularly among women, the incidence in British samples in the early 1980s rising from about 1 per 1000 for both sexes at 55 years to 30 per 1000 at 85 years among females and 15 per 1000 for males (Figure 1.3) (Boyce and Vessey, 1985). A rise in age-specific incidence has occurred during the last three decades in Britain, Scandinavia and the United States (Melton, O'Fallon and Riggs, 1987; O'Brant *et al.*, 1989). In England and Wales, age-specific hip fracture rates in both sexes roughly doubled during 1955–75 (Law, 1990). Recent evidence suggests that the rise in incidence rates has slowed since 1979 in England and Wales (Spector, Cooper and Fenton Lewis, 1990) and no

increase in rates was reported in Saskatchewan during 1976–85 (Ray *et al.*, 1990). There are strong seasonal, ethnic and national variations in the frequency of fractures.

Most hip fractures are associated with falls which themselves have complex causes related

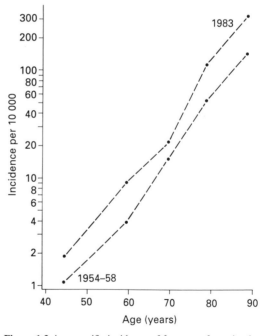

Figure 1.3 Age-specific incidence of fracture of proximal femur among females, City of Oxford, 1954–58 and 1983. (The incidence rates are as reported by Boyce and Vessey (1985) Table 1, and Knowelden, Buhr and Dunbar (1964). They have been plotted at the estimated mean ages of irregular age-groups, using 1961 and 1981 sex-specific age distributions for the City of Oxford from the England and Wales census)

to age, cognizance, body weight and domestic circumstances – a large proportion of falls occur on stairs. Only a minority of falls produce fractures, although the probability increases with age, and this may be associated with bone mass and the severity of osteoporosis. Research into falls suggests that by identifying and eliminating environmental risks in the home, one-quarter to one-third of all fall-related accidents could be prevented (Rubinstein, 1983).

The reasons for the rising incidence (over and above those produced by the changing age structure) are not clear, although several hypotheses recur in the literature. Increases in tobacco smoking among women may have reduced age-specific bone density. Inactivity is also implicated in decreasing bone mass and the reduced number of manual occupations and more sedentary life styles may therefore be factors (Law, 1990). Increased (multiple) medication may have increased the likelihood of falls or decreased the effectiveness of people's accident-avoiding actions (Cooper, 1989). It has been found that when allowance is made for the risk of falling, osteoporosis is clearly implicated as a determinant of hip fracture in those aged 50–74 years and that other factors are influential at older ages (Cooper *et al.*, 1987).

If recent cohorts have experienced less stress to their joints at work or in the home, the prevalence of osteoarthrosis may have fallen (Felson, 1988). The complexities of the relationships between physical activity throughout adult life, bone-mass, arthritic pain, medication, agility in old age, the propensity to fall, and the likelihood of fractures from falls may have to be unravelled before the recent epidemic of femoral neck fractures is understood. Almost all hip fractures are presented and they must be among the best recorded disorders of old age. As a result, clear evidence of temporal changes in incidence and of cohort differentials has been revealed. One positive return should be a widespread acceptance that the frequency of fractures in the future cannot reliably be predicted exclusively on the basis of age-structure change. For this condition at least premonitions of an overwhelming burden of treatment based solely on the growth of the elderly population will not be convincing. A strong database and the fecundity of the present debate also suggest that aetiological and epidemiological research will progress in understanding the reasons for the rising incidence of femoral neck fractures during the 1960s and 1970s and for stability more recently.

Conclusion

While the growth of the 60 years and over population in Britain has abated during the 1980s and will not again be substantial until the early decades of the next century, recent falls in late-life mortality have accentuated the increase in the numbers of people aged 75 years and over. The adjustment of the nation's social services and pensions funds required during the coming decades is modest compared with those we have already achieved and with those faced in other countries. The health services face rapidly growing demands for specific treatments for old people, but not always exclusively because of the changing age structure. Cohort changes in exposure to risk factors and the changing expectations of physicians and their patients are also altering treatment loads, not always upwards.

Rapid advances in research have recently been made in models of the implications of cause-specific mortality change but their utility is restricted by data deficiencies. Forecasts remain dependent on cross-sectional data and understandings. Little information is available on cohort changes and their implications and, to improve the power of health status models, more attention needs to be given to longitudinal changes, such as health habits, awareness and expectations, exposure to risk factors and disease prevalence. There is gathering support for large-scale and long-term health surveys and panel studies.

In Britain good quality official demographic and cause-of-death data enable useful forecasts to be made of regional and local population change. Age and sex-specific incidence and prevalence rates for a condition, its degree and its treatment needs can readily be combined with population forecasts for any area. The smaller the area, the greater the instability of the vital rates and particularly of the migration component of population change. Forecasts for small areas should therefore be ranges and for relatively short periods. These can be extended to individual hospital catchments to provide valuable indicative forecasts at least for the short term.

Projection methodology and the epidemiology of age-dependent disorders have made considerable strides in recent years. The recommended 'standard' mortality predictions are based, at least in part, on well tested time series models although subjective guesswork is still employed (Olshansky, 1988). Readily diagnosed and normally presented conditions such as femoral neck fractures have produced the fullest longitudinal incidence data. Such information may bring forward formal time series models of incidence and prevalence. The refinement and integration of demographic and epidemiological methods and data in recent years have proceeded rapidly and with many benefits to clinical science and service management. Great caution still needs to be exercised however when using population and case-load forecasts, particularly for the population of extreme old age.

References

Alderson, M. (1988) Demographic and health trends among the elderly. In *The Ageing Population: Burden or Challenge* (eds N. Wells and C. Freer), Macmillan, Basingstoke, pp. 87–103

Alderson, M. and Ashwood, F. (1985) Projections of mortality rates for the elderly. *Pop. Trends*, **42**, 22–29

Benjamin, B. (1989) Demographic aspects of ageing. *Ann. Hum. Biol.*, **16**, 185–235

Bergmann, K. (1985) Epidemiological aspects of dementia and considerations in planning services. *Dan. Med. Bull.*, **32**, (Suppl. 1), 84–91

Bond, J. (1987) Psychiatric illness in later life: a study of prevalence in a Scottish population. *Int. J. Geriat. Psychiat.*, **2**, 39–57

Boyce, W.J. and Vessey, M.P. (1985) Rising incidence of fracture of the proximal femur. *Lancet*, **i**, 150–151

Cooper, C. (1989) Osteoporosis – an epidemiological perspective: a review. *J. Roy. Soc. Med.*, **82**, 753–757

Cooper, C., Barker, D.J.P., Morris, J. and Briggs, R.S.J. (1987) Osteoporosis, falls and age in fracture of the proximal femur. *Br. Med. J.*, **295**, 13–15

Felson, D.T. (1988) Epidemiology of hip and knee osteoarthritis. *Epidemiol. Rev.*, **10**, 1–28

Freer, C. (1990) Screening the elderly. *Br. Med. J.*, **300**, 1447–1448

Fries, J.F. (1980) Aging, natural death and the compression of morbidity. *N. Engl. J. Med.*, **303**, 130–136

Fries, J.F. (1989) The compression of morbidity: near or far. *Milbank Q.*, **67**, 208–232

Grundy, E. (1987) Retirement migration and its consequences in England and Wales. *Ageing Soc.*, **7**, 57–82

Hall, R.G.P. and Channing, D.M. (1990). Age, pattern of consultation and functional disability in elderly patients in one general practice. *Br. Med. J.*, **301**, 424–428

Hayflick, L. (1987) Origins of longevity. In *Modern Biological Theories of Aging* (eds H. R. Warner *et al.*), Raven, New York, pp. 21–34

Hendricks, J. and Hendricks, C.D. (1986) *Aging in Mass Society: Myths and Realities*, Little, Brown & Co., Boston

Hunter, D., Kalache, A. and Warnes, A.M. (1988) *Health Promotion for Elderly People*, King's Fund Institute, London

Jorm, A.F. (1987) *Understanding Senile Dementia*, Croom Helm, London

Kannisto, V. (1988) On the survival of centenarians and the span of life. *Pop. Stud.*, **42**, 389–406

Katzman, R. (1988) Alzheimer's disease as an age dependent disorder. In *Research and the Ageing Population* (ed. J. Evered), Wiley, Chichester, pp. 69–79

Kinsella, K. (1988) *Aging in the Third World, International Population Reports P–95*, No. 79, United States Bureau of the Census, Washington DC

Knowelden, J., Buhr, A.J. and Dunbar, O. (1964) Incidence of fractures in persons over 35 years of age. *Br. J. Prevent. Soc. Med.*, **18**, 130–141

Koizumi, A. (1982) Toward a healthy life in the 21st century. In *Population Aging in Japan: Problems and Policy Issues in the 21st Century* (ed. T. Kuroda), Population Research Institute, Nihon University, Tokyo, pp. 1–19

Law, C.M. and Warnes, A.M. (1984) The elderly population of Great Britain: locational trends and policy implications. *Trans. Inst. Br. Geogr., New Series*, **9**, 37–59

Law, M. (1990) An epidemic of hip fracture. *Roy. Soc. Med., Curr. Med. Lit. Orthop.*, **3**, 67–69

Manton, K.G. (1986) Cause specific mortality patterns among the oldest old: multiple cause of death trends, 1968–1980. *J. Gerontol.*, **41**, 313–327

Manton, K.G. and Soldo, B.J. (1985) Dynamics of health changes in the oldest old: new perspectives and evidence. *Milbank Mem. Fund Q.: Hlth Soc.*, **63**, 206–285

Martin, L. (1988) The aging of Asia. *J. Gerontol.*, **43**, S99–113

Melton, L.J., O'Fallon, W.M. and Riggs, B.L. (1987) Secular trends in the incidence of hip fractures. *Calcif. Tissue Int.*, **41**, 57–64

Myers, G.C. (1985) Aging and worldwide population change. In *Handbook of Aging and the Social Sciences* (eds R.H. Binstock and E. Shanas), Van Nostrand Reinhold, New York, pp. 173–198

O'Brant, K.J., Bengner, U., Johnell, O., Nilsson, B.E. and Sernbo, I. (1989) Increasing age-adjusted risk of fragility fractures: a sign of increasing osteoporosis in successive generations? *Calcif. Tissue Int.*, **44**, 157–167

Office of Population Censuses and Surveys (1983) *Census 1981, Great Britain, Migration Tables*, Part 1 (100%) Tables. HMSO, London

Office of Population Censuses and Surveys (1985) *Population Trends*, No. 45, Table 20, HMSO, London

Office of Population Censuses and Surveys (1987) *Population Projections 1985–2025*, HMSO, London

Office of Population Censuses and Surveys (1989a) *Population Projections 1987–2027* HMSO, London

Office of Population Censuses and Surveys (1989b) *Mortality Statistics 1987*: General Tables 1 and 3, HMSO, London

Olshansky, S.J. (1988) On forecasting mortality. *Milbank Q.*, **66**, 482–530

Organization for Economic Cooperation and Development (1990) *Health Care Systems in Transition: The Search for Efficiency*, OECD, Paris, Tables 50–55

Ray, W.A., Griffin, W.R., West, R., Strand, L. and Melton, L.J. (1990) Incidence of hip fracture in Saskatchewan, Canada. *Am. J. Epidemiol.*, **131**, 502–509

Rosenwaike, I. (1985) *The Extreme Aged in America*, Greenwood, Westport, CT

Rubinstein, L. (1983) Falls in the elderly: a clinical approach. *West. J. Med.*, **138**, 273–275

Spector, T.D., Cooper, C. and Fenton Lewis, A. (1990) Trends in admissions for hip fracture in England and Wales, 1968–85. *Br. Med. J.*, **300**, 1173–1174

Stillwell, J., Boden, P. and Rees, P.H. (1990) Trends in internal net migration in the UK: 1975–86. *Area*, **22**, 57–65

Torrey, B.B., Kinsella, K. and Taeuber, C.M. (1987) *An Aging World. International Population Reports p–95, No. **78***, US Bureau of the Census, Washington DC

United Nations Organization (1985) *The World Aging Situation: Strategies and Policies*, UNO, New York

Warnes, A.M. (1987) The ageing of Britain's population: geographical dimensions. *Esp. Pop. Soc.*, **2**, 317–327

Warnes, A.M. (1989a) Elderly people in Great Britain: variable projections and characteristics. *J. Care Elderly*, **1**, 7–10

Warnes, A.M. (1989b) The ageing of populations. In *Human Ageing and Later Life* (ed. A.M. Warnes), Arnold, London, pp. 47–66

Warnes, A.M. (1989c) Geographical perspectives on dementia. In *Innovative Trends in Psychogeriatrics* (eds J. Wertheimer, P. Baumann, M. Gaillard and P. Schwed), Karger, Basel pp. 1–12

Wing, S., Casper, M., Davis, W. *et al.* (1990) Trends in the geographic inequality of cardiovascular disease mortality in the United States, 1962–82. *Soc. Sci. Med.*, **30**, 261–266

2

The economic implications of an ageing population

Richard J. Fordham

Introduction

The ageing of a population results in major implications for both health service utilization and expenditure. These are a challenge to all health professionals but especially to those who must bear the brunt of any anticipated change in workload. During this century orthopaedic surgeons in the Western world have shifted their attention from dealing predominantly with the consequences of infectious disease in younger adults, e.g. osteomyelitis and tuberculosis, to the treatment of the sequelae of those degenerative conditions of the musculoskeletal system which declare themselves principally in the elderly, e.g. osteoarthrosis and osteoporosis-related fractures. Since such degeneration is highly correlated with age it follows that the older the average age of patients seen the more work of this nature is likely to be encountered. The most obvious challenge in planning orthopaedic services for an ageing population is, therefore, to devise strategies to meet the potentially burgeoning demand within the resources available.

While some might argue that the only solution to this problem is to have more resources, the inescapable fact of scarcity remains, i.e. individuals and society always have more wants and perceived needs than available resources can ever satisfy. The problem of scarcity will frequently require difficult choices to be made with regard to the allocation of resources. Health care is not exempt from this dilemma even if it is sometimes believed that it

should have priority over other human activities. Realistically there can only be a finite number of resources for health care and decisions regarding which treatments to offer and to whom have to be made. Such decisions are made daily by clinicians although this is not necessarily recognized. It is impossible to offer each patient every conceivable investigation or treatment that may theoretically benefit them. Usually the clinician must ask himself if the treatment or test is 'worth doing' by intuitively weighing up the expected benefits relative to its costs and potential complications.

Rationing of scarce health care resources is therefore inevitable although there has only been overt recognition of this problem by clinicians in recent years (Klein, 1984). Rationing has usually been implemented through waiting lists, particularly in public health care systems which are 'free' to the user at the point of consumption (Horvath, 1990). However, this method is neither necessarily 'fair' nor efficient. In the light of the expected increase in workload described above the logistic problems facing orthopaedic and geriatric departments will be legion. The proposition will be advanced in this chapter that consideration of the costs and benefits of alternative treatment programmes is perhaps the only rational way to decide priorities between competing demands on limited resources. This approach is both equitable and ethical in that it gives priority to patients on the basis of need. It also recognizes that a responsibility exists to use resources efficiently not only for current patients but also for those waiting for care.

The scale of the economic problem of ageing

There is no doubt that the unprecedented problem of containing health expenditures in 'developed' countries in recent years is due, at least in part, to the ageing population structure which most of these countries face. Other factors such as inflation and the increasing use of high technology procedures also contribute significantly to this problem. The vast majority of the elderly population are able to function independently if appropriate support in a suitable environment is provided (Horrocks, 1986). However, those elderly patients who do require health services often make disproportionate use of them. In England the rate of discharge per 10 000 population from acute hospitals increases rapidly with age, especially after 55 years (see Figure 2.1). In addition between 1979 and 1985, discharge rates have been increasing among the older age groups as the population has aged, although they have remained constant for all other ages groups (OPCS, 1987) (Figure 2.2). In Britain, expenditure per head on health care doubles over the age of 65 years and at 75 and over is nearly five times as great as below retirement age (Tinker, 1984).

Utilization rates and expenditure rates are strongly correlated with increasing age in other countries too. For example in the United States, per capita rates of health care expenditures also rise sharply after 55 years (Barer *et al.*, 1987) such that those over 65 years who in 1980 made up 11% of the population absorbed 29% of the total health expenditure (Davidson and Marmor, 1980). In Canada 9% of the elderly population consume 43% of the total acute hospital beds (Roos and Shapiro, 1984) and in Australia, though the elderly comprise 10% of the population they consume approximately 40% of the total health care bill.

In England, evidence from the annual 'Hospital In-patient Enquiry' (HIPE) performed on a 10% sample of patients in non-psychiatric hospitals suggests that the orthopaedic workload has been increasing in the 1980s due, among other factors, to the ageing population structure. Discharge rates for those patients categorized as suffering from 'diseases of the musculoskeletal system and connective tissue', i.e. International Classification of Diseases groups 710–739 (ICD–9, 1975), increased overall from approximately 44 per 10 000 in 1979 to 60 per 10 000 in 1985. Those discharge rates within this diagnostic group which increased the fastest were for those conditions commonly associated with old age including osteoarthrosis and femoral neck fractures. Predictably this has led to increasing numbers of total hip replacements and operations for hip fractures being undertaken (OPCS, 1987). These trends are confirmed by the author's own findings in a recent survey of the Yorkshire Regional Health Authority. Of the 10 most common orthopaedic diagnoses treated in 1988/89 the first three conditions were associated in general with the older age groups, i.e. 'fractured neck of femur', 'osteoarthrosis and allied disorders' and 'arthropathies and related disorders' (all diagnostic groups according to ICD–9). Similarly, the most common orthopaedic operations performed were found to be 'open reduction of fractured neck of femur

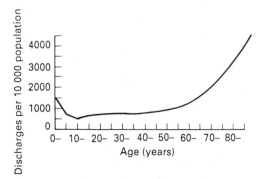

Figure 2.1 Hospital discharge rates by age group, England, 1985 (*Source*: based on Office of Population Censuses and Surveys, 1987)

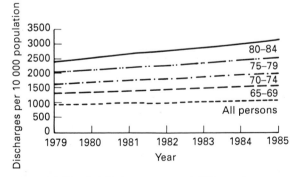

Figure 2.2 Hospital discharge rates per 10 000 population—comparison of all persons and age groups 65 years and over (*Source*: based on Office of Population Censuses and Surveys, 1987)

using pin and plate', 'total prosthetic replacement of hip joint' and 'prosthetic replacement of head of femur'.

The older age groups within our population are making increasing demands on acute hospital services and approximately one-fifth of all medical and surgical beds in England and Wales are occupied by patients over the age of 75 years (OPCS, 1977). The problem is particularly experienced on the orthopaedic wards where many of the older patients have significant coexisting conditions which require medical as well as surgical input. They also have greater social problems which may delay discharge from hospital. As the population ages it is becoming less appropriate to distinguish services for the elderly from acute services and it has been argued cogently that acute and geriatric specialties should be integrated (Grimley Evans, 1987). In orthopaedics, despite the relatively low proportion of admissions of elderly patients (approximately 5%) relative to all ages, this group consumes approximately 25–30% of available resouces, and it is appropriate for orthopaedic and geriatric specialties to liase closely to secure ways of reducing unnecessary duplication and utilization of resources.

The health-related costs of an ageing population

The 'direct' costs to the health sector of caring for an ageing population manifest themselves in budgets in which expenditures are increasingly being concentrated on elderly clients. Many examples of planning for future services for the elderly can be found in the 'strategic plans' of Health Authorities. These plans enumerate expected utilization rates, changes in patterns of provision, expenditure and quality of services over a 10-year period. For example, in the Trent Regional Health Authority's plan, *Better Health for Trent*, an increase in expenditure on the elderly is projected from 9.5% of the total budget to 11% over the period 1983 to 1993. In terms of service provision this means a 14% increase in hospital beds in addition to the replacement of 3000 unsatisfactory geriatric beds, 752 new day places, 1800 new acute/assessment beds, one extra consultant in geriatric medicine per district and £122 million on capital expenditure.

In addition to meeting extra hospital costs, there are also the other direct costs of maintaining sick elderly people in the community (preferably in their own homes) and out of hospital. These costs fall both on health and social service agencies. For the most disabled patients community health care may include day hospitals, home nursing, home helps and domiciliary physiotherapy. For other patients appropriate domestic modifications may be indicated but for some alternative accommodation, such as sheltered housing, may be necessary. In 1987/88 local authorities in England spent £2350 million on community care, £1183 million on residential care and £1167 million on domiciliary and day care facilities (DHSS, 1989). In a recent review of community care (DHSS, 1988) a diversity of funding and organizational structures was found to have contributed to the inefficient delivery of community care. It has been recommended therefore that a single local authority in each community be made responsible for the coordination of non-institutional based care including the assessment of an individual's need for services (DHSS, 1989).

In addition, some community costs are borne by patients and their families. For example, some may use their life-savings to pay for nursing home accommodation or convert capital assets, such as their homes, into income for such purposes. Economists refer to these as 'indirect costs'. A major problem of estimating the costs of community care is valuing the sacrifices borne by patients themselves and by those caring for them. These are predominantly spouses and close family who may spend a considerable number of hours per week attending to their needs. The value of this 'productive labour' is often ignored in costing community care schemes because the carers tend to be 'non-wage earners' and their time is frequently regarded as 'free'. Even where a carer is a 'wage-earner' participating in the labour market, forgone opportunities for higher wages and overtime are rarely taken into consideration. Future studies should take account of the market value of domestic labour, accommodation and materials needed for home care. Evidence from economists working in this field shows that community care can be a more cost-effective solution than institutionalized hospital care depending on the circumstances of the patient. However, policy-makers need to recognize the limitations of community care for the housebound living alone and the very disabled living with relatives unable to cope in the long term (Boldy and Canvin, 1985; Wright, 1987).

Perhaps the greatest costs to the elderly however are the less easily measured, more intangible costs associated with the reduction in well-being, health status and independence arising from injury and illness. This is the 'disutility' of the disease *per se*. A disability-free and pain-free remainder of life is valued by the elderly (as it is by other age groups), for the potential to enjoy life in all its consumption, productive and investment opportunities. In this regard health economists have developed the concept of the 'quality-adjusted-life-year' (QALY) (Williams, 1985) to take account of the quality of additional years of life obtained from treatment programmes. This would seem particularly relevant for the elderly where extending life has sometimes been seen as a 'trade-off' between extra years and quality of life. A good programme should attempt to maximize both.

New technology and changing demand

Although advancing technology is sometimes perceived as a panacea to the demands made on health services by the changing population structure, it is more probable that it has been an overall net contributor to these problems. Technology allows some procedures to be performed faster, more accurately and often with better outcomes for patients. It also allows resources to be used more intensively, generates further demands and expectations for procedures that hitherto were unavailable or not feasible so creating new problems to be solved.

A good example of this phenomenon is joint replacement surgery. Refinements in anaesthesia, implant design and surgical technique now allow these procedures to be offered in some of the most technically demanding situations previously considered not amenable to a surgical solution. Arthroplasties such as total hip replacement are now routine procedures in most orthopaedic departments, whereas 25 years ago they were considered experimental and limited to a few research centres. Knee replacement surgery has become widely available in the last few years although it is still unevenly distributed between districts. Other joints, such as the shoulder, elbow and ankle have proved more

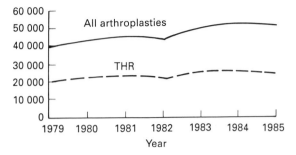

Figure 2.3 Number of arthroplasties and total hip replacements (THR) performed, England 1979–85 (*Source*: based on Office of Population Censuses and Surveys, 1987)

difficult to mimic artificially but are being developed in a few specialized centres.

In 1967 there were approximately 5000 total hip replacements performed in England and Wales compared with 10 years later when the figure had leapt to approximately 20 000 (Laing and Taylor, 1982). By 1985 (the last year for which HIPE data is available), this rate of increase had slowed down considerably such that only 24 000 such arthroplasties were being performed per year (OPCS, 1987) (see Figure 2.3). It should be remembered however that these figures are an underestimate of the real workload since they do not include operations undertaken in the private sector where, it has been estimated, in the UK 26% of all hip arthroplasties are performed (Nicoll *et al.*, 1984). In addition, significant regional disparities of a factor of 7 to 1 have been shown to exist (Laing and Taylor, 1982). However, international comparisons show that the rate of hip replacement is much lower for England and Wales (289 per million population) than in the United States (538 per million) (Melton *et al.*, 1982a). This may be due in part to differences in the age structure and underlying risk factors of the two populations.

New technologies on the other hand may improve the potential for preventive measures and may reduce the high cost of resources used in treating conditions associated with degenerative change. For example, as was shown in the previous chapter the incidence of fractures of the proximal femur increases exponentially after age 65 years and it has been estimated that the rate doubles every 5 years thereafter (Jensen, 1980). The age-specific rate also appears to have increased in the UK (Boyce and Vessey, 1985) and in the US (Melton, *et al.*, 1982b). It has been estimated that the direct hospital costs of fractured hip, which account for 20% of orthopaedic bed use in England and Wales, is approximately $304 million per year (1987/88 prices) (Royal College of Physicians, 1989). In the United States the national cost of this injury has been estimated at $884 million (Owen *et al.*, 1980) and in Australia the direct costs of osteoporotic fractures have recently been estimated to be approximately $160 million (Salkeld and Leeder 1990) (all figures in US dollars).

Osteoporosis, one of the major underlying risk factors of hip and other bone fractures in the elderly, has been shown to be at least partly amenable to treatment by drug therapy (Weiss *et al.*, 1980). However, a major question which arises is whether it is cost-effective to introduce this therapy in a systematic way following screening of asymptomatic women. This is because of both the high costs of detection and treatment of this condition. Some preliminary work suggests this approach would not be cost-effective in all women (Weinstein, 1980) but only for those in high risk factor categories. Should new technology provide cheaper screening and therapeutic alternatives it may then become possible to minimize both the huge costs and suffering described above resulting from osteoporosis-related fractures.

The way forward

The Duthie Report (DHSS, 1981) reviewed orthopaedic services in the light of the increasing waiting times for elective procedures and highlighted a number of problems facing orthopaedic departments. These included inefficient utilization of operating theatres, poor discharge planning, longer than expected lengths of inpatient stay for routine conditions, variability in length of stays between hospitals and poor waiting list management. The report concluded that resources for orthopaedic departments had increased in the 10 years prior to 1981 at the same rate as other surgical specialties but there still remained large scope for improvement in the way services were organized. It was concluded that a plea for more resources could not necessarily be justified until greater efficiency in the use of existing resources was achieved.

One of the greatest challenges facing orthopaedic departments now and in the forseeable

future is the expected increase in the volume of work described above together with its prioritization. An imperative for future policy is to look for solutions within the level of existing resources which deal effectively with increasing demand. This may lead to some essential but very difficult choices having to be made and will require some decisions to be based more on cost-effectiveness criteria rather than simply on clinical criteria alone. Two major approaches must therefore be considered.

First, the outcomes of treatments must be evaluated more carefully in order to determine the likely net benefits to elderly patients seeking orthopaedic treatment. Too often in the past orthopaedic care has been input-orientated and has assessed success or failure of interventions on very limited dimensions of outcome, e.g. technical failure, infection, re-admission. While these are important they overlook the ultimate purpose of intervention which is the restoration of the patient's 'normal' everyday level of functioning. Second, if treatment is to be provided, ways of improving the process of care must be found as there still appears to be wide variations in management practices, even among common conditions where the greatest use of resources is made.

The largest scope for the prioritization of workload in orthopaedics is in elective surgery where both the surgeon and the patient quite often have the luxury of some time and relatively normal health to review the 'pros' and the 'cons' of operative intervention. The area of trauma is obviously less amenable to this discussion process. Some ranking of priorities on waiting lists for elective surgery currently does take place usually in terms of the 'urgency' with which admissions are arranged to occur, e.g. 'immediately' (i.e. if necessary, displace another elective patient); 'urgent' (i.e. with in the next few weeks) and 'non-urgent' (i.e. routine). However, these definitions can be interpreted differently by different clinicians. This kind of prioritization system is purely ordinal in nature and does not normally have any cardinal or interval properties. That is, the system does not allow one to answer questions such as 'how much *more* urgent is Joe Blogg's case than Mary Smith's or does surgeon A have higher priority cases on his waiting list than surgeon B etc?

The answer may involve moving to an outcome-orientated system whereby the likely functional improvements derived from treatment would be compared with the patients' need for operation as judged by objective criteria bestowed with true interval properties. This is opposed to existing systems where patients' needs are assessed subjectively on different criteria by different surgeons.

A possibly more rational approach to the prioritization of waiting lists has been proposed by Williams, (1985). He argues for using the 'quality-adjusted-life-years' methodology for assessing the relative needs of patients for elective surgery. In his view treatment is indicated if the expected outcome is either an extension to life expectancy, an improvement in the quality of life or some combination of these two dimensions, i.e. a life year adjusted for quality. Using this method it is theoretically possible to prioritize waiting lists in a cardinal ranking system based on a score of 'quality-adjusted-life-years' for each patient. This may be a more efficient way to maximize health benefits in the face of limited resources. Of course in practice there are many practical problems with such a system but some preliminary work has been undertaken by economists to determine the expected net benefits (in terms of quality-adjusted-life-years) from treatment of some common general surgical conditions 1 year earlier than would have otherwise occurred (Gudex *et al.*, 1990).

The second area requiring policy consideration is the reduction of unnecessary utilization of resources both in hospital and in the community. By 'unnecessary' is meant those activities which show no demonstrable contribution to the net benefit produced by the treatment. These might include extra bed days for the sake of hospital convenience, extra investigations of the 'nice to know' variety and unquestioned policies based on convention rather than proven efficacy.

Policies which have been developed in recent years to improve the throughput of patients and produce better outcomes include the introduction of preadmission assessment clinics for elective cases, early and planned discharge, collaborative care such as that practised in orthogeriatric units, community care schemes and day case surgery. Perhaps the most interesting of these have been those which address the growing problem of increased hospital utilization by elderly patients, particularly those with femoral neck fractures. A number of alternative solutions to this problem have been proposed based on different philosophies.

The two main approaches have been collaborative 'orthogeriatric' care, either in jointly managed wards or using a liaison service and the early discharge approach. The latter approach concentrates on minimal hospital intervention, early mobilization and postoperative community care. Several variants on these two themes have been promulgated and are described in detail in chapter 17. However, evidence regarding outcomes and particularly costs is still sparse (Currie, 1989). All these schemes involve the commitment of considerable formal and informal resources but only a few such studies have included satisfactory costing methodologies (Fordham *et al.*, 1986). None have investigated how costs are distributed between different sectors and similarly none have considered the wider social costs. Furthermore, it is not known whether such schemes offer any long-term advantages over conventional management.

Conclusion – the need for economic evaluation

Economics has been described as the science of scarcity. It is concerned with society's productive potential and particularly with what is produced, how it is produced and for whom. The key notion which underlines the discipline is the concept of 'opportunity cost' which is true cost of goods and services produced in terms of the forgone benefits or sacrifices in their next best use. This is distinct from the financial or bookkeeping notion of costs which only show what is spent in monetary terms. Decisions regarding commitment of resources involve trade-offs or 'opportunity costs'. Thus, if society is going to use its resources efficiently then it should seek to satisfy its needs with the minimum of opportunity cost or sacrifice. Unless we minimize the sacrifices involved in using resources we are depriving others of some benefit and are acting inefficiently. It is therefore essential that the costs of all procedures are determined accurately as well as the likely benefits that these will bring about.

Only when benefits are shown to exceed costs or the benefit-cost ratio is demonstrated to be greater in one programme compared with another will we find ourselves managing our limited health care resources efficiently. Due in part to the complexity of our health care systems, we still know relatively little about either costs or benefits and how inputs combine with other inputs to produce outputs. In many cases we are still trying to define the main goal of health services. For example, is it prolonging the life of an infirm elderly patient with hip fracture at any cost or is it improving the quality of that patient's remaining life?

Summary

Elderly patients make disproportionate demands on health care resources and in particular on the most expensive of these, the hospital services. This problem is compounded by the ageing of the population structure and by the mixed blessings brought about by advances in technology.

It is inevitable that there will always be too few resources to satisfy all needs and improved management techniques will be necessary, including more satisfactory methods of prioritization as well as the development of techniques to ensure the delivery of health care at minimum cost. One such approach may be the introduction of collaborative programmes such as the combined orthogeriatric service but other options are available, such as early discharge schemes. However, prior to their widespread and uncontrolled implementation they require to be carefully evaluated in terms of their cost effectiveness.

References

Barer, M.L., Evans, R.G., Hertzman, C. and Lomas, J. (1987) Ageing and health care utilisation: new evidence on old fallacies. *Soc. Sci. Med.*, **10**, 851–862

Better Health for Trent – A Plan for Action, 1983/4 – 1993/4, Services for the elderly

Boldy, D. and Canvin, R. (1985) Community care of the elderly in Britain: Value for money? *Home Hlth Care Serv. Q.*, **5**, 109–121

Boyce, W.J. and Vessey, M.P. (1985) Rising incidence of fracture of the proximal femur. *Lancet*, **i**, 150–151

Currie, C.T. (1989) Hip fractures in the elderly: beyond the metal work – cooperation between orthopaedic surgeons and geriatricians should pay off. *Br. Med. J.*, **298**, 473–474

Davidson, S.M. and Marmor, T.R. (1980) *The Cost of Living Longer*, Lexington Books, MT

Department of Health and Social Security (1981) Report to the Secretary of State for Social Services: *Orthopaedic services: waiting time for out-patient appointments and in-patient treatment* (Chairman: Professor R.B. Duthie), HMSO, London

Department of Health and Social Security (1988) Report to the Secretary of State for Social Services: *Community Care: Agenda for Action* (Chairman: Sir Roy Griffiths) HMSO, London

Department of Health and Social Security (1989) *Caring for people – community care in the next decade and beyond*, Cm 849, HMSO, London

Fordham, R., Thompson, R., Holmes, J. and Hodkinson, C. (1986) A cost-benefit study of geriatric–orthopaedic management. Centre for Health Economics, University of York, Discussion paper 14

Grimley Evans, J. (1987) Integration of geriatric with general medicine. *Hosp. Update*, **13**, 205–212

Gudex, C., Williams, A., Jourdan, M., Mason, R., Maynard, J., O'Flynn, R. and Randall, M. (1990) Prioritising waiting lists. *Hth Trends*, **22**, 103–108

Horrocks, P. (1986) The components of a comprehensive district health service for elderly people – a personal view. *Age Ageing*, **15**, 321–342

Horvath, D.G. (1990) The ethics of resource allocation. *Med. J. Aust.*, **153**, 437–438

International Classification of Diseases (1975) *Manual of the international statistical classification of diseases, injuries, and causes of death*, 9th revision with UK amendments and extensions. Geneva, World Health Organization

Jensen, J.S. (1980) Incidence of hip fractures. *Acta Orthop. Scand.*, **5**, 511–513

Klein, R. (1984) Rationing health care. *Br. Med. J.*, **289**, 143–144

Laing, W. and Taylor, D. (eds) (1982) *Studies of Current Health Problems – Hip Replacement and the NHS*, Office of Health Economics, London

Melton, L.J. III, Stauffer, R.N., Chao, E.S. and Ilstrup, D.M. (1982a) Rates of total hip arthroplasty – a population based study. *N. Engl. J. Med.*, **307**, 1242–1245

Melton, L.J., Ilstrup, D.M., Riggs, B.L. and Beckenbaugh, R.D. (1982b) Fifty year trend in hip fracture incidence. *Clin. Orthop.*, **162**, 144–149

Nicoll, J.P. Thomas, K.L. Williams, B.T. and Knowelden, J. (1984) Contribution of the private sector to elective surgery in England and Wales. *Lancet*, **ii**, 89–92

Office of Population Censuses and Surveys for Government Actuary's Department (1977) *Hospital in-patient enquiry*, HMSO, London

Office of Population Censuses and Surveys for Government Actuary's Department (1987) OPCS Monitor (MB4 87/1) *Hospital in-patient enquiry (England) – trends 1979–85*, HMSO, London

Owen, R., Melton, L.J., Gallagher, J.C. and Riggs, B.L. (1980) The national cost of acute care of hip fractures associated with osteoporosis. *Clin. Orthop.*, **150**, 172–176

Roos, N.P. and Shapiro, E. (1984) The Manitoba longitudinal study on ageing: preliminary findings on health care utilisation by the elderly. *Med. Care*, **19**, 644–657

Royal College of Physicians of London (1989) *Fractured Neck of Femur – Prevention and Management*, London

Salkeld, G. and Leeder, S. (1990) Osteoporosis and its costs to Australia. *Proceedings of the Public Health Association of Australia's Annual Conference*, Hobart, September

Tinker, A. (1984) *The Elderly in Modern Society*, London, Longman

Weinstein, M.C. (1980) Estrogen use in postmenopausal women – cost, risks and benefits. *N. Engl. J. Med.*, **303**, 308–316

Weiss, N.S., Ure, C.L. Ballard, J.H. *et al.* (1980) Decreased risk of fractures of the hip and forearm with post-menopausal use of estrogen. *N. Engl. J. Med.*, **303**, 1195

Williams, A. (1985) The economics of coronary artery by-pass grafting. *Br. Med. J.*, **291**, 326–329

Wright, K. (1987) *Cost-effectiveness in community care*, Discussion Paper 33 Centre for Health Economics and Health Economics Consortium, University of York

3

General medical problems of the elderly patient

William E. Bagnall

Introduction

When considering the medical management of elderly people in a hospital setting it is most important to remember that they are people first and foremost, ill second and temporarily, and elderly last and least. It is very easy to be misled by the frail and dependent appearance of an elderly person admitted to hospital into adopting a passive approach that would not be countenanced in a younger age group. Each patient, no matter how old or frail, has the right to an accurate diagnosis, a clearly thought-out scheme of investigation, and a management plan designed to restore maximum independence as quickly as possible. The environment of the orthopaedic ward should encourage the attainment of these clinical goals by providing a setting in which all members of the team are aware of the special needs of the elderly patient and are able to contribute equally to the treatment programme based on a personalized assessment of need.

With the increasing proportion of time that the oldest members of society require from the orthopaedic services, it is relevant in this chapter to consider the basic principles that govern medical assessment, investigation and management of the elderly patient in hospital.

Basic principles of assessment

Assessing elderly patients requires an understanding not only of the presenting medical problem but also of the many interrelated factors that have led to admission to hospital. Without this appreciation a satisfactory clinical outcome culminating in an early return to the community is unlikely to be achieved.

Illnesses in old age are frequently multiple, may present in atypical fashion and are often precipitated by events which may in themselves appear trivial. Independent living in old age is a precarious business associated with risks which are usually well accepted by the elderly person. The aim of therapeutic intervention is to minimize these risks without replacing them by the anathema of custodial care. The failure of the support network, be it relative, friend or statutory organization, may tempt the elderly person out of necessity to undertake an activity that leads to a fall. Even if a fracture is not sustained, the resulting loss of confidence may lead rapidly to reduced mobility, incontinence, confusion and finally to hospital admission. An appreciation of the interplay of environmental factors such as these is vital to the understanding of the response of the elderly person in hospital.

Admission to hospital is a daunting experience for anyone; for the elderly person it may be a nightmare. The transition from 'home' with its security, privacy and known hazards, to the institution with its noise, unfamiliar routines and plethora of strange faces and uniforms can, at the very least, be disturbing. It is not surprising, therefore, that during the first few days in hospital the elderly patient may become frightened, disorientated and confused. Mild nocturia may be normal for some elderly patients who may have difficulty transferring to and from a hospital bed in the semi-gloom. They may find it impossible to use a urinal lying down and they may be unable to find a poorly signposted toilet, thereby running the risk of being labelled a 'confused wanderer'. Older people, particularly, are upset by the loss of dignity that all too frequently accompanies hospital admission. Bed screens are often too short or ill fitting and this may cause embarrassment when dressing or using a bedside commode. Ward routines should ideally place the patient at the centre of activity, strive to maintain a daily programme that is as 'normal' as possible and be conducted with a sensitive, non-patronizing approach. Older patients are all too commonly addressed by their first names without their consent, or discussed from the end of the bed as if they are uninvolved onlookers. At worst they may be disregarded altogether. Whereas young patients may be happy to spend 2 or 3 weeks in hospital dressed in night attire, elderly people generally respond badly and may become depersonalized, readily adopting the role of 'patient'.

It is essential to enquire of elderly patients on admission to hospital their normal daily routine, dietary preferences and specific requirements. They should be encouraged to wear their own clothes and shoes and be given their usual aids to daily living. The management plan should be agreed in consultation with the patient and relatives and not simply imposed. In general, elderly patients need repeated reassurance and a sympathetic approach if their confidence is to be gained and kept. All doctors need to be aware of these basic issues, they are not merely the concern of nursing and paramedical staff. Moreover, unless the clinician plays a major and constructive part in the multidisciplinary assessment, the contribution of all other members of the team will be greatly diminished.

Presentation of disease

Although almost the whole range of clinical pathology occurs in the elderly age group, certain disease processes, particularly those with a long gestation, tend to predominate. These include cardiovascular disease in all its various manifestations (Agner, 1981) and cancer, particularly of the gastrointestinal tract and bronchus. Other disabling disorders frequently encountered are osteoarthrosis, hiatus hernia, diverticular disease, cholelithiasis and, of course, Alzheimer-type dementia.

Unfortunately, many common conditions present in atypical fashion in elderly patients or may remain undetected until revealed, to the chagrin of the clinician, by the pathologist at autopsy. Conditions such as confusion and incontinence should *never* be regarded as diagnoses but purely as symptoms in search of a cause.

Cardiovascular disease

Although ischaemic heart disease is common (WHO, 1979) and may present in classic form in old age, it often appears in quite non-specific fashion. Precordial chest pain suggestive of myocardial ischaemia may be short-lived or atypical in distribution. Myocardial infarction can occur in the absence of any history of chest pain (Pathy, 1967) and may simply be discovered on routine electrocardiography, or during the investigation of falls or hypotension. Severe ischaemia, myocardial or peripheral, may remain undetected simply because the patient is limited in activity to walking within a small flat. General weariness, increasing fatigue and anorexia, although non-specific symptoms, may indicate developing cardiac failure. These symptoms in association with established cardiac failure may indicate the insidious onset of bacterial endocarditis. More substantial evidence of cardiac decompensation in the form of cardiac enlargement, pleural effusions and elevation of the jugular venous pulse should be sought before assigning the patient to a drug regimen that may be long term.

Oedema of the lower limbs is often not of cardiac origin and arises due to a combination of dependent posture, obesity, venous insufficiency and hypoalbuminaemia. Treating hypostatic oedema with diuretics has the potential for unleashing a torrent of incontinence in addition to causing renal embarrassment and gross electrolyte disturbance.

Respiratory disease

Many of the traditional indicators of an acute chest infection, cough, pyrexia, dyspnoea and chest pain may be absent in the elderly patient. 'Failure to progress', hypotension and acute confusion may be the only unhelpful clues. One of the few useful indicators is an elevation of that frequently overlooked component of the observation chart, the respiratory rate (McFadden *et al.*, 1982). All too often a perfunctory auscultation reveals the ubiquitous basal crackles that are then labelled as 'infection/failure' and treated with antibiotics, diuretics and bronchodilators for good measure. A good quality chest radiograph is an essential part of the examination of any patient with suspected respiratory or cardiac disease, both in the initial assessment and as an aid to monitoring progress.

Studies of airways reversibility and steroid responsiveness may help to clarify the aetiology of expiratory wheeze by identifying and separating that important group of patients who have late-onset asthma from the majority with chronic obstructive pulmonary disease.

An all too common autopsy finding in elderly patients is undiagnosed pulmonary embolism and infarction. The symptoms and signs, often far from florid, may be dismissed as trivial; a slowly resolving pneumonia, a transient dysrhythmia or episodes of atypical chest pain may be the only clues to raise suspicion in the mind of the clinician.

Gastrointestinal disease

Peptic ulceration is common in old age as is gastric cancer. The symptoms may be indistinguishable and demand visual (and preferably tissue) diagnosis before being masked by the administration of H_2 antagonists. Perforation of a hollow viscus in the elderly patient may occur without the expected signs of shock and peritonism. Similarly, severe sepsis in the biliary tract or in a colonic diverticulum may be present with only the most trivial of clinical findings. Acute surgery in elderly patients carries a high mortality, especially in those aged over 75 years (Blake and Lynn, 1976). Any unexpected deterioration in the well-being of an elderly patient, particularly if associated with confusion and hypotension, should prompt a thorough and urgent examination together with appropriate investigation.

Neurological disease

Although stroke illness is common in old age, it would be an injustice to commit all neurological abnormalities to the diagnostic dustbin of 'cerebrovascular disease'. Slowly growing cerebral tumours may mimic vascular disease and, moreover, may present without the features of raised intracranial pressure because of co-existent cerebral atrophy (Sharr, 1989). Chronic subdural haematoma can also present insidiously as progressive cerebral compression (O'Neill, 1989).

The precipitating event may be minimal cerebral trauma or, on occasion, haemorrhage due to vascular abnormality or disturbance of haemostasis (Loew and Kivelitz, 1976). Disproportionate incontinence, confusion and ataxia may be the signs of so-called 'normal pressure hydrocephalus' (Adams *et al.*, 1965) and respond to ventriculoperitoneal shunting. Florid Parkinson's disease is easy to identify, but the early stages are readily overlooked and the patient assumed to be 'slow' or uncooperative.

Renal and metabolic disease

The interrelationship between ageing and disease is nowhere better demonstrated than in the control of the internal metabolic environment. The ageing kidney is smaller and less efficient than in young adult life (McLachlan, 1978; Bone, 1988). The glomerular filtration rate (GFR) falls progressively throughout life at a rate of approximately 10 ml/min of GFR per decade and is a sign of true renal ageing (Rowe *et al.*, 1976). In addition, basal energy requirements reduce with age, musculoskeletal mass shrinks, and total body water, principally in the intracellular space, falls. In spite of the age-related reduction in creatinine clearance, the level of serum creatinine, which correlates with muscle energy balance, may remain unchanged and therefore give a grossly misleading impression of renal function (Rowe *et al.*, 1976).

The overall effect of these changes is to blunt the normal homeostatic response to alterations of salt, water and energy balance. Elderly patients, whose sensation of thirst may be impaired (Miller *et al.*, 1982), are therefore prone to dehydration and alteration in sodium metabolism when stressed by illness, fluid and calorie deprivation or the nephrotoxic effects of drugs. The clinical presentation of these changes may be non-specific but includes confusion and hypotension. The superimposition of infection, especially of the urinary tract, on the diminished renal reserve of old age can lead to a rapid reduction in renal function and the development of uraemia.

Chronic renal failure may frequently be associated with small contracted kidneys but it is essential to exclude a reversible obstructive uropathy. Similarly, the conjunction of impaired renal function, anaemia and proteinuria should alert the clinician to the possibility of myeloma (Defronzo *et al.*, 1975).

Abnormalities of glucose handling following an oral glucose tolerance test are common in elderly patients (Butterfield, 1964; Andres, 1971), many of whom will not progress to clinical disease. True diabetes mellitus, however, is not a benign condition in the elderly in whom there is a major risk of macrovascular and metabolic complications (Pirart, 1978) and whose risk of microvascular disease may be greater even than that of younger adults (Caird et al., 1969). The onset of new diabetes in old age may be insidious; balanitis, candidiasis and pruritus vulvae may be indicators for investigation, but polyuria in the presence of a urinary tract infection or symptoms of prostatism may pass unsuspected. Urinalysis for glycosuria is often unhelpful as a monitoring aid due to the elevation of renal threshold, and short-term glycaemic control is therefore best assessed by frequent blood glucose measurements. Supplementary evidence regarding control in the previous 3 weeks may be obtained by estimating fructosamine levels and in the previous 2–3 months by measuring glycosylated haemoglobin (Bunn, 1981).

Hypothyroidism is second only to diabetes as an endocrine disorder of old age with a prevalence in hospitalized patients of 2–4% (Jefferys, 1972). Clinical diagnosis may be difficult with many suspected patients turning out to be obese and depressed rather than hypothyroid. The disease may often be uncovered in the investigation of angina, anaemia or cardiac failure. Because treatment is not urgent, except in rare cases of myxoedema coma, and because intercurrent disease and trauma may affect protein binding, it is desirable to defer estimation of serum T4 and TSH levels until any acute illness is over. In hyperthyroidism, the brunt of the disease is again borne by the cardiovascular system in the form of angina, cardiac failure and atrial fibrillation; rarely do the classic features of exophthalmos, goitre and tremor appear. Just occasionally, a withdrawn, lethargic cachectic condition is produced, so-called apathetic hyperthyroidism (Thomas, Mazaferri and Skillman, 1970).

The history

Taking an accurate and comprehensive history from an elderly person is an exercise that may require patience of biblical proportions. It is always important to seek corroborative evidence from family, friends, community health services and social services personnel. The collation of this information ensures that the clinical condition is viewed in context and that the proposed management plan is soundly based.

Simply communicating effectively may be the greatest hurdle. One or more of the following 'difficult d's' may inhibit the process: deafness, dysarthria, dysphasia, dysphonia, dyskinesia, depression, drugs, dementia, dialect, disorientation, dentures and disinterest. It is essential to differentiate between them and seek alternative methods of communication wherever possible.

Many elderly people exhibit a degree of benign forgetfulness which, although not clinically significant, may nevertheless necessitate the use of direct questioning – particularly in the review of systems. Anecdotes and homilies abound in the 'telling of the story' and may be grossly misleading. Symptoms may be minimized or dismissed altogether if not actually present at the time of the interview.

A detailed social and domestic history is mandatory if a satisfactory discharge is to be achieved. This is not simply the responsibility of the social worker; clinicians need to be able to evaluate all the background factors in the formulation of the management plan. A long list of discharge support services which may, in any event, be unnecessary is no substitute for a thorough appraisal of the needs of the individual begun on admission. Of special importance are the layout of the home environment including stairs, type of heating, the position of bathroom and toilet, distances between the principal rooms, possibility of adaptation for wheelchair use and the availability of kitchen appliances. A list of formal and informal carers should be obtained and their contribution within the support network analysed. It is important to maintain a dialogue with the principal carers from the beginning of the admission; not only to ensure effective communication, but also to pre-empt the possibility of discharge delay due to the carers withdrawing their support. An enquiry should be made into the normal routine of the patient and particular attention drawn to the use of dentures, hearing aids, spectacles, walking aids and footwear. Finally, it is essential to obtain a detailed history of current drug therapy and to verify this with the carers and the family doctor who may provide useful information on compliance.

The examination

General

The medical examination should be conducted on traditional lines although it may need to be carried out piecemeal rather than by system. In the community many elderly people seem to be clad in innumerable layers of clothing whatever the weather, usually with no visible means of clinical access! In hospital this is less of a problem but it is important to perform the necessary detailed examination while maintaining the privacy and dignity of the patient.

With advancing years the skin becomes thin, inelastic and atrophic. So-called senile purpura is common on the extensor surfaces of the hands and arms following minimal trauma. They do not change colour as may other purpuric lesions and are of little clinical significance although the patient may need reassurance as to their benign nature. Assessing the haemoglobin from skin pallor and conjunctivae is notoriously inaccurate as is gauging the state of hydration from skin turgor in the limbs; the skin over the cheek may be a more useful guide. If the skin of the abdominal wall is cold then hypothermia should be suspected and the rectal temperature measured. Laxity in the ligaments of the wrist may give rise to 'apparent' ulnar deviation which may then be misdiagnosed as rheumatoid arthritis. A variety of minor foot afflictions including onychogryphosis, calluses and corns may be the 'sole' cause of impaired mobility.

Cardiovascular signs

Unilateral elevation of the jugular venous pulse, usually on the left side, may occur due to compression of the innominate vein by a tortuous aorta; this usually disappears on inspiration. In some elderly patients, usually women, a forceful carotid pulsation is visible above the right clavicle due to an unfolded aorta; this may be mistaken for a carotid aneurysm.

The blood pressure should always be taken with the patient both lying and standing. Postural hypotension is a frequent finding in old age and has many causes including infection, haemorrhage, autonomic neuropathy, ischaemic vascular disease and drugs. Occasionally, symptoms of postural hypotension occur only after the patient has walked. In this situation it is important to check the blood pressure after exercise. Other common cardiovascular findings such as atrial fibrillation and cardiac failure are often attributed to ischaemic heart disease without adequate evidence and the ambiguous nature of ankle oedema has already been discussed.

Thoracic signs

Senile kyphosis may make interpretation of signs in the chest difficult. Basal crackles may not be pathologically significant in a semi-recumbent patient who is unable to take deep breaths and whose cooperation may be limited. These problems merely serve to underline the necessity of high quality chest radiography in the examination of the respiratory system.

Elderly women not infrequently fail to notice breast lumps until they are very large or symptomatic; those that do find them often do not mention the fact spontaneously. Examination of the breast is, therefore, an essential component of the chest examination.

Abdominal signs

In examining the abdomen care must be given to positioning the patient correctly, particularly where obesity obscures the bony landmarks. Warm hands and the ability to distract the patient's attention help to avoid the apparent 'peritonism' that frequently follows the imperative to relax. Although abdominal aortic aneurysm is not rare, it is possible to palpate a normal sized aorta in thin patients. Distinguishing faecal masses from visceral tumours may be difficult especially over the line of the colon. Repeated examination over several days together with abdominal radiographs may help resolve this issue. Rectal examination is mandatory in all patients. Faecal impaction, rectal and prostatic neoplasm and urinary retention are all regularly encountered in the older age group and should be identified with the minimum of discomfort.

Neurological signs

Neurological examination is potentially a lengthy exercise often executed badly. Rather than a poor attempt at the full examination it is often better (in the absence of a history suggestive of neurological disease) to perform an 'exclusion' assessment. This should consist of testing visual acuity and the cranial nerves; upper limb drift, grip and finger movement; straight leg raising and dorsiflexion of the feet; touch, pinprick and position sense in the hands and feet; all tendon reflexes and plantar responses; and observation of the gait. If this procedure is combined with mental state assessment most important neurological abnormalities will be detected (George, 1989).

One of the major difficulties in the examination of the nervous system is in differentiating pathological change from normal ageing. A number of studies have attempted to clarify this position, often with conflicting results (Critchley, 1931; Prakash and Stern, 1973; Potvin *et al.*, 1980). The following are some of the findings in normal elderly people in which there is concordance between the authors. The pupil becomes irregular and less reactive to light with age; the small muscles of the hand tend to atrophy but power may be preserved; an essential tremor, particularly involving the head, is common; balance may be impaired when standing on one leg; the loss of the abdominal reflexes, but not necessarily the ankle reflexes, is frequently found; and diminution of vibration sense in the lower limbs is almost universal.

Apart from these findings, neurological abnormalities in elderly people should be subject to the same evaluation as in the young. To ascribe them to ageing alone may not only perform a great disservice to the patient, but also stifle the urge to discover the true identity of, as yet, undiagnosed pathology.

Mental assessment

The examination of an elderly patient is incomplete without an assessment of mental function. Confusional states, depression and dementia are all common and need to be differentiated from each other. Confusion is no more of a diagnosis than chest pain and the range of possible causes embraces most of medicine. Some of those that have particular relevance to elderly patients are listed in Figure 3.1. The commonest causes are infective: chest, urinary, wound and pressure sores, constipation, drugs, hypotension, minor stroke and change of routine. Confusional episodes may be superimposed on a dementing illness in which case the cause of the acute episode may be quite trivial. If investigation of acute confusion fails to identify a clinically

acceptable cause, then the possibility of underlying dementia should be considered. In addition to the medical history and direct questioning, it may be useful to administer a mental state questionnaire to evaluate mental performance on a semi-quantitative basis (Table 3.1).

The 10-question test (Hodkinson, 1972) may be a valuable aid to monitoring progress, while the 'mini-mental status' examination of Folstein *et al.* (1975) is more comprehensive and assesses orientation, memory, language and spatial construction.

Functional assessment

Functional assessment and rehabilitation are covered elsewhere in this book but it is important to stress the message of Devas (1974) that one of the most important physical signs in the practice of orthopaedic surgery in the elderly population is to see the patient walk and undertake the activities of daily living. A number of rating scales are available to assess formally the ability of a patient to wash, dress, cook, walk and attend to personal hygiene. The ideal scale should be validated over a range of disabilities, be reproducible and sensitive to minor change in function. Although not hierarchical one of the most widely used assessment scales is the Barthel index (Mahoney and Barthel, 1965).

Although much of the functional assessment is likely to be carried out by therapists, nursing staff and social workers the clinician must be able to communicate with the other professionals on equal terms if a clear, coordinated management plan is to be formulated.

Investigation

General

There is a tendency to under-investigate older patients. This nihilistic attitude may stem either from an ageist view or from the approach that the patient is too frail for the investigation or that the result will not alter management. If there is a reasonable chance that investigation will lead to a treatment regimen that will alleviate, if not cure, the patient's symptoms then it should be actively considered. Appropriate investigation is acceptable, the pursuit of academic interest alone, however, is not. Because of the non-specific way in which many illnesses

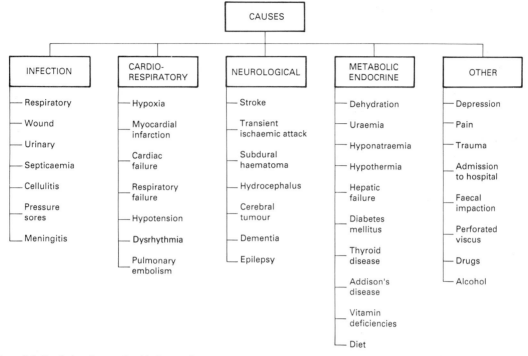

Figure 3.1 Confusional states in elderly people

Table 3.1 Ten-question mental test score

1. Patient's age
2. Time of day to nearest hour
3. Give an address, ask patient to repeat it, recall later
4. Present year
5. Name of hospital
6. Recognition of two persons
7. Date of birth
8. Year of First (Second) World War
9. Name of monarch/prime minister
10. Ask patient to count backwards from 20 to 1

Score 1 point for each correct answer.
Re-test periodically and record in patient's notes.

present in old age it is easy to justify a number of screening investigations for all new admissions. These should include: haemoglobin, full blood count and film; electrolytes, urea and creatinine clearance; blood sugar, calcium and albumin; electrocardiograph, chest radiographs, urinalysis and culture. Because of the occurrence of mixed haematological deficiency it may also be necessary to measure B_{12}, folate and ferritin levels. Plasma T4 and TSH may also be appropriate but can wait until after the acute episode of illness is over. Further investigations will be dictated by initial results, clinical progress and further assessment.

The fall

One of the most important investigations in orthopaedic surgery is the analysis of the cause of the fall that may have resulted in injury.

Falling is such a common problem in old age that the incidence of fracture of the femoral neck rises to one in four women by the age of 90 years (Evans, Prudham and Wandless, 1979). Figure 3.2 gives an outline of some of the more common medical and environmental factors precipitating falls. This is not an exclusive list and there may be considerable overlap between the conditions with premonitory symptoms and those without. It is always necessary to determine whether there are environmental factors involved that may be corrected in order to prevent recurrent falling. Many falls are multifactorial, e.g. vitamin D deficiency leading to osteomalacia with pathological changes in the bone, and myopathy resulting in proximal weakness, gait disorder and a tendency to instability. If an unsuitable walking frame and loose carpets are added to the equation falls are almost inevitable.

The falls that carry the highest morbidity are invariably those occurring unwitnessed indoors. In this situation the elderly person is likely to be

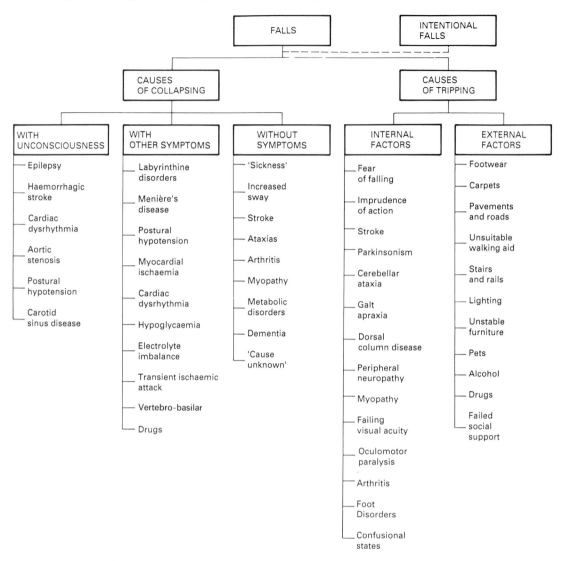

Figure 3.2 Causes of falls in elderly people

living alone, housebound and physically frail and disabled. Porter *et al.* (1990) suggest that those most at risk from hip fracture are elderly women with osteoporosis complicated by cognitive impairment and above average mobility. The implication being that they are more likely to fall through imprudence. Isaacs (1985) suggests that those patients who fall and lie on the floor for 1 h or more without being able to rise experience a 50% mortality within 3 months of the fall. This is the group of elderly patients who tend to have recurrent falls and for whom the scheme of rehabilitation and aftercare needs particularly careful and unhurried planning.

Occasionally, falling may be the result of a deliberate act on the part of the elderly person (Young *et al.*, 1987). In this situation there is often quite severe psychological or psychiatric illness.

Management

General

Nowhere should the meaning of the word 'holistic' be better encapsulated than in the multidisciplinary management of the elderly patient in the orthopaedic unit. The urgency of fracture fixation and the intensity of subsequent rehabilitation have been well documented elsewhere in this book. It is, however, the balance of care that is all important. The complete assessment of the patient and her illness; her aspirations, hopes and fears, all need to be seen in the context of the various treatment options, likely outcomes and risks. Elderly people are still occasionally denied the most appropriate treatment on the grounds of age and frailty. The consequences of this judgmental approach are to be seen languishing in continuing care wards or nursing homes.

Failure to thrive is a condition found not only in infancy; the elderly patient when denied access to active intervention or stimulation may rapidly lose heart and the will to live. The personal and financial risks of prevarication or conservative treatment may easily outweigh those of early surgery. For many patients death is not the worst outcome of illness but prolonged pain, disability, dependence and despair may well be.

The environment in which elderly patients are treated is clearly important. They need to feel secure and yet private; to have personal space and, at the same time, companionship. There are few sights quite as degrading as a group of elderly patients clad in ill-fitting night attire, restrained in tilt-back chairs complete with dangling catheter bags, clustered around the ward television on full volume, gazing in breakfast-stained bewilderment at an Open University astrophysics lesson. Elderly patients function best with their own clothes and shoes; they require beds and chairs of the correct height, and they need their own dentures, spectacles, aids to daily living and a ward timetable adjusted to their normal domestic pattern. During the first days of admission while the clinical plan is being formulated and executed the discharge date should also be anticipated, discussed and planned so that the different strands of care can be brought together at the appropriate point. It is this therapeutic optimism and conviction that characterizes the success of many orthopaedic-geriatric units.

Diet and fluids

Dietary habits and patterns of eating change with increasing age. Elderly people often eat only one main meal per day supplemented by snacks and drinks. It becomes increasingly difficult to achieve a diet that is balanced nutritionally when energy input falls below 1800 kcal/day. If social isolation, poverty and poor health are superimposed on a diet that is already borderline malnutrition may supervene.

Hospital catering departments are not always known for their sensitivity to the needs of their clients and elderly patients may be especially disadvantaged by meals that are inappropriate in content, quantity, presentation and timing. Dietetic help should be sought in planning a diet that is nutritionally balanced, attractively presented and delivered to allow some flexibility of meal times.

Older patients for reasons already described have a tendency to develop dehydration and electrolyte imbalance. Fluid input/output charts can be grossly inaccurate and need to be supplemented by regular weighing. This is appropriate not only for patients requiring extra fluids but also for those in cardiac failure whose therapeutic regimen is being adjusted. The imperative to 'push fluids' is generally meaningless, the total daily requirement needs to be stated clearly together with the frequency of administration.

Bladder, bowels and skin

Although the detailed investigation and treatment of urinary incontinence is outside the scope of this book, a simplified approach to the problem is given in Figure 3.3. It is essential to pre-empt difficulties by trying to promote continence.

The normal pattern of micturition of the patient should be noted, toilets well signposted and lit, urinals and commodes supplied where necessary, hypnotics and diuretics withdrawn if possible, fluids encouraged and chronic constipation with faecal impaction treated. The patient should be reassured that the problem, if acute, is likely to be short-lived and treatable. Drug treatment with anticholinergics or calcium antagonists should only be given after acute temporary and mechanical causes have been excluded. Pads, sheaths and catheters, appropriately used, may allow the patient to lead a life with dignity and self respect and should not be withheld simply because they are thought to represent therapeutic failure. No one with incontinence, irrespective of cause, should have to struggle on without hope of improvement,

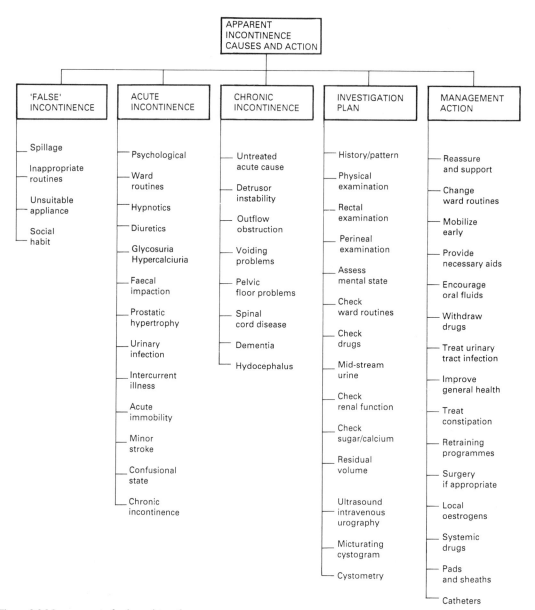

Figure 3.3 Management of urinary incontinence

understanding or a remedy that allows the problem to be coped with.

Many elderly people seem preoccupied with their bowels and the need to open them daily. Bowel symptoms, however functional they might appear, must be taken seriously. Chronic constipation is very common and may lead to faecal impaction with overflow diarrhoea, urinary retention and incontinence, and confusion.

The importance of the rectal and abdominal examination has already been stressed, supplemented, if necessary, by plain abdominal radiographs. An adequate fluid intake is essential to maintain normal bowel action together with an increased intake of dietary fibre. It is folly, however, to treat established constipation and faecal impaction with fibre supplements, as this will only compound and compact the problem.

In this situation the best line of approach is by giving oral fluids and a faecal softener together with suppositories and enemas.

A particular problem of elderly patients following surgery is the tendency to develop pressure necrosis of the skin overlying bony prominences. Both in clinical and financial terms this is a problem that is far better to prevent than to treat. It calls for vigilance on the part of the nursing staff together with an agreed unit policy on pressure sore prevention and management. Enforced immobility, over-sedation, dehydration, malnutrition and anaemia are all contributory factors.

The cornerstone of effective prevention is 2-hourly turning. Other measures such as the use of pads, creams and sprays are of dubious value; but the use of the large-celled ripple mattress has been shown to be of benefit (Bliss, McLaren and Exton-Smith, 1967). The management of established pressure sores is essentially that of maintaining the general health and nutrition of the patient; debriding the infected area of slough, keeping it clean and dry and allowing granulation to occur. The case for packing deep pressure sores with a variety of condiments, best kept where they belong in the kitchen cupboard, has yet to be made.

Medical care in elderly surgical patients

Although most authorities suggest that surgery in elderly patients has a higher morbidity and mortality than in the young, there is no consensus as to the precise level of additional risk that age, as an independent variable, bestows on surgery. One of the difficulties is in distinguishing the effects of age from the pathology that accompanies it; in some cases this may be quite impossible. Surgery within 3 months of a myocardial infarction is said to be associated with a re-infarction rate of 30% (Steen, Tinker and Tarhan, 1978) and postoperative myocardial infarction has a 50% mortality rate (Goldman *et al.*, 1978). It is reasonable, therefore, to postpone elective surgery for 3–6 months after a myocardial infarction.

Fit elderly people have less reserve than fit younger people (Goldman, 1983; Seymour, 1983) and there are age-related changes to pulmonary function, particularly a reduction in vital capacity and PO_2 (Sorbini *et al.*, 1968). There is consequently a higher risk of postoperative hypoxia and confusion. Patients with significantly impaired respiratory function may need blood gas analysis and spirometry and may then require local or spinal anaesthesia.

The incidence of postoperative thromboembolic disease increases with age (Morrell, Truelove and Barr, 1963) with hip surgery a particularly high risk procedure.

While prevention of thromboembolic disease is highly desirable, there is no consensus as to the best approach. Early mobilization, external compression, low-dose heparin, dextran and modified-dose warfarin have all been suggested as prophylactics. While low-dose heparin has been shown to be effective in medical and general surgical patients (Halkin *et al.*, 1982) this is not the case in orthopaedic patients, and a more intensive approach using adjusted-dose heparin or modified dose warfarin has been suggested (Trulock, 1988). The use of low molecular weight heparins has more recently been reported (SICOT, 1990) as conferring protection as effective as other regimens but with an improved side-effect profile. To achieve a high probability of excluding suspected thromboembolic disease a sequence of investigation may be required beginning with Doppler ultrasound or impedance plethysmography and culminating in venography and radionuclide ventilation-perfusion (V/Q) scanning.

The blood sugar of elderly diabetic patients is often best controlled during the perioperative period by means of intravenous dextrose and insulin administered by syringe driver. In this way smaller doses of insulin can be titrated against the requirement to keep blood glucose from rising above 12 mmol/l, a level which is considered safe at this traumatic time (Bagdade, Root and Bulger, 1974). The same policy is advisable if sepsis occurs postoperatively.

Finally, the surgical procedure should be discussed with the patient and family; not only to confirm the appropriateness of the clinical action, but also to warn that in the immediate postoperative period there may be confusion, disorientation and even hallucination. These changes are common after surgery (Heller *et al.*, 1970) and preoperative awareness of them may help dispel postoperative anxiety.

Conclusion

This chapter outlines some of the particular difficulties and problems involved in the medical assessment and management of the elderly patient in the orthopaedic unit. It is important for all doctors, in whichever branch of adult medicine they practise, to have a working knowledge of the needs of their elderly clients. A sound clinical knowledge base is fundamental, teamwork is vital, but therapeutic optimism and the willingness to look beneath the surface wrinkles to the person within are essential to a successful outcome.

References

Adams, R.D., Fisher, C.M., Hakim, S., Ojemann, R.G. and Sweet, W.H. (1965) Symptomatic occult hydrocephalus with 'normal' cerebrospinal fluid pressure. A treatable syndrome. *N. Engl. J. Med.*, **273**, 117–126

Agner, E. (1981) Possible previous myocardial infarction and intermittent claudication during the eighth decade. A longitudinal epidemiological study. *Acta Med. Scand.*, **210**, 271–276

Andres, R. (1971) Ageing and diabetes. *Med. Clin. N. Am.*, **55**, 835–846

Bagdade, J.D., Root, R.K. and Bulger, R.J. (1974) Impaired leukocyte function in patients with poorly controlled diabetes. *Diabetes*, **23**, 9–15

Blake, R. and Lynn, J. (1976) Emergency abdominal surgery in the aged. *Br. J. Surg.*, **63**, 956–960

Bliss, M.R., McLaren, R. and Exton-Smith, A.N. (1967) Preventing pressure sores in hospital: controlled trial of a large-celled ripple mattress. *Br. Med. J.*, **1**, 394–397

Bone, J.M. (1988) Nephrology in the older patient. In *Advances in Geriatric Medicine*, (eds F.I. Caird and J.G. Evans), Pitman, London, vol 7, p. 20

Bunn, H.F. (1981) Evaluation of glycosylated haemoglobin in diabetic patients. *Diabetes*, **30**, 613–617

Butterfield, W.J.H. (1964) Summary of the results of the Bedford diabetes survey. *Proc. Roy. Soc. Med.*, **57**, 196–200

Caird, F.I., Pirie, A. and Ramsell, T.G. (1969) *Diabetes and the Eye*, Blackwell Scientific, Oxford and Edinburgh

Critchley, M. (1931) The neurology of old age. Clinical manifestations in old age. *Lancet*, **i**, 1221–1230

Defronzo, R.A., Humphrey, R.L., Wright, J.R. and Cooke, C.R. (1975) Acute renal failure in multiple myeloma. *Medicine*, **54**, 209–223

Devas, M. (1974) Geriatric orthopaedics. *Br. Med. J.*, **1**, 190–192

Devas, M. (1977) In *Geriatric Orthopaedics*, (ed. M. Devas), Academic Press, London, p. 1

Evans, J.G., Prudham, D. and Wandless, I. (1979) A prospective study of fractured proximal femur: incidence and outcome. *Publ. Hlth*, **93**, 235–241

Folstein, M.F., Folstein, S.E. and McHugh, P.R. (1975) Mini-mental status. A practical method for grading the cognitive state of patients for the clinician. *J. Psychiat. Res.*, **12**, 189–198

George, J. (1989) The neurological examination of the elderly patient. In *The Clinical Neurology of Old Age* (ed. R. Tallis), John Wiley, Chichester, p.67

Goldman, L., Caldera, D.L., Southwick, F.S., Nussbaum, S.R. Murray, B. O'Malley, T.A. *et al.* (1978) Cardiac risk factors and complications in non-cardiac surgery. *Medicine*, **57**, 357–370

Goldman, L. (1983) Cardiac risks and complications of noncardiac surgery. *Ann. Intern. Med.*, **98**, 504–513

Halkin, H. Goldberg, J., Modan, M. and Modan, B. (1982) Reduction of mortality in general medical in-patients by low-dose heparin prophylaxis. *Ann. Intern. Med.*, **96**, 561–565

Heller, S.S., Frank, K.A., Malm, J.R., Bowman, F.O., Harris, P.D., Charlton, M.H. and Kornfeld, D.S. (1970) Psychiatric complication of open-heart surgery; a re-examination. *N. Engl. J. Med.*, **283**, 1015–1020

Hodkinson, H.M. (1972) Evaluation of a mental test score for the assessment of mental impairment in the elderly. *Age Ageing*, **1**, 233–238

Isaacs, B. (1985) Falls. In *Practical Geriatric Medicine* (eds A.N. Exton-Smith, and M.E. Weksler), Churchill Livingstone, Edinburgh, p. 154

Jefferys, P.M. (1972) The prevalence of thyroid disease in patients admitted to a geriatric department. *Age Ageing*, **1**, 33–37

Loew, F. and Kivelitz, R. (1976) Chronic subdural haematomas. In *Handbook of Clinical Neurology* (eds P.J. Vinken and G.W. Bruyn), **24**, 297

McFadden, J.P., Price, R.C., Eastwood, H.D. and Briggs, R.S. (1982) Raised respiratory rate in elderly patients; a valuable physical sign. *Br. Med. J.*, **284**, 626–627

McLachlan, M.S.F. (1978) The ageing kidney. *Lancet*, **ii**, 143–145

Mahoney, F.I. and Barthel, D.W. (1965) Functional evaluation: the Barthel index. *Rehabilitation*, **14**, 61

Miller, P.D., Krebs, R.A., Neal, B.J. and McIntyre, D.O. (1982) Hypodipsia in geriatric patients. *Am. J. Med.*, **73**, 354–356

Morrell, M.T., Truelove, S.C. and Barr, A. (1963) Pulmonary embolism. *Br. Med. J.*, **II**, 830–835

O'Neill, P. (1989) Cranio-cerebral trauma. In *The Clinical Neurology of Old Age* (ed. R Tallis), John Wiley, Chichester, p. 285

Pathy, M.S. (1967) Clinical presentation of myocardial infarction in the elderly. *Br. Heart J.*, **29**, 190–199

Pirart, J. (1978) Why don't we teach and treat diabetic patients better? [editorial] *Diabet. Care*, **1**, 139–140

Porter, R.W., Miller, C.G., Grainger, D. and Palmer, S.B. (1990) Prediction of hip fracture in elderly women: a prospective study. *Br. Med. J.*, **301**, 638

Potvin, A.R., Syndulko, K., Tourtellotte, W.W., Lemmon, J.A. and Potvin, J.H. (1980). Human neurological function and the ageing process. *J. Am. Geriat. Soc.*, **28**, 1–9

Prakash, C. and Stern, G. (1973) Neurological signs in the elderly. *Age Ageing*, **2**, 24–27

Rowe, J.W., Andres, R., Tobin, J.D., Norris, A.H. and Shock, N.W. (1976) The effect of age on creatinine clearance in men: a cross sectional and longitudinal study. *J. Gerontol.*, **31**, 155–163

Seymour, D.G. (1983) The geriatrician in the general surgical ward – Dundee. In *Advances in Geriatric Medicine, 3* (eds F.I. Caird and J.G. Evans), London, Pitman, pp. 163–171

Sharr, M (1989) Tumours of the nervous system. In *The Clinical Neurology of Old Age* (ed. R Tallis), John Wiley, Chichester, p. 235

SICOT (1990) Societé Internationale de Chirurgie Orthopedique et de Traumatologie. 18th World Congress, Montreal, Canada

Sorbini, C.A., Grassi, V., Solinas, E. and Muiesan, G. (1968) Arterial oxygen tension in relation to age in healthy subjects. *Respiration*, **25**, 3–13

Steen, P.A., Tinker, J.H. and Tarhan, S. (1978) Myocardial reinfarction after anaesthesia and surgery. *J. Am. Med. Ass.*, **239**, 2566–2570

Thomas, F.B., Mazaferri, E.L. and Skillman, T.G. (1970) Apathetic thyrotoxicosis: a distinct clinical and laboratory entity. *Ann. Intern. Med.*, **72**, 679–685

Trulock, E.P. (1988) Approaches to deep venous thrombosis and pulmonary embolism in ageing patients. *Geriatrics*, **43**, 101–102

Young, J.B., Belfield, P.W., Bagnall, W.E. and Mulley, G.P. (1987) Deliberate falls in the elderly. *Age Ageing*, **16**, 123–124

World Health Organization (1979) *Wld Hlth Stat. Ann.*, WHO, Geneva

4

Changes in the clinical pharmacology of drugs with age

Jeffrey K. Aronson

Although ageing is a universal phenomenon the rate at which different people age is not uniform. This observation is particularly important with regard to prescribing drugs for the elderly, since it is one's aim to give patients dosages of drugs which are most appropriate for their condition, i.e. dosages which will produce maximum likely benefits with minimum likely risks. Since individuals age at different rates, there will be greater variability in optimum dosage regimens among older people than among younger people.

Unfortunately, most of the information which relates to the effects of drugs in elderly people comes from studies in which comparisons have been made between groups of elderly people on the one hand and groups of younger people on the other. There are few studies of the ways in which dosage requirements gradually change as ageing occurs. This means that in practice one has to recommend dosage regimens for the *average* elderly person and trust to the prescriber to individualize the dosage regimen for each patient based on that patient's response. Clearly this is difficult to perform successfully since in 1980 a multi-centre study involving 2000 admissions to 42 geriatric units in the United Kingdom showed that about 1 in 10 of all patients were admitted solely or partly because of adverse drug interactions – the reasons for which will be described in detail below. Extrapolation of these figures suggests that up to 15 000 elderly hospital admissions are made each year in the United Kingdom which are due at least in part to suboptimal prescription in this particularly vulnerable age group (Woodhouse, 1991).

The ways in which dosage regimens in elderly people vary from those in younger people can be considered under two broad headings – changes in the disposition (pharmacokinetics) of drugs with age and changes in the responses of individuals to drugs. This chapter starts by reviewing the ways in which changes of these sorts can affect drug therapy in elderly people on average and ends by discussing the ways in which recommended average dosage regimens can be tailored to the requirements of the individual.

Changes in the disposition of drugs with age

There are four major aspects to the disposition of drugs: administration, absorption, distribution, and elimination. All of these may be affected by advancing age, but the extent to which they affect drug therapy differs.

Drug administration

Elderly people may have difficulty in swallowing drugs and occasionally tablets may stick in the oesophagus and cause local damage, e.g. Slow-K and emepronium bromide. This can be avoided by advising elderly patients to 'wash down' their tablets well. Other practical considerations in the self-administration of drugs by elderly people are mentioned at the end of this chapter.

Absorption and systemic availability

The extent to which a drug reaches the systemic circulation after oral administration (the systemic availability or bioavailability) depends on the rate at which it is absorbed and the extent to which it is metabolized in the liver after absorption (so-called first-pass metabolism).

Although there are many changes in the function of the gut with ageing, such as reduced gastric acidity and emptying rate, reduced transit time and a reduced area of the mucosa available for absorption, there is little evidence that any of these changes causes any important alteration in either the rate or the extent of absorption of drugs in elderly people. However, if absorption after oral administration is the rate-limiting step determining the half-life of the drug then in some circumstances a slowing of the rate of absorption, which in other circumstances may be clinically unimportant, may lead to a prolongation of the apparent half-life of the drug. This may in turn lead to greater accumulation of the drug than would have been expected had the rate of absorption been normal.

In contrast, there may be important changes in the presystemic metabolism of some drugs in elderly people, because of reduced liver blood flow. For this reason the amounts of certain drugs reaching the systemic circulation may be increased in elderly people. These drugs include chlormethiazole (Matiron *et al.*, 1976), morphine (Baillie *et al.*, 1989) and propranolol (Castleden and George, 1979). The effects of such changes have been shown in relation to nifedipine (Figure 4.1) (Robertson *et al.*, 1988). In a group of elderly volunteers plasma concentrations of nifedipine after a single oral dose were higher than in young volunteers and the apparent half-life was prolonged in elderly people from 3.8 to 6.7 h. The difference between the young and elderly people was greater after oral than after intravenous administration (*cf.* Figures 4.1a and 4.1b).

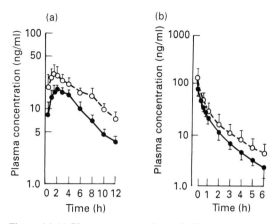

Figure 4.1 (a) Plasma concentrations of nifedipine after the oral administration of 10 mg of a sustained-release formulation in young (●) and elderly (○) volunteers. (b) Plasma concentrations of nifedipine after the intravenous administration of 2.5 mg in young (●) and elderly (○) volunteers. (From Robertson *et al.*, 1988, with permission)

total body fat, a fall in total body water and a fall in the masses of major organs such as the liver and kidney. Thus, the extent to which drugs may be distributed to the tissues may be reduced in the cases of some drugs. For example, the extent of distribution of digoxin is reduced in the elderly, partly because digoxin is not distributed into body fat and partly because elderly people tend to have renal impairment which is associated with a reduced distribution of digoxin to the tissues. The reasons for this are not clear (Aronson, 1983). Since the apparent volume of distribution of a drug influences the loading dose required, this means that in elderly patients the prescriber should start with lower dosages of drug than would generally be used in younger people.

Changes in drug distribution

There are two facets of drug distribution which should be considered, changes in the distribution of a drug to body tissues and changes in the binding of drugs to plasma proteins.

Changes in tissue distribution

There are many changes in the composition of the body with ageing which may influence the distribution of drugs to body tissues. These include a fall in lean body mass, an increase in

Changes in protein binding

There is a fall in plasma albumin concentration with age and this leads to reduced protein binding and hence to an increase in the unbound concentration of drugs in the plasma. This is clinically important only for drugs which are extensively bound to plasma albumin, principally warfarin, phenytoin and tolbutamide. Although the concentrations of another major binding protein, alpha₁-acid glycoprotein, are also reduced with ageing this change seems to have little clinical implication.

Changes in drug metabolism

With age there is reduced liver size, reduced hepatic microsomal oxidative enzyme activity and a reduced ability of liver enzymes to respond to inducing stimuli. The effects of reduced liver blood flow with age have been referred to above in relation to reduced first-pass metabolism and thus the increased systemic availability of some drugs.

Drug metabolism is conventionally considered to take place in two phases. So-called phase 1 metabolism involves a variety of oxidative transformations including hydroxylation, deamination, dealkylation, sulphoxidation, desulphuration and dehalogenation. These reactions are all dependent on a system known as the mixed function oxidase system and the activity of that system falls with age. So-called phase 2 reactions are conjugation transformations such as acetylation, methylation, glucuronidation, and sulphation. In contrast to phase 1 reactions these change hardly at all with age.

There are many examples of drugs whose metabolism by oxidation has been shown to fall with increasing age. These include diazepam (Macklon *et al.*, 1980), quinidine (Ochs *et al.*, 1978), theophylline (Antal *et al.*, 1981), propranolol (Castleden and George, 1979), nortriptyline (Dawling, Crome and Braithwaite, 1980) and nifedipine (Figure 4.1) (Robertson *et al.*, 1988). Since reduced clearance of drugs by impaired metabolism causes an increase in both the steady-state concentrations of the drug for a given dose and the time it takes to reach steady state, dosages of these drugs should be reduced in elderly people.

Changes in renal drug elimination

Since glomerular filtration rate declines with age elderly people have a reduced rate of clearance of drugs which are eliminated unchanged by the kidneys. These include digoxin, aminoglycoside antibiotics, procainamide and lithium.

In all these cases dosages should be less for elderly people than for younger people, since the elderly are likely to clear these drugs at a slower rate and will therefore tend to accumulate the drugs. They will therefore have higher steady-state plasma concentrations and will take a longer time to reach steady state.

There are other drugs which are cleared by the kidneys and whose elimination is slowed in renal failure. These include many antibiotics such as

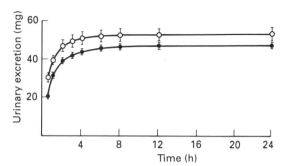

Figure 4.2 The mean cumulative excretion of frusemide in the urine during the 24 h after intravenous injection of 80 mg in young (○) and elderly (●) volunteers. (From Andreasen *et al.*, 1983, with permission)

the penicillins and cephalosporins. However, because those drugs have a high toxic:therapeutic ratio there is less need to be careful about dosages than for drugs which have a low toxic:therapeutic ratio. Nevertheless, in cases of severe renal impairment it may be necessary to reduce the dosages of these usually safe drugs.

In the case of diuretics poor renal function may lead to reduced drugs effects, since some diuretics act from the luminal side of the nephron. This has been shown in the case of frusemide (Figure 4.2) which does not gain such ready access to its site of action in elderly patients because of reduced renal excretion (Andreasen *et al.*, 1983).

Changes in the pharmacological effects of drugs with age

The elderly tend to be more sensitive to the actions of some drugs for at least two reasons. First, there may be changes in the normal physiological mechanisms whereby homoeostasis is preserved and the response to a drug which alters a physiological function may therefore be affected. Second, there may be changes in either the number or the nature of the specific receptors through which a drug exerts its action. In some cases both mechanisms may play a part.

Changes in physiological function affecting responses to drugs

Blood pressure

Elderly people have greater difficulty in maintaining blood pressure than younger people and they may therefore be more sensitive to the vasodilatory effects of drugs such as the nitrates and the calcium antagonists (Doherty, 1986). This means that not only will elderly patients require, on average, lower dosages of antihypertensive drugs, but they will also be more sensitive to the adverse effects of other drugs on the cardiovascular system including phenothiazines, L-dopa and diuretics (whether used as antihypertensives or not, since they reduce plasma volume).

Cerebral function

Elderly patients are more susceptible to the adverse effects of drugs which act on the brain for reasons which are not fully understood. This means that they are more likely to suffer the adverse effects of drugs such as the phenothiazines (e.g. chlorpromazine), lithium, the benzodiazepines (e.g. diazepam), antihistamines and alcohol.

Posture

Elderly individuals have more difficulty in maintaining an upright posture than younger people. This means that drugs which act on the brain may more readily cause them to fall (Rae *et al.*, 1987).

Body temperature

Elderly people have problems in maintaining their body temperature. They are therefore more likely to develop hypothermia after drug overdose, particularly with drugs which act on the brain.

Changes in receptors

Changes in receptor number or nature occur in the elderly. For example, there is an alteration in the sensitivity of the heart to cardiac glycosides, such as digoxin, which may be related to a reduction in the number of sodium/potassium pumps in the cell membranes or to a change in the susceptibility of those pumps to inhibition by cardiac glycosides (Kelly, Copeland and McDevitt, 1983). Similarly, the elderly have reduced amounts of clotting factors and are therefore more sensitive to the actions of the oral anticoagulants (Shepherd *et al.*, 1977). The effects of benzodiazepines on the brain are greater in elderly people than in younger people, perhaps because of changes in the specific receptors in the brain which mediate the actions of these drugs (Cook, Flanagan and James, 1984).

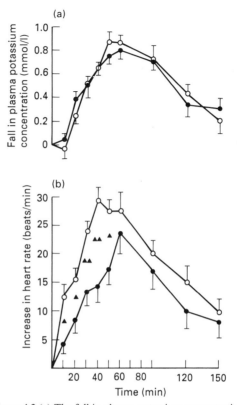

Figure 4.3 (a) The fall in plasma potassium concentrations after the intravenous administration of terbutaline to young (○) and elderly (●) subjects. (b) The increase in heart rate after the intravenous administration of terbutaline to young (○) and elderly (●) subjects. (Adapted from Kendall *et al.*, 1982, with permission)

In some cases both of these types of mechanism, changes in physiological processes and changes in receptors, may play a part. The increase in the effects of the calcium antagonists in elderly individuals provides an example of a combination of these two different types of mechanism, because of changes in the blood pressure-controlling mechanisms and alterations in the susceptibility of calcium channels to their antagonists (Robertson *et al.*, 1988).

Another interesting example of the ways in which drugs can affect the young and old differently is the action of terbutaline on cardiovascular and other functions. Terbutaline causes less of an increase in heart rate in elderly people than in young people but the fall in potassium concentration which it causes is the same in the two groups (Figure 4.3) (Kendall *et al.*, 1982). These actions arise through complex mechanisms, but they illustrate that one cannot generalize about actions of drugs in the elderly.

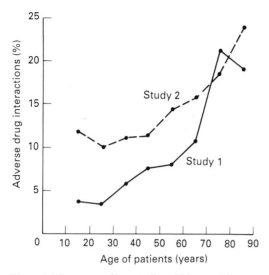

Figure 4.4 Summary of two studies which report increases in adverse drug interactions with age. (Royal College of Physicians, 1984)

There is some controversy about the extent to which the elderly are more or less sensitive to drugs than their younger counterparts. However, as with changes in drug disposition with ageing, it is wise to assume from the outset that the elderly are likely to be more sensitive to the actions of drugs than younger people and to start treatment with lower dosages. If the response is suboptimal the dosage can subsequently be increased. However, if the dose is too high drug toxicity may occur and toxicity may be difficult to treat and can significantly complicate the overall management.

Drug interactions

Adverse drug interactions are more commonly seen in older patients but the magnitude of this problem has only been recognized relatively recently. Surveys in the United Kingdom, the USA and Sweden show that the incidence of adverse drug interactions increases with advancing age (Figure 4.4) (Royal College of Physicians, 1984). Similarly, the death rate due to this form of iatrogenic disease also rises with age (Adelstein and Loy, 1979). Unfortunately those patients who survive do not necessarily recover fully after cessation of treatment.

Elderly patients are not inherently more susceptible to adverse drug interactions than younger ones and the above observations may simply be a reflection of the disproportionate number of prescriptions that have to be endured by the aged members of our population. For example, in 1980 the elderly were dispensed twice as many prescriptions as the national average (Office of Health Economics, 1980). Similarly, whereas only one-third of 21 to 24-year-old patients take prescribed medication during a 2-week period this figure rises to nearly three-quarters in the 75 years and over age groups (Dunnel and Cartwright, 1972). Similarly, in a random study of people over 65 years of age living at home 28% took no medication, 37% took one to three prescribed drugs and 15% took four or more; 85-year-olds were more likely to take more drugs than people aged 65–74 years.

Because virtually all adverse drug interactions are due to changes in the disposition of one drug by another, such interactions may be exacerbated by conditions such as pre-existing renal or hepatic impairment or reduced protein binding. For example, the renal elimination of lithium is reduced by thiazide diuretics – if there is pre-existing renal impairment this effect may become more pronounced.

The uses of non-steroidal anti-inflammatory drugs in elderly people

Since this book concerns itself primarily with the comprehensive orthopaedic care of the elderly individual it is necessary to discuss the non-steroidal anti-inflammatory drugs (NSAIDs) separately.

Changes in the disposition of NSAIDs

Aspirin may have greater effects in elderly patients than in younger ones for two reasons. First, it is highly protein bound and second, it is metabolized by aspirin esterase, the activity of which may be reduced in the elderly. However, it should be noted that this reduction in esterase activity is not an effect of ageing *per se*, but is related to the frailty of the individual (Williams *et al.*, 1989). This observation underlines the remarks made at the beginning of this chapter that treatment should be tailored to the requirements of each individual, whether old or young.

Other NSAIDs, such as indomethacin and naproxen, are also highly protein bound and the changes in protein binding which can occur with age may affect their disposition. In addition, almost all of these drugs are metabolized in the liver. However, they are generally not subject to the effects of liver impairment on the systemic availability of drugs and there seems to be little effect of impaired metabolism on the disposition of NSAIDs.

Although it may appear paradoxical that changes in renal function can alter the disposition of drugs which are largely eliminated by hepatic metabolism, this has been shown to be the case with some of the NSAIDS. This is because some of the metabolites of these compounds are unstable and can be deconjugated to form the parent drug again. Thus, if these metabolites accumulate because of renal impairment, more of the parent drug can be formed. There is also evidence that inactive enantiomers of some of these compounds can be converted to active forms and, if there is accumulation of the inactive forms, that too may enhance the actions of these drugs (Brater, 1988).

Adverse effects of NSAIDs

Ulcerogenic effects

There is evidence that the risk of peptic ulceration with consequent haemorrhage and perforation is increased in the elderly (Somerville, Faulkner and Langman, 1986; Walt *et al.*, 1986). The risk is not uniform with different NSAIDs and those associated with the lowest risk are ibuprofen, diclofenac, sulindac and flurbiprofen (Committee on Safety of Medicines, 1986).

There is evidence that misoprostol, a prostaglandin E analogue, can reduce the risk of anti-inflammatory drug-induced gastric ulcers (Graham, Agrawal and Roth, 1988). There is also evidence that misoprostol can reduce the risk of duodenal ulceration in patients taking aspirin (Langman, Morgan and Worrall, 1985). However, this preparation should not be used routinely in all patients taking a NSAID, but should be reserved for those in whom there is known to be an increased risk of peptic ulceration and in whom NSAID therapy is thought to be mandatory. In individuals at risk of duodenal as opposed to gastric ulceration some suggest the use of a histamine (H_2) receptor antagonist. It is not yet clear whether these types of therapy will cause a reduction in the risk of haemorrhage or perforation from formed ulcers.

Renal damage

NSAIDs can cause renal damage, typically in the form of acute interstitial nephritis. Since renal function is in any case impaired in the elderly, they are likely to run a higher risk of renal damage from these drugs. There is some evidence that sulindac is less likely to cause renal impairment and it may therefore be used in individuals in whom it is felt that this is a particular risk (Clive and Stoff, 1984). It is, however, not normally considered as a first-line NSAID.

Sodium and water retention

All of the NSAIDs can cause retention of sodium and water which can result in oedema and cardiac failure. The risk of this may be increased in elderly people (Van der Ouweland and Gribnau, 1988). Unfortunately treatment with diuretics may exacerbate the problem since potassium-wasting diuretics may cause hyponatraemia in these circumstances (Goodenough and Loutz 1988) and potassium-sparing diuretics may increase the risk of renal damage.

A practical approach to prescribing for the elderly

From all these observations some simple principles emerge which may be used in tackling the problem of prescribing drugs for the elderly.

First, because renal and/or hepatic elimination of drugs may be reduced in the elderly one can expect that the half-life of any drug so affected will be prolonged (see for example, Figure 4.1). This means that it will take longer to reach a steady state during repeated administration of the drug and one may therefore have to wait longer in elderly people before a therapeutic effect occurs (if a loading dose is not given) than one would in younger people. In addition, impairment of renal or hepatic elimination of drugs will lead to a greater degree of accumulation of those drugs and thus to higher steady-state plasma drug concentrations once a steady state has been reached. The problems that can arise from this can be avoided by using lower maintenance dosages of drugs in elderly people.

The extent to which drug dosages should be reduced if there is renal impairment can be judged by measurement of the creatinine clearance, based on which there are simple methods for altering the dosages of relevant drugs (Grahame–Smith and Aronson, 1984). However, there is no equivalent simple test of impaired liver function in relation to drug metabolism and in such cases changes in dosage have to be made empirically.

Second, a reduction in the apparent volume of distribution of the drug will also give rise to an increase in its half-life with the consequences outlined above. Furthermore, if the apparent volume of distribution of a drug is lowered it is wise to use lower *loading* doses than normal, if loading doses are to be given at all.

Third, increased sensitivity to a drug will mean that the patient will respond to a greater extent for a given dose or plasma concentration of that drug. For this reason it is always prudent to start at the lower end of the dosage range and slowly increase the dose while monitoring for therapeutic and adverse effects. Of course, this is a general principle which applies to drug therapy in patients of all ages, but it is one which should be applied with particular care to elderly people.

In addition to all these factors, there are some simple practical points which may make drug therapy difficult in the aged patient. First, elderly people may find tablets difficult to swallow. Second, they may have difficulty in opening bottles, particularly those which are intended to be 'child-proof'. Third, they may not be able to read the instructions on the bottle, either because of poor eyesight or because of difficulties in comprehending novel ideas. Fourth, they may comply poorly with therapy; this may be due to difficulties in communication which may be exacerbated by poor memory and hearing.

Simple measures may obviate these problems. For example, many patients benefit from being given written instructions and one should also make sure that instructions written on medicine bottles are in simple language (e.g. 'heart tablets', 'water tablets') and in large print. Sometimes one may have to offer patients the choice of an elixir if they cannot swallow tablets. Informing relatives about the need for therapy and the type of therapy being used may also be helpful.

When prescribing drugs for elderly people consider the following questions.

Is your prescription really necessary?

Unnecessary prescribing occurs commonly. For example, patients with senile dementia are not infrequently treated with cerebral vasodilators. However, there is little evidence that this kind of treatment is of any benefit whatsoever and some evidence that it may do harm by diverting blood from poorly-perfused areas of the brain. Similarly, the prescription of so-called 'tonics' containing vitamins and minerals without any evidence of deficiencies of those substances is clearly unnecessary. Broad-spectrum antibiotics for acute diarrhoea are generally not required and may even cause prolongation of the illness.

It is not always easy to decide whether or not treatment is necessary in an individual but it helps if the question is considered on each occasion of prescribing.

Which drug should be prescribed?

This question has three facets relating to the therapeutic class of drug, the group of drugs within that therapeutic class and the particular drug within that group. Although in general the therapeutic class of drug is obvious (for example, an antibiotic for an infection) it may at times be more difficult to choose. For example, one might have to consider a choice of a diuretic, a positive inotropic drug, a vasodilator, or an ACE inhibitor in the treatment of cardiac failure. However, this choice is one which is generally not influenced by age.

In contrast, when one comes to choose a group of drugs within the therapeutic class, age may play a part in one's decision. For example, when choosing an antibiotic it is generally better to avoid the tetracyclines, since they tend to accumulate in patients with renal impairment and can cause nausea and vomiting, with consequent acute renal failure in a patient with pre-existing renal damage. Similarly, when choosing a particular drug in a therapeutic group of drugs one may be influenced by the age of the patient. For example, if one felt that one was forced to use a tetracycline to treat an infection in an elderly patient one might choose doxycycline since of all the tetracyclines it is the least likely to accumulate in the individuals with renal impairment.

In choosing a drug one may also be influenced by other preparations the patient is taking in view of the need to avoid adverse drug interactions. Since elderly patients are more likely to be taking multiple drugs when compared with younger patients this becomes more of a consideration when prescribing for this age group.

Common important drug interactions

Drug interactions occur when one drug alters the effects of another. Usually such interactions result in an adverse effect, although on occasion it may be beneficial, e.g. the interaction of ACE inhibitors and diuretics in the treatment of hypertension

In this description of drug interactions I shall refer to the drug which causes an interaction the 'precipitant' drug and the drug whose effects are altered the 'object' drug.

Drug interactions can be classified according to their mechanism:

1. Pharmacokinetic interactions
   (a) Altered absorption
   (b) Altered protein binding
   (c) Altered metabolism
   (d) Altered excretion

2. Pharmacodynamic interactions
   (a) Direct interactions
   (b) Indirect interactions

Pharmacokinetic interactions involving drug absorption and protein binding are usually of little clinical significance and will not be discussed further. In contrast, interactions which occur by other mechanisms are often important.

The metabolism of a drug in the liver may be either stimulated ('induced') or inhibited by another drug. In the former case the precipitant drug increases the activity of drug-metabolizing enzymes and reduces the effects of the object drug. If higher dosages are not given undertreatment will result. Conversely, if higher dosages of the object drug are prescribed and the precipitant drug is then withdrawn there may be toxicity due to the object drug. An example is the increased dosage requirements of warfarin when an enzyme-inducing drug is given, e.g. phenytoin; when the inducer is withdrawn warfarin dosages must be reduced in order to avoid bleeding. Examples of interactions due to enzyme induction are listed in Table 4.1.

Inhibition of drug metabolism commonly causes toxicity due to warfarin and phenytoin.

Table 4.1 Drug interactions due to induction of drug metabolism (decreased effects of the object drugs)

Precipitant drug(s)	Object drug(s)
Alcohol	Coumarin anticoagulants, phenytoin
Barbiturates	Chlorpromazine, corticosteroids, coumarin anticoagulants, doxycycline, phenytoin
Carbamazepine	Phenytoin
Dichloralphenazone	Warfarin
Glutethimide	Coumarin anticoagulants
Griseofulvin	Warfarin
Orphenadrine	Chlorpromazine
Phenytoin	Corticosteroids, coumarin anticoagulants, tolbutamide
Rifampicin	Coumarin anticoagulants, tolbutamide

Important examples of this type of drug interaction are listed in Table 4.2.

If a precipitant drug inhibits the renal excretion of an object drug the action of the object drug will be enhanced and toxicity may occur. For example, thiazide diuretics inhibit the excretion of lithium and may cause lithium toxicity. Important interactions of this kind are listed in Table 4.3.

Direct pharmacodynamic interactions occur when two drugs which act at the same site are given together. Usually this type of interaction results in potentiation of the effects of each drug. A common example of this type of interaction, a list of which is given in Table 4.4a, is the effect of alcohol in patients who are taking drugs which act on the brain, e.g. benzodiazepines, antihistamines. Patients taking drugs of this sort should be advised that even the smallest amount of alcohol may make it unsafe for them to operate machinery or to drive. Occasionally a direct interaction may cause antagonism of the effects of the object drug as in the reversal of the effects of opiates by naloxone.

Indirect pharmacodynamic interactions (Table 4.4b) occur when the precipitant drug has some effect which in turn alters the action of the object drug. For example, drugs which can cause peptic ulceration may precipitate toxicity due to anticoagulants by providing a site for bleeding.

Conclusion

The elderly should not be considered as a homogeneous group of patients to be contrasted with

Table 4.2 Drug interactions due to inhibition of drug metabolism (increased effects of the object drugs)

(a) Inhibition of the mixed function oxidases

Precipitant drug(s)	Object drug(s)
Azapropazone	Phenytoin, warfarin
Chloramphenicol	Phenytoin, tolbutamide, warfarin
Cimetidine	Diazepam, propranolol, warfarin
Isoniazid (slow acetylators)	Phenytoin
Imidazoles (e.g. metronidazole, ketoconazole)	Alcohol, warfarin
Sulphinpyrazone	Warfarin

(b) Inhibition of specific metabolic enzymes

Precipitant drug(s)	Enzyme	Object drug(s)
Allopurinol	Xanthine oxidase	Azathioprine, 6-mercaptopurine
Carbidopa and benserazide	Dopa decarboxylase	L-dopa
Disulfiram	Alcohol dehydrogenase	Alcohol
MAO inhibitors	Monoamine oxidase	Amine-containing foods (see below), amphetamine

(c) Amine-containing foods which may interact with MAO inhibitors

Cheese (matured, especially Cheddar; cream and cottage cheeses are safe)
Meat or yeast extracts
Some wines
Unfresh protein (especially hung poultry or game; canned or frozen foods are safe if eaten immediately after opening or thawing)
Caviare

Table 4.3 Drug interactions involving altered drug excretion

Precipitant drug(s)	Object drug(s)	Result
Activated charcoal	Tricyclic antidepressants, phenobarbitone	Enhanced excretion rate of object drug
Thiazide diuretics	Lithium	Lithium retention
Loop diuretics	Gentamicin	Nephrotoxicity
Probenecid	Penicillin	Penicillin retention
Probenecid	Chloroquine	Retinopathy
Salicylates (low dose)	Sulphinpyrazone	Decreased uricosuric effect
Salicylates (low dose)	Methotrexate	Methotrexate retention
Quinidine, verapamil, spironolactone, amiodarone	Digoxin	Digoxin retention

younger people. They are individuals and require individual management. Dosage regimens are generally best established in each case by starting with low doses (whether loading or maintenance dosages) and slowly increasing the dosage in search of a therapeutic effect, monitoring the patient's clinical progress. Monitoring therapy may be helped by carrying out

Table 4.4 Pharmacodynamic drug interactions

Precipitant drug(s)	Object drug(s)	Result
(a) Direct		
Aminoglycosides, quinidine, quinine	Depolarizing muscle relaxants	Enhanced skeletal muscle relaxation
Centrally-acting drugs	Centrally-acting drugs	Potentiation
β-adrenoceptor antagonists	Verapamil	Arrhythmias, asystole, heart failure
Physostigmine	Tricyclic antidepressants	Reversal of anticholinergic effects
Naloxone	Opiate analgesics	Reversal of opiate effects
Vitamin K_1	Coumarin anticoagulants	Diminished anticoagulation
Anabolic steroids Clofibrate Corticosteroids Oestrogens Tetracyclines	Warfarin	Increased anticoagulation
(b) Indirect		
Class I antiarrhythmic drugs and amiodarone	Class I antiarrhythmic drugs and amiodarone	Increased risk of cardiac arrhythmias
Drugs affecting platelet adhesiveness (e.g. non-steroidal anti-inflammatory drugs)	Anticoagulants	Impaired haemostasis
Drugs causing gastrointestinal bleeding (e.g. non-steroidal anti-inflammatory drugs)	Anticoagulants	Increased chance of bleeding
Drugs causing fibrinolysis (e.g. streptokinase)	Anticoagulants	Impaired haemostasis
Drugs causing potassium loss (e.g. diuretics)	Cardiac glycosides Antiarrhythmic drugs Sulphonylureas	Increased effects Decreased effects Decreased effects
Drugs causing hypercalcaemia (e.g. calcium salts, vitamin D)	Cardiac glycosides	Increased effects
Drugs causing fluid retention (e.g. non-steroidal anti-inflammatory drugs)	Diuretics	Decreased effects
β-adrenoceptor antagonists	Vasodilators	Improved control of hypertension/angina

simple measures of the pharmacodynamic actions of drugs (e.g. the exercise heart rate in patients taking beta-blockers and the international normalized ratio (INR) in patients taking warfarin) or by measuring the plasma drug concentration (e.g. in the cases of digoxin, theophylline, phenytoin and lithium).

An excellent compilation of information on the use of drugs in the elderly is to be found in Denham and George (1990).

References

Adelstein, A and Loy, P. (1979) Fatal adverse effects of medicines and surgery. *Pop. Trends*, **17**, 17–22

Andreasen, F., Hansen, U., Husted, S.E. and Jansen, J.A. (1983) The pharmacokinetics of frusemide are influenced by age. *Br. J. Clin. Pharm.*, **16**, 391–397

Antal, E.J., Kramer, P.A., Mercik, S.A., Chapron, D.J. and Lawson, I.R. (1981) Theophylline pharmacokinetics in advanced age. *Br. J. Clin. Pharm.*, **12**, 637–645

Aronson, J.K. (1983) Clinical pharmacokinetics of cardiac glycosides in patients with renal dysfunction. *Clin. Pharmacokin.*, **8**, 155–178

Baillie, S.T., Bateman, D.N., Coates, P.E. and Woodhouse, K.W. (1989) Age and the pharmacokinetics of morphine. *Age Ageing*, **18**, 258–262

Brater, D.C. (1988) Clinical pharmacology of NSAIDs. *J. Clin. Pharm.*, **28**, 518–523

Castleden, C.M. and George, C.F. (1979) The effect of ageing on the hepatic clearance of propranolol. *Br. J. Clin. Pharm.*, **7**, 49–54

Clive, D.M. and Stoff, J.S. (1984) Renal syndromes associated with non-steroidal anti-inflammatory drugs. *N. Engl. J. Med.*, **310**, 563–572

Committee on Safety of Medicines (1986) CSM update. Non-steroidal anti-inflammatory drugs and serious gastrointestinal adverse effects – 2. *Br. Med. J.*, **292**, 1190–1191

Cook, P.J., Flanagan, R. and James, I.M. (1984) Diazepam tolerance; Effect of age, regular sedation and alcohol. *Br. Med. J.*, **289**, 351–353

Dawling, S., Crome, P. and Braithwaite, R. (1980) Pharmacokinetics of single oral doses of nortriptyline in depressed elderly hospital patients and young healthy volunteers. *Clin. Pharmacokin.*, **5**, 394–401

Denham, M.J. and George, C.F. (eds) (1990) Drugs in old age. New perspectives. *Br. Med. Bull.*, **46**, 1–299

Doherty, J.R. (1986) Aging and the cardiovascular system. *J. Autonom. Pharm.*, **6**, 77–84

Dunnel, K. and Cartwright, A. (1972) *Medicine Takers, Prescribers and Hoarders*, Routledge, Kegan and Paul, London

Goodenough, G.K. and Loutz, L.J. (1988) Hyponatremic hypervolemia caused by drug-drug interaction mistaken for syndrome of inappropriate ADH. *J. Am. Geriat. Soc.*, **36**, 285–286

Graham, D.Y., Agrawal, N.M. and Roth, S.H. (1988) Prevention of NSAID-induced gastric ulcer with misoprostol: multicentre, double-blind, placebo-controlled trial. *Lancet*, **ii**, 1277–1280

Grahame–Smith, D.G., Aronson, J.K. (1984) *The Oxford textbook of clinical pharmacology and drug therapy*, Oxford University Press, Oxford, pp. 46–47

Kelly, J.G., Copeland, S. and McDevitt, D.G. (1983) Erythrocyte cation transport and age: effects of digoxin and furosemide. *Clin. Pharm. Ther.*, **34**, 159–163

Kendall, M.J., Woods K.L., Wilkins, M.R. and Worthington, D.J. (1982) Responsiveness to β-adrenergic receptor stimulation: the effects of age are cardioselective. *Br. J. Clin. Pharm.*, **14**, 821–826

Langman, M.J.S., Morgan, L. and Worrall, A. (1985) Use of anti-inflammatory drugs by patients admitted with small or large bowel perforations and haemorrhage. *Br. Med. J.*, **290**, 347–349

Macklon, A.F., Barton, M., James, O. and Rawlins, M.D. (1980) The effect of age on the pharmacokinetics of diazepam. *Clin. Sci.*, **59**, 479–483

Matiron, R.L., Learoyd, B., Barber, J. and Triggs, E.J. (1976) The pharmacokinetics of chlormethiazole following intravenous administration in the aged. *Eur. J. Clin. Pharm.*, **10**, 407–415

Ochs, H.R., Greenblatt, D.J., Woo, E. and Smith, T.W. (1978) Reduced quinidine clearance in elderly persons. *Am. J. Cardiol.*, **42**, 482–485

Office of Health Economics (1980) *Effects of Prescription Charges*, OHE briefing, December, p. 13

Rae, W.A., Griffin, M.R., Schaffner, W., Baugh, D.K. and Melton, L.J. (1987) Psychotropic drug use and the risk of hip fracture. *N. Engl. J. Med.*, **316**, 363–369

Robertson, D.R.C., Waller, D.G., Renwick, A.G. and George, C.F. (1988) Age-related changes in the pharmacokinetics and pharmacodynamics of nifedipine. *Br. J. Clin. Pharm.*, **25**, 297–305

Royal College of Physicians (1984) Medication for the elderly; report of a working party. *J. Roy. Coll. Phys. Lond.*, **18**, 7–17

Shepherd, A.M.M., Hewick D.S., Moreland, T.A. and Stevenson, I.H. (1977) Age as a determinant of sensitivity to warfarin. *Br. J. Clin. Pharm.*, **4**, 315–320

Somerville, K., Faulkner, G. and Langman, M. (1986) Non-steroidal anti-inflammatory drugs and bleeding peptic ulcer. *Lancet*, **i**, 462–464

Van der Ouweland, F.A. and Gribnau, F.W.A. (1988) Congestive heart failure due to non-steroidal anti-inflammatory drugs in the elderly. *Age Ageing*, **17**, 8–16

Walt, R., Katschinski, B., Logan, R., Ashley, J. and Langman, M. (1986) Rising frequency of ulcer perforation in elderly people in the United Kingdom. *Lancet*, **i**, 489–492

Williams, F.M., Wynne, H., Woodhouse, K.W. and Rawlins, M.D. (1989) Plasma aspirin esterase; the influence of old age and frailty. *Age Ageing*, **118**, 39–42

Woodhouse, K. (1991) Adverse drug reaction is bitter pill for elderly. *Hosp. Doctor*, **C11**, 37

5

Anaesthetic considerations in the elderly patient

Stephen R. Swindells

The majority of anaesthetic procedures performed in the UK are delivered to middle-aged and elderly patients and this bias towards the elderly is set to become even more marked as the demographic features of our population change with an increased number of aged individuals. The physiology and pharmacological needs of the elderly are significantly different and quite distinct from those of younger adults and it maybe difficult on purely clinical grounds to assess the functional reserve of the cardiorespiratory system in an aged patient. This is because many such individuals are relatively immobile due to their orthopaedic condition and rarely exercise sufficiently to stress their cardiorespiratory system during their normal activities of daily living. In addition to the physiological changes of ageing (Figure 5.1) there are specific disease processes which are more prevalent in the elderly and which have implications with regard to anaesthesia.

Before describing the pre-, peri- and postoperative anaesthetic considerations in the elderly patient it is first necessary to outline those physiological changes and specific diseases which have relevance to the anaesthetist.

Physiological changes in the cardiovascular system with ageing

Through life the healthy heart increases in weight and this may relate to the gradual concomitant increase in body mass (Smith, 1928). Similarly, the cardiothoracic ratio increases slightly but stays within normal limits in the absence of cardiovascular disease (Potter *et al.*,

1982). Cavity size remains stable with age but left ventricular wall thickness may increase by up to 30% (Gardin *et al.*, 1977; Gerstenblith *et al.*, 1977). The ability of the heart to increase in weight or size is not altered by age and it is possible that when and if cardiac atrophy occurs it is no more than a reflection of the general weight loss associated with chronic disease.

Though the valves of older people tend to thicken and sometimes calcify, this does not necessarily indicate a functional disorder (Wong, Tei and Shah, 1983). There is an increased tortuosity of the coronary arteries of little clinical significance (Hutchins *et al.*, 1977) but the incidence of atherosclerotic plaques is related to, but probably not a result of, ageing (McMillan and Lev, 1961). With age the peripheral arteries thicken, calcify and subsequently dilate, resulting in an increase in lumen diameter. The aorta demonstrates this to the greatest degree and these changes within it influence left ventricular function during the ejection phase. The loss of elasticity in part explains the development of systolic hypertension with the increased pulse pressure so often seen in the aged population. There is also an increased left ventricular output impedance and workload which may explain the age-related increase in left ventricular wall thickness.

Resting cardiac output probably does not fall with age in health (Granath, Jonsson and Strandell, 1964; Proper and Wall, 1972; Rodenheffer, 1984) but the heart's response to catecholamines in terms of inotropic and chronotropic activity is diminished (Weisfeldt, 1981). Similarly, cardiac muscle responsiveness to all receptor-mediated inotropes including digitalis glycosides decreases (Gerstenblith *et al.*, 1975; Lakatta *et*

45

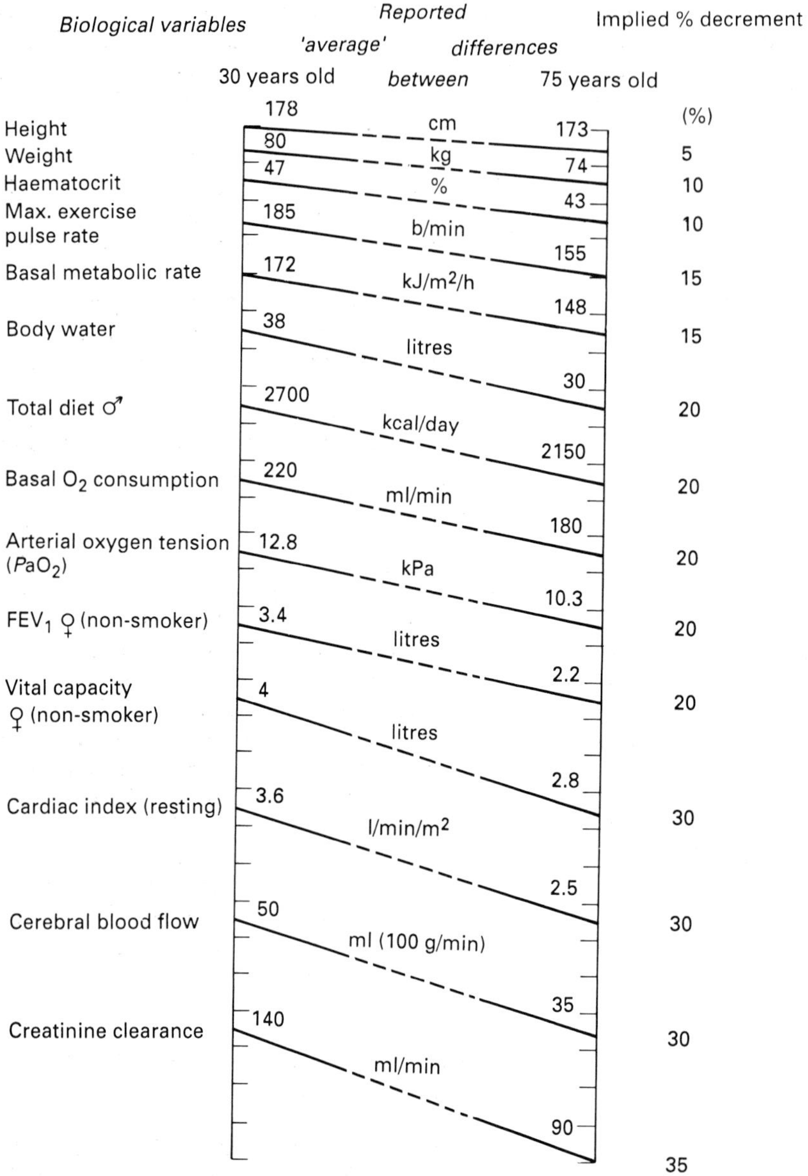

Biological variables	'average' 30 years old	Reported differences between	Implied % decrement 75 years old	(%)
Height	178	cm	173	
Weight	80	kg	74	5
Haematocrit	47	%	43	10
Max. exercise pulse rate	185	b/min	155	10
Basal metabolic rate	172	$kJ/m^2/h$	148	15
Body water	38	litres	30	15
Total diet ♂	2700	kcal/day	2150	20
Basal O_2 consumption	220	ml/min	180	20
Arterial oxygen tension (PaO_2)	12.8	kPa	10.3	20
FEV_1 ♀ (non-smoker)	3.4	litres	2.2	20
Vital capacity ♀ (non-smoker)	4	litres	2.8	20
Cardiac index (resting)	3.6	$l/min/m^2$	2.5	30
Cerebral blood flow	50	ml (100 g/min)	35	30
Creatinine clearance	140	ml/min	90	30
				35

Figure 5.1 Changes in some relevant physiological parameters with age. (From Davenport, 1988)

al., 1975), but this is not the case with calcium which does not require a specific receptor. With advancing age there is an increase in the threshold of stimulation of the cardiac autonomic nerves required to elicit an effect. This includes the cardiac response to hypoxia and hypercarbia via the chemoreceptors and to postural and blood pressure changes via the baroreceptors which are attenuated with age (Kronenberg and Drage, 1973). There is also a reduction in vagal influence with reduced responsiveness to the effects of atropine.

Cardiac output and the arteriovenous oxygen content difference are the two principal determinants of maximum oxygen consumption (VO_2max). The latter is approximately 45 ml/kg/min in a physically fit healthy adult and declines at a rate of 1.0 ml/kg/min per year. Buskirk and

Hodgson (1987) have suggested that if extrapolated this natural decline would lead to a situation in which the oxygen consumption associated with the basal metabolic rate would exceed VO_2max at the age of 110 years. Similarly, the oxygen demand of 7 ml/kg/min associated with a major operation could not be met after the age of 102 years.

It is clear that in terms of oxygen delivery the cost of major surgery is no greater than a slow walk and that any patient who can accomplish this can deliver enough oxygen to his tissues to undergo major surgery aerobically though this may not be the case at the extremes of senescence. The cardiac and respiratory pathologies described below have a far greater impact on VO_2max than the physiological changes associated with ageing and have to be considered when assessing fitness or otherwise of an elderly patient to undergo anaesthesia and surgery. There is no doubt that physical exercise will improve an individual's oxygen delivery ability and it is desirable that elderly people should participate in a regular programme of exercise, especially of the weight-bearing variety. However, in practice it is often difficult and impractical to encourage an elderly patient with orthopaedic problems to undertake such a programme. In these patients the single most effective way of improving oxygen delivery capability is the correction of anaemia even if this may not be a permanent adjustment, e.g. the treatment of the chronic anaemia of rheumatoid disease by blood transfusion 2 or 3 days preoperatively.

Cardiovascular disease in the aged

The diagnosis of cardiac disease in the asymptomatic patient is difficult but postmortem studies indicate that coronary atherosclerosis is common in the elderly (White, Edward and Dry, 1950). Risk factors such as smoking and hypertension are difficult to separate from age-related intimal changes of the blood vessels and ageing itself is seen as a greater risk factor than either smoking or hypertension (Pooling Project Research Group, 1978).

Myocardial infarction is associated with a high mortality in the elderly (Schnur, 1954; Williams *et al.*, 1976) and is of the order of 30–80% with a much higher incidence of complications such as congestive cardiac failure, pulmonary oedema and low output states (Zeman and Rodstein, 1960; Williams *et al.*, 1976). Congestive heart failure occurs in the elderly more frequently than is generally realized (McKee *et al.*, 1971), since the associated sedentary lifestyle masks the incidence of symptoms which in a younger person would accompany exercise and activity. Ischaemic heart disease causes most congestive cardiac failure followed by hypertension and valvular disease (Pomerance, 1976). There is little evidence that age itself produces congestive failure.

Valvular changes in the elderly are common (Wong, Tei and Shah, 1983; Bloor, 1982) and include calcific aortic stenosis and mitral valve prolapse. They do not seem to limit most patients although there may be an increased risk of endocarditis in certain circumstances. Atrial fibrillation is present in about 10% of the elderly population in hospital and can occur without other evidence of cardiac disease. Prolongation of the PR interval on electrocardiogram is frequently seen in aged patients and may be related to cellular changes in the sinoatrial node (Davies and Pomerance, 1972). Left axis deviation occurs as a result of left ventricular wall thickening (Fisch, 1981). The incidence of complete heart block is low and is associated with calcification of the mitral or aortic valve rings. Various degrees of heart block can be associated with previous aortic valve surgery and with inferior myocardial infarction.

Physiological changes in the respiratory system with ageing

Dyspnoea on exertion in the elderly is frequently due to a reduction in vital capacity related both to increased rigidity of the thoracic cage as well as emphysema occurring as part of a general tissue atrophy (see Figure 5.1). Emphysema may also be a feature of chronic respiratory disease such as chronic bronchitis or asthma. Loss of elastic recoil may well be responsible for the observation that airway closure occurs at increasing lung volume with advancing age (Holtz, Bake and Oxhoj, 1976).

This critical relationship between closing volume and functional residual capacity is more marked in the supine and head-down positions (Editorial, 1972). The increase in volume at which dependent zones cease to ventilate increases the ventilation/perfusion mismatch with age and causes a decrease in arterial oxygenation with age (Lablanc, Ruff and Milic-Emili, 1970). Rhonchi are common in the elderly without any underlying pulmonary disease but crepitations are usually a sign of incipient pneumonia or congestive cardiac failure.

Respiratory bronchioles and alveolar ducts undergo progressive enlargement in later life and this is associated with a decrease in alveolar surface area (Ryan *et al.*, 1965). Increased residual volume results in a reduction in vital capacity with age (Muiesan, Sorbini and Grassi, 1971) but the total lung capacity may be unaffected. This is because the effects of a relatively rigid chest wall with reduced muscle strength are offset by the reduced static recoil of the lung.

After the age of 40 years the intrinsic properties of the lung have an increasing influence on residual volume. For example, as elastic recoil forces of the lung decrease the stability of the terminal airways is reduced resulting in airway closure occurring at higher lung volume and an increased residual volume (Leith and Mead, 1967). Airway closure occurs in the lung bases at progressively greater lung volume or closing volume. When the closing volume moves into the tidal volume range airway closure at the bases may occur during ordinary breathing (Edelman *et al.*, 1968).

Changes in carbon dioxide production are matched by changes in alveolar ventilation and this remains constant in health irrespective of age. When airway closure in the lung bases begins to occur in the aged lung in the tidal volume range a low ventilation and high perfusion state is created. This reduces the partial pressure of oxygen in the capillaries in these particular regions of the lung.

With ageing there is a progressive fall in arterial oxygenation (Sorbini *et al.*, 1968) associated with changes in ventilatory control resulting in a significant reduction in the body's physiological responses to hypoxia and carbon dioxide (Kronenberg and Drage, 1973). Although the tension of oxygen in the arterial blood of the elderly is decreased at rest this is rarely a significant reduction and oxygen delivery to tissues is unimpaired at rest. There is a reduced cardiovascular response (Gerstenblith, Lakatta and Weisfeldt, 1976) to respiratory gas disturbance in the elderly with a progressive

decline in maximal heart rate and maximal oxygen uptake (Davies, 1972).

Systematic exercise training in the elderly (DeVries, 1970; Adams and DeVries, 1973) increases work capacity and reduces resting heart rate. It seems that oxygen delivery by the cardiovascular system is the limiting factor in determining maximal oxygen consumption (Robinson, 1964) rather than limited lung function. The decreased maximal cardiac output accounts for the decreased maximal aerobic work that the elderly can perform (Robinson, 1964; Davies, 1972; Gerstenblith, Lakatta and Weisfeldt, 1976)

Respiratory disease in the aged

Healthy individuals even at an advanced age may have no respiratory symptoms and it is clear that it is the cardiovascular system which limits physical capability and not the respiratory system. However, the age-related changes described above deplete the enormous functional reserve of the respiratory system resulting in marked and unexpected oxygen desaturation in the presence of superimposed respiratory disease. Furthermore, this situation may be worse in the recumbent position frequently assumed postoperatively. Similarly, the elderly patient may fail to respond appropriately when metabolic demands increase carbon dioxide production, e.g. pyrexia and postoperative catabolic states, resulting in a rising arterial carbon dioxide tension and an acute respiratory acidosis. They may also not respond adequately to those situations which affect the efficiency of ventilation or of oxygen transfer because of increased physiological dead space or shunt fraction. Such disorders include pulmonary embolism, postoperative atelectasis, pneumonia and pulmonary oedema. Furthermore, the impaired cardiac response to falling arterial oxygenation increases the chances of hypoxic tissue damage.

Elderly patients developing respiratory failure may not manifest the usual clinical signs of tachypnoea and tachycardia and it is essential to look for the more subtle signs of blood gas disturbance such as mental confusion or agitation. Careful assessment by oximetry and blood gas analysis with appropriate oxygen therapy will improve the outcome.

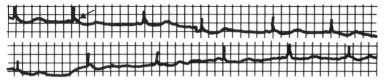

Figure 5.2 Electrocardiogram (lead II) showing four features of hypothermia, i.e. sinus bradycardia, the 'J' wave (arrowed), shivering (muscle tremor) artefact and prolongation of the QT interval. (From Schamroth, 1990)

Other relevant physiological changes

Renal and hepatic function are less efficient with age and blood urea levels are often elevated. Though renal function may be adequate, there is a loss of reserve together with an impaired ability to excrete drugs which may result in confusion (Leading article, 1972).

There is a general lowering of the metabolic rate in the aged possibly due in part to the reduction in the amount of active tissue and its replacement by relatively inert fibrous and connective tissue. Body temperature regulation may be abnormal in the elderly with body temperature related to ambient temperature in some circumstances (MacMillan *et al.*, 1967; Fox *et al.*, 1973). The use of a low reading thermometer is essential for the initial assessment of elderly trauma patients especially in the Accident and Emergency department. Low core temperatures may be associated with loss of or lowered conscious level mimicking a stroke and cardiac arrhythmia including ventricular fibrillation. In hypothermia there is a characteristic electrocardiographic appearance of sinus bradycardia with J waves at the junction of the QRS and ST segment (Figure 5.2).

Hypothyroidism may occur in up to 2.3% of elderly patients and non-specific clinical presentation is common (Bahemuka and Hodgkinson, 1975). Less than one-third show typical signs and symptoms and psychiatric manifestations such as depression may be seen. These patients can be unduly sensitive to anaesthetic and sedative drugs.

The pharmacology of anaesthetic drugs in the elderly

Adverse drug reactions are frequently recorded in elderly patients (Hurwitz, 1969) which may be due in part to inappropriate prescription and poor compliance. Age-related pharmacokinetic and pharmacodynamic factors must also be considered (Crooks, Shepherd and Stevenson, 1975) and are discussed fully in Chapter 4. They include alterations in drug handling, absorption, distribution and elimination as well as altered receptor/tissue sensitivity and impaired homeostatic mechanisms. Absorption of drugs from the gastrointestinal tract may be delayed or incomplete resulting in oral administration of drugs being less reliable than parenteral medication. The lower serum albumin associated with age results in an increase in free drug in the plasma so that the actions of some of the muscle relaxants and thiopentone will be exaggerated. A decreased lean body mass will cause an alteration in the volume of distribution of thiopentone in the fat depots prolonging its clinical action. Reduced elimination by the liver and kidneys leads to an increased sensitivity to those drugs such as gallamine and pancuronium which depend on renal excretion for their elimination. There is some evidence that differences in receptor/tissue sensitivity may account for some of the increased drug sensitivities in the elderly, e.g. the increased degree of analgesia in the elderly patient given morphine or pentazocine for the relief of postoperative pain (Bellville *et al.*, 1971). Usually the nature of the response to a drug is unaltered though the degree of response is exaggerated. The delerium following the use of hyoscine and oral barbiturates is probably the only example of alteration in the type of response to anaesthetic drugs found in the elderly (Dundee, 1977).

There is a growing tendency in orthopaedic practice, especially where elderly patients are concerned, to use non-steroidal anti-inflammatory drugs (NSAIDs) rather than opiates for postoperative analgesia. This facilitates mobilization by eliminating drug-induced dizziness and respiratory depression is not produced. It must be remembered, however, that NSAIDs such as diclofenac can cause renal impairment especially in dehydrated patients or in those with poor fluid intake. Those rheumatoid patients taking methotrexate should be assessed carefully as its half-life is prolonged by diclofenac. There are also associated interactions with digoxin, lithium and diuretics (with increased risks of renal impairment).

Preoperative assessment and consent

With advances in anaesthesia and the realization of the importance of adequate preoperative preparation and postoperative care, many aged patients can now benefit from orthopaedic surgery though the mortality does increase with age (Ochsner, 1967). Where an operation is an emergency as, for example, in the arrest of haemorrhage, speed in bringing the patient to theatre is of the utmost importance. Less obvious is the case of the elderly patient with hip fracture. In this instance, extreme haste is not vital but conversely any delay results in a deterioration of the patient's overall condition (Davie, MacRae and Malcolm–Smith, 1970). One must, therefore, balance expeditious timing with the need to ensure adequate preoperative preparation of the elderly patient against the hazards of delayed surgery (Villar, Allen and Barnes, 1986).

When assessing an elderly patient for anaesthesia and surgery chronological age is of less importance than the 'biological age' which takes into account the significance of any pathological changes in the cardiovascular, pulmonary and other important systems. In my view, the most valuable component in the assessment of cardiorespiratory status is the history and any potential benefit to be obtained by invasive monitoring should be balanced against the risks involved. The major problem in assessing the cardiac and respiratory reserve in an elderly orthopaedic patient is the fact that mobility is often limited by musculoskeletal disorders rather than the cardiovascular or respiratory systems themselves. Background exercise levels, general physical fitness and aerobic capacity may be chronically low and sometimes are associated with and exacerbated by obesity.

The aim of orthopaedic surgery is to assist elderly patients to improve the quality of their life either by increasing mobility and/or by reducing the level of pain associated with a particular activity. Less commonly, but of no less importance, orthopaedic intervention is to limit damage and save life in an elderly trauma victim. In this situation, there is less opportunity to make a full social assessment and to consider the details of their lifestyle. It is my belief that most elderly patients are far more concerned about their independence and ability to enjoy life rather than with their longevity. When consent for treatment is obtained it should be informed but on occasion the patient may feel that surgery is not worth having at his or her advanced age. The discussion should include alternatives to surgery, if any, and an appraisal of what may happen without surgery. One should adopt a 'risks and rewards' philosophy which obviously means a discussion about morbidity and mortality and appropriate advice should be given to the patient in the light of a full physical, mental and social assessment. Individual patients may persist in their attitude that 'the doctor knows best'; someone has to make an executive decision in these cases but this should only be done after discussion with the full surgical team. This includes the nursing staff who in these circumstances often act as the patient's advocate and often provide a well-balanced view in any debate.

There is an unfortunate tendency to treat some elderly patients like children and this may take the form of discussing consent with the relatives. One must always keep the patient's best interests at heart and strike a balance between confidentiality and the natural desire to inform and communicate with the family. If one forms an impression that, because of a patient's mental status, informed consent is not obtainable then it is proper to discuss the situation with those caring for the patient and the next of kin. It is not uncommon that they are asked to sign a consent form and the legal significance of this is discussed fully in Chapter 19.

A significant proportion of elderly patients are deaf and it is a sad fact that many physicians and surgeons tend to confuse deafness with daftness! This problem can be further compounded in a surgical environment when the patient's hearing aid, spectacles and dentures are removed preoperatively. Such an action certainly contributes to disorientation with confusion and adds to the difficulty of nursing the patient in the recovery phase. Furthermore, the routine removal of a patient's dentures adds to his/her embarrassment as does the use of a short and inadequately fitting theatre gown. There is no reason why a patient should not retain his hearing aid, spectacles and dentures when preparing for a surgical procedure under local anaesthesia. Similarly, when the operation is performed under general anaesthesia the aids should only be removed in the anaesthetic room at a suitable moment in the proceedings and should be returned to the patient as soon as convenience and safety permits following recovery from anaesthesia. The patient must be transferred to and from theatre in a suitable gown and covered with sheets that confer a degree of modesty commensurate with the patient's age.

If a patient is depressed, then a feeling of low self-esteem may influence his decisions. A refusal of a treatment option may well be a rational decision at the time but may be influenced by a temporary state of depression. Surgery may have to be postponed in these situations and reviewed later. A positive attitude to surgery and the subsequent mobilization regime is of the utmost importance in the elderly patient and will undoubtedly confer a beneficial influence on the outcome.

Appropriate investigations

Preoperative screening tests, even those considered to be routine by the surgical and nursing staff, can be most worrying for an elderly patient. It can be very tiring to be transported around the hospital for radiographs, electrocardiograms and blood tests, especially when in pain and a full explanation of such procedures should be provided. A full blood count is useful in all elderly patients prior to surgery as unsuspected anaemia is not uncommon especially in those taking NSAIDs. If the anaemia is chronic and not marked then transfusion may not be necessary especially if there is good cardiorespiratory function. Overzealous transfusion may cause circulatory overload and it may be more appropriate to treat the anaemia by other means postoperatively (Lloyd, 1971; Watson–Williams, 1979).

Preoperative chest radiography has no predictive value in the assessment of risk of postoperative problems but does provide a baseline for comparison later. Unsuspected neoplastic lesions may be discovered and this may alter the approach to planned surgery (Seymour, Pringle and Shaw, 1982). Fifty to 80% of elderly patients have an electrocardiographic abnormality and its preoperative recording is helpful for postoperative comparison (Seymour, Pringle and MacLennan, 1983). Unfortunately, the electrocardiogram is of little value in predicting which patients will experience postoperative cardiac problems.

A study by Del Guercio and Cohn (1980) on patients aged 65 years and over suggests that invasive investigations including Swan–Ganz catherization was of significant benefit to the outcome of the patient following surgery. They found that using these complicated techniques the 3-month mortality in patients undergoing surgery for hip fracture was reduced from 30% to 3% and they attributed this to the preoperative adjustments to the cardiopulmonary system that were based on the findings of these invasive investigations. Such a finding requires confirmation by other workers but this type of approach in general would be seen in the United Kingdom as highly unconventional and would certainly be associated with significant cost implications. Aggressive intervention has a place in the management of the elderly (Paton, 1981) but one experiences a natural caution and suspicion of those invasive procedures in which the investigation itself is either associated with a significant risk or is inordinately unpleasant. It must always be remembered that apparently fit, asymptomatic subjects may have hidden pathology and that a sensible balance must be found between bland acceptance of this situation and the value of information which might be gleaned from invasive investigative procedures with their attendant risks (Goldman *et al.* 1977; Djokovic and Hedley-White, 1979). Information must be useful in terms of improving the preoperative state, the assessment of risk and the planning of perioperative management. Any other information obtained is for academic reasons only and may well be recorded only after endangering the elderly and often frail patient's condition.

The reliable and yet conventional assessment of pulmonary function in terms of risk and outcome from surgery is not easy and Nunn has suggested that the patient's subjective account of dyspnoea may be the best indicator of risk (Nunn *et al.*, 1988). Preoperative respiratory treatment is useful but may have to be prolonged to be really effective in certain conditions. For example, in smokers 6–8 weeks of therapy are required for an improvement to occur in bronchorrhoea, cilial action, cerebral circulation (Jones *et al.*, 1987) and carboxyhaemoglobin levels (Roger *et al.*, 1985).

Intraoperative care and monitoring

Advancing age, relative immobility and steroid administration are associated with osteoporosis and an increased liability to fracture. Similarly, degenerative joint conditions may be present with contractures and stiffness and atrophy of the skin may allow minor trauma to result in lacerations and skin flaps. Meticulous care is therefore needed in positioning and protecting all elderly patients on the operating table (and subsequently in the recovery area) when their protective reflexes may be obtunded by anaesthesia. The head and neck may be affected by rheumatoid disease with instability of the cervical spine and stiffness of the temporomandibular joints creating intubation problems. These, however, should have been anticipated preoperatively.

For long operations the use of a warming blanket and temperature probe is recommended and whenever a limb is positioned to facilitate access it must rest easily on a support. This must be appropriately padded to prevent high point loading which is of particular importance to the radial and ulnar nerves which are easily injured. The use of a tourniquet needs careful thought with an appreciation that higher than usual inflation pressures may be needed to overcome the effect of systolic hypertension. This is associated with greater risk of trauma to those structures compressed by the tourniquet and in this situation a wide cuff is beneficial (Muirhead and Newman, 1986; Newman and Muirhead, 1986). There is little place in the author's practice for the use of bilateral tourniquets in the elderly because of the potential problems associated with an increase in preload on the heart when they are applied. Similarly, elderly patients demonstrate a limited ability to cope with the low afterload due to reactive hyperaemia when they are removed.

In all patients the prime aim of the anaesthetist is to maintain an adequate tissue oxygen supply but especially to the heart, brain and kidney. There are several factors involved with this including PaO_2, haemoglobin content and saturation and tissue blood flow. Cerebral blood flow is affected by both mean arterial pressure and intracranial pressure and may be reduced by occult carotid artery disease. The diameter of the cerebral vessels is important and is reduced by a falling $PaCO_2$ which can be produced if the lungs are overventilated during anaesthesia. Autoregulatory mechanisms maintain cerebral blood flow with falling mean arterial pressure to a certain critical level which is increased in hypertensive subjects.

The combination of hypocarbia and hypotension in the elderly patient has the potential for seriously affecting cerebral oxygen supply. Hypotensive techniques should therefore be used with extreme caution in the elderly as there is no effective way of ensuring that the cerebral perfusion is adequate in these circumstances. Irreversible cerebral damage may occur and may only be diagnosed postoperatively as irreversible mental deterioration or stroke. The anaesthetist should also be aware that profound hypotension and even death can occur during the course of joint arthroplasty when acrylic cement is inserted under pressure. Similarly, marked hypotension may occur when an anaesthetized patient is raised into a semi-sitting position to facilitate shoulder surgery.

It is essential that systolic arterial pressure is controlled accurately and normal oxygen and carbon dioxide levels maintained. A fall in $PaCO_2$ from 5.5 kPa to 2.5 kPa may reduce cerebral blood flow by up to 60% and peroperative monitoring should therefore include capnography and oximetry.

Regional versus general anaesthesia

The most salient feature of a regional anaesthetic technique is that it considerably simplifies anaesthesia since the single injection of one drug provides for most or all of the requirements of surgery especially in those orthopaedic operations involving a limb. The conscious state is preserved allowing the airway and its protective reflexes to be maintained. The profound analgesia produced means that opioid requirements are low or non-existent thus reducing the risk of central respiratory depression. There are features of regional anaesthesia which would seem to be advantageous and some epidemiological studies suggest that the morbidity and, possibly, mortality of surgery and anaesthesia may be decreased by the wide use of regional techniques. For example, McLaren, Stockwell and Reid (1978) demonstrated a lower mortality from hip fracture in the elderly treated with regional anaesthesia but this has not been confirmed by other groups (Valentin *et al.*, 1986). A more detailed analysis by McKenzie, Wishart and Smith (1984) showed that femoral neck fracture surgery performed under general anaesthesia was associated with a greater cumulative mortality than that performed under regional anaesthesia when the measurement was made at 2 weeks. By 6 weeks following the surgery the two groups of patients did not differ significantly.

Postoperative hypoxaemia (McKenzie *et al.*, 1980) and bronchopneumonia (McLaren, 1982) have been shown to be decreased by the wider use of regional anaesthesia as have the thromboembolic complications associated with hip replacement (Thorburn, Louden and Vallance, 1980; Bodig, 1982). Whether this is due to increased mobility as a result of better analgesia and reduced opioid requirements or due to increased limb blood flow or even because of a direct effect of absorbed local anaesthetic on platelet stickiness is debatable.

A recent study comparing general and local anaesthetic techniques in patients over 60 years of age indicated that cognitive and functional competence were not detectably impaired when attention was paid to the known perioperative influences on mental function (Jones *et al.*, 1990). When possible local anaesthesia should be used as a sole technique to avoid some of the adverse effects of sedative drugs and general anaesthetic agents.

The practical application of regional anaesthetic techniques to the elderly orthopaedic patient can be categorized into three broad groups. First, the regional blockade may be used as the only form of anaesthesia to facilitate the surgery and a prime example of this would be arthroplasty of either the hip or knee. Other examples would be the use of brachial plexus blockade (Winnie, 1984) or Bier's block anaesthesia for procedures such as manipulation of Colles' fracture and Dupuytren's fasciectomy. Thompson, Newman and Semple (1988) have shown that brachial plexus anaesthesia for upper limb surgery is safe even in the elderly and is successful in 95% of attempted cases though some augmentation by associated nerve blocks, local infiltration, etc. may be necessary.

A second application is the combination of regional anaesthesia with basal sedation and this technique is frequently administered for surgery for femoral neck fracture in a patient who is confused and agitated and who cannot be relied upon to cooperate with the surgery under regional anaesthesia alone.

A third use for regional anaesthesia would be the provision of postoperative pain relief. A successful block can give total abolition of pain and if a long-acting agent such as bupivacaine is used complete pain relief may be achieved for more than 10 h. This obviates the need to use opiate drugs or even NSAIDs. Good practical examples of this would be the use of a ulnar nerve block for postoperative pain relief following Dupuytren's fasciectomy of the little and ring fingers and of course a median nerve block at the wrist can be added if the fasciectomy involves the middle or index fingers. Blocks of the femoral and lateral cutaneous nerve of thigh can be performed separately or as part of the so-called Winnie triple block (Winnie *et al.*, 1973) to give good pain relief following total hip arthroplasty. They can also be administered prior to the application of a Thomas' splint for femoral shaft fracture or following intramedullary nailing of such a fracture. Intermetatarsal blocks are easy to administer and are possibly more successful than the ankle block for pain relief following bunion and toe surgery. Finally, the management of chest pain due to multiple rib fractures must be included. The severe lancinating pain inhibits the respiratory effort leading rapidly in the elderly to the development of bronchopneumonia which can be fatal. Multiple intercostal nerve blocks are remarkably effective in controlling this pain and reducing the requirement for potent analgesics. Intrapleural installation techniques have recently been described which may be easier to use than indwelling thoracic epidural catheters for prolonged analgesia (Knottenbelt *et al.*, 1991).

The place for intensive care and high dependency units

Age *per se* is not relevant to the provision of intensive care or high dependency facilities and, indeed, advanced age may be a specific indication for such treatment. The use of the facility should be for specific reasons and preferably be pre-planned following preoperative discussion with the patient and family. Invasive cardiovascular monitoring can be an advantage in some of the situations already described so leading to a reduction in morbidity and, perhaps, mortality.

The ready availability of well-trained staff and appropriate equipment mean that pain control can be readily achieved in the high dependency or intensive care unit. This can be effected by means of opioid infusions, patient-controlled analgesic techniques and even continuous epidural or brachial plexus infusions (Helm and Newman, 1991).

Facilities for repeated blood gas analysis and oximetry will be available allowing the careful control of oxygen therapy. This has been shown by Jones *et al.* (1985) to be needed for much longer periods postoperatively than has previously been recognized. The hypoxaemia of basal atelectasis or early bronchopneumonia may be difficult to detect clinically in an elderly patient especially one in a postoperative phase. Similarly, opiates may induce a more profound hypoxaemia due to hypoventilation and cough suppression (Carroll, 1974). In such conditions hypoxaemia should be readily detected in a high dependency or intensive care unit in which continuous monitoring is practised.

Conclusion

In conclusion it is axiomatic that anaesthesia is no more than a part of the overall therapeutic package offered to the elderly orthopaedic patient. To minimize risk, anaesthesia has to be especially tailored and adapted to the individual patient bearing in mind the physiological and pathological constraints discussed above. One must be at times pragmatic about the extent to which patients are exposed to various tests and investigations prior to surgery but one must not have a closed mind to the possibility that audit may show a need constantly to evaluate and update ideas concerning the optimization of patient care (Davenport, 1991).

References

Adams, G.M., DeVries, H.A. (1973) Physiological effects of an exercise training regimen upon women aged 52–79. *J. Gerontol.*, **28**, 50–55

Bahemuka, M. and Hodgkinson, H.M. (1975) Screening for hypothyroidism. *Br. Med. J.*, **2**, 601–603

Bellville, J.W., Forrest, W.H., Miller, E. and Brown, B.W. (1971) Influence of age on pain relief from analgesics. *J. Am. Med. Ass.*, **217**, 1835–1841

Bloor, C.M. (1982) Valvular heart disease in the elderly. *J. Am. Geriat. Soc.*, **30**, 466–478

Bodig, J. (1982) Thromboembolism and blood loss; continuous epidural block versus general anaesthesia with controlled ventilation. *Reg. Anesth.*, **7**, S84

Buskirk, E.R. and Hodgson, J.L. (1987) Age and aerobic power: the rate of change in men and women. *Fed. Proc.*, **46**, 1824–1829

Carroll, D. (1974) Sleep, periodic breathing and snoring in the aged; control of ventilation in the ageing and diseased respiratory system. *J. Am. Geriat. Soc.*, **22**, 307–315

Crooks, J., Shepherd, A.M.M. and Stevenson, I.H. (1975) Drugs and the elderly, the nature of the problem. *Hlth Bull.*, **33**, 222–227

Davenport, H.T. (1988) *Anaesthesia and the Aged Patient*, Blackwell Scientific, Oxford

Davenport, H.T. (1991) Anaesthetics and elderly patients: the new frontier. *Br. Med. J.*, **303**, 870–871

Davie, I.T., MacRae, W.R. and Malcolm–Smith, N.A. (1970) Anaesthesia for the fractured hip, a survey of 200 cases. *Anaesth. Analg. Curr. Res.*, **49**, 165–170

Davies, C.T.M. (1972) The oxygen transporting system in relation to age. *Clin. Sci.*, **42**, 1–13

Davies, M.J. and Pomerance, A. (1972) Quantitiative study of ageing changes in the human sinoatrial node and internodal tracts. *Br. Heart. J.*, **34**, 150–152

Del Guercio, L.R.M. and Cohn, J.D. (1980) Monitoring operative risk in the elderly. *J. Am. Med. Ass.*, **243**, 1350–1355

DeVries, H.A. (1970) Physiological effects of an exercise training regimen upon men aged 52–88. *J. Gerontol.*, **25**, 325–336

Djokovic, J.L., Hedley–Whyte, J. (1979) Prediction of outcome of surgery and anaesthesia in patients over 80. *J. Am. Med. Ass.*, **242**, 2301–2306

Dundee, J.W. (1977) Response of the elderly to drugs used by the anaesthetist. *Symposium on drugs and the elderly*, Dundee

Edelman, N.H., Mittman, C., Norris, A.H. *et al.* (1968) Effects of respiratory pattern on age differences in ventilation uniformity. *J. Appl. Physiol.*, **24**, 49–53

Editorial (1972) Airway closure. *Br. J. Anaesth.*, **44**, 633

Fisch, C. (1981) Electrocardiogram in the aged: an independent marker of heart disease? *Am. J. Med.*, **70**, 4–6

Fox R.H., MacGibbon, R., Davies, L. and Woodward, P.M. (1973) Problem of the old and the cold. *Br. Med. J.*, **1**, 21–24

Gardin, J.M., Henry, W.L., Savage, D.D. *et al.* (1977) Echocardiographic evaluation of an older population without clinically apparent heart disease. *Am. J. Cardiol.*, **39**, 277

Gerstenblith, G., Lakatta, E.G., Weisfeldt, M.L. (1976) Age changes in myocardial function and exercise response. *Prog. Cardiovasc. Dis.*, **19**, 1–21

Gerstenblith, G., Spurgeon, H. A., Froelich, J. P. *et al.* (1975) Diminished inotropic response of the aged myocardium to cathecholamines. *Circ. Res.*, **36**, 262–269

Gerstenblith, G., Frederiksen, J., Yin, F.C.P. *et al.* (1977) Echocardiographic assessment of normal adult ageing population. *Circulation*, **36**, 273–278

Goldman, L. *et al.* (1977) Multifactorial index of cardiac risk in non cardiac surgical procedures. *New Engl. J. Med.*, **297**, 845–850

Granath, A., Jonsson, B. and Strandell, T. (1964) Circulation in healthy old men, studied by right heart catheterisation at rest and during exercise in supine and sitting positions. *Acta Med. Scand.*, **176**, 425–446

Helm, R. and Newman, R.J. (1991) Personal communication

Holtz, B., Bake, B. and Oxhoj, H. (1976) Effect of inspired volume on closing volume. *J. Appl. Physiol.* **41**, 623–630

Hurwitz, N. (1969) Predisposing factors in adverse reactions to drugs. *Br. Med. J.*, **1**, 536–539

Hutchins, G.M., Buckley, B.H., Miner, M.M. (1977) Correlation of age and heart weight with tortuosity and caliber of normal human coronary arteries. *Am. Heart. J.*, **94**, 196–202

Jones, J.G. *et al.* (1985) Episodic post operative oxygen desaturation; the value of added oxygen. *J. Roy. Soc. Med.*, **78**, 1019–1022

Jones, M.J.T. *et al.* (1990) Cognitive and functional competence after anaesthesia in patients aged over 60; controlled trial of general and regional anaesthesia for elective hip or knee replacement. *Br. Med. J.*, **300**, 1683

Jones, R.M. *et al.* (1987) Smoking and anaesthesia. *Anaesthesia*, **42**, 1–2

Knottenbelt, J.D., James, M.F. and Bloomfield, M. (1991) Intrapleural bupivacaine analgesia in chest trauma: a randomised, double-blind controlled trial. *Injury*, **22**, 114–116

Kronenberg, R.S. and Drage, G.W. (1973) Attenuation of the ventilatory and heart rate responses to hypoxia and hypercapnia with ageing in normal man. *J. Clin. Invest.*, **52**, 1812–1819

Lablanc, P., Ruff, F. and Milic-Emili, J. (1970) Effect of age and body position on "airway closure" in man. *J. Appl. Physiol.*, **28**, 448

Lakatta, E., Gerstenblith, G., Angel, C.S. *et al.* (1975) Diminished inotropic response of aged myocardium to catecholamines. *Circ. Res.*, **36**, 262–269

Leading article (1972) Drugs and the elderly mind. *Lancet*, **ii**, 126

Leith, D.E., and Mead, J. (1967) Mechanisms determining residual volume of the lungs in normal subjects. *J. Appl. Physiol.*, **23**, 221–227

Lloyd, E.L. (1971) Serum iron levels and haematological status in the elderly. *Geront. Clin.*, **13**, 246–255

McKee, P.A., Castelli, W.P., McNamara, P.M., *et al.* (1971) The natural history of congestive heart failure: The Framlington Study. *N. Engl. J. Med.*, **285**, 1441–1446

McKenzie, P.J. *et al.* (1980) Comparison of the effects of spinal anaesthesia and general anaesthesia on postoperative oxygenation and perioperative mortality. *Br. J. Anaesth.*, **52**, 49

McKenzie, P.J., Wishart, H.Y. and Smith, G. (1984) Long-term outcome after repair of fractured neck of femur. Comparison of subarachnoid and general anaesthesia. *Br. J. Anaesth.*, **56**, 581–585

McLaren, A.D. (1982) Mortality studies: a review. *Reg. Anesth.*, **7**, 5172

McLaren, A.D., Stockwell, M.C. and Reid, V.T. (1978) Anaesthetic techniques for surgical correction of fractured neck of femur. A comparative study of spinal and general anaesthesia in the elderly. *Anaesthesia*, **33**, 10

McMillan, J.B. and Lev. M. (1961)The ageing heart: myocardium and epicardium. In *Biological Aspects of Ageing* (ed. N.W. Shock) Colombia University Press, New York, pp. 163–173

MacMillan, A.L. *et al.* (1967) Temperature regulation in survivors of accidental hypothermia in the elderly. *Lancet*, **ii**, 165–169

Muiesan, G., Sorbini, C.A. and Grassi, V. (1971) Respiratory function in the aged. *Bull. Physiol. Pathol. Resp.*, **7**, 973–1009

Muirhead, A. and Newman, R.J. (1986) A low pressure tourniquet system for the lower limb. *Injury*, **17**, 53–54

Newman, R.J. and Muirhead, A. (1986) A safe and effective low pressure tourniquet. A prospective evaluation. *J. Bone Joint Surg.*, **68B**, 625–628

Nunn, J.F. *et al.* (1988) Respiratory criteria for fitness for surgery and anaesthesia. *Anaesthesia*, **43**, 543–551

Ochsner, A. (1967) Is risk of indicated operation too great in the elderly? *Geriatrics*, **22**, 121–130

Paton, A. (1981) Aggressive intervention, therapeutic arrogance and mania for measurement. *World Med.*, **16**, 66–68

Pomerance, A. (1976) Pathology of the myocardium and valves. In *Cardiology in Old Age* (eds Caird, F.I., Dall, J.L.C., Kennedy, R.D.). Plenum Press, New York, pp. 11–55.

Pooling Project Research Group (1978) Relationship of blood pressure, serum cholesterol, smoking habits, relative weight and electrocardiogram abnormalities to incidence of major coronary events: final report of the Pooling Project. *J. Chron. Dis.*, **31**, 201–306.

Port, S., Cobb, F.R., Coleman, R.E. *et al.* (1980) Effect of age on the response of the left ventricular ejection fraction to exercise. *N. Engl. J. Med.*, **303**, 1133–1136

Potter, J.F., Elahi, D., Tobin, J.D. *et al.* (1982) Effect of ageing on the cardiothoracic ratio of men. *J. Am. Geriat. Soc.*, **30**, 404–409

Proper, R. and Wall, F. (1972) Left ventricular stroke volume measurements not affected by age. *Am. Heart J.*, **83**, 843–845

Robinson, S. (1964) Physical fitness in relation to age. In New York, *Ageing of the Lung: Perspectives* (ed. L. Chander) Moyer Grune & Stratton, pp. 287–301

Rodeheffer, R.J. *et al.* (1984) Exercise cardiac output is maintained with advancing age in healthy human subjects. *Circulation*, **69**, 203–213

Roger, R.K. *et al.* (1985) Abstention from cigarette smoking improves cerebral perfusion among elderly chronic smokers. *J. Am. Med. Ass.*, **253**, 2970–2974

Ryan, S.F., Vincent, T.N., Mitchel, R.S. *et al.* (1965) Ductectasia: An asymptomatic pulmonary change related to age. *Med. Thorac.*, **22**, 181–187

Schamroth, L. (1990) *An Introduction to Electrocardiography*, 75th. edn, Blackwell Scientific, Oxford, p. 139

Schnur, S. (1954) Mortality rates in acute myocardial infarction: III. The relationship of patients age to prognosis. *Ann. Intern. Med.*, **41**, 294–298

Seymour, D.G., Pringle, R. and Shaw, J.W. (1982) The role of the routine preoperative chest x-ray in the elderly general surgical patient. *Postgrad. Med. J.*, **58**, 741–745

Seymour, D.G., Pringle, R. and MacLennan, W.J. (1983) The role of the routine preoperative electrocardiogram in the elderly surgical patient. *Age Ageing*, **12**, 97–104

Smith, H.L. (1928) The relationship of the weight of the heart to the weight of the body and weight of the heart to age. *Am. Heart. J.*, **4**, 79–93

Sorbini, C.A., Grassi, V., Solinas,E. *et al.* (1968) Arterial oxygen tension in relation to age in healthy subjects. *Respiration*, **25**, 3–13,

Thompson, A.M., Newman, R.J. and Semple, J.C. (1988) Brachial plexus anaesthesia for upper limb surgery, a review of eight years experience. *J. Hand Surg.*, **13B**, 195–198

Thorburn, J., Louden, J.R. and Vallance, R. (1980) Spinal and general anaesthesia in total hip replacement; frequency of deep venous thrombosis. *Br. J. Anaesth.*, **58**, 1117

Watson–Williams, E.J. (1979) Hematological and hemostatic considerations before surgery. *Med. Clin. N. Am.*, **63**, 1165–1189

Weisfeldt, M.L. (1981) Presbycardia. *Johns Hopkins Med. J.*, **149**, 203–208

White, N.K., Edward, J.E. and Dry, T.J. (1950) The relationship of the degree of coronary atherosclerosis with age in men. *Circulation*, **1**, 645–654.

Williams, B.O. *et al.* (1976) The elderly in a coronary unit. *Br. Med. J.*, **2**, 451–453

Winnie, A.P. (1984) *Plexus Anesthesia*. Vol I. *Perivascular Technique of Brachial Plexus Blockade*. Churchill Livingstone, London

Winnie, A.P., Ramamurthy, S. and Durrani, Z. (1973) The inguinal paravascular technique of lumbar plexus anaesthesia: the '3 in 1' block. *Anaesth. Analg.*, **52**, 989–996

Wong, M., Tei, C. and Shah, P.M. (1983) Degenerative calcific valvular disease and systolic murmurs in the elderly. *J. Am. Geriat. Soc.*, **31**, 156–163

Valentin, N. *et al.* (1986) Spinal or general anaesthesia for surgery of the fractured hip. A prospective study of mortality in 578 patients. *Br. J. Anaesth.*, **58**, 284

Villar, R.N., Allen, S.M. and Barnes, S.J. (1986) Hip fractures in healthy patients: operative delay versus prognosis. *Br. Med. J.*, **293**, 1203–1204

Zeman, F.D. and Rodstein, M. (1960) Cardiac rupture complicating myocardial infarction in the aged. *Arch. Intern. Med.*, **105**, 431

6

Arthritis surgery in the elderly

Ian F. Goldie

Arthritis in the elderly tends to be either degenerative – osteoarthrosis – or inflammatory, of which the commonest type is rheumatoid disease. Other joint conditions also cause symptoms including septic, crystal and psoriatic arthropathies.

Definitions

Osteoarthrosis

A comprehensive definition of osteoarthrosis must include the following feature:
Clinical – joint pain, tenderness, limitation of movement, crepitus, deformity and effusion.
Pathological – patchy loss of cartilage (particularly in areas of increased load), subchondral sclerosis, cysts and marginal osteophytes.
Radiographical – radiographic demonstration of the above pathological features.
Histological – fragmentation of cartilage, cloning of chondrocytes, crystal deposition, remodelling and evidence of repair.
Biomechanical – alteration of tensile, compressive and shear properties of cartilage as well as its hydraulic permeability.
Biochemical – reduction in proteoglycan concentration, alteration in aggregation of proteoglycans, variation in collagen fibre size and increased synthesis and degradation of matrix molecules.

As osteoarthrotic changes are characterized by a number of degenerative phenomena the term 'degenerative joint disease' has been coined. This phrase, however, gratuitously specifies an aetiology and may cause semantic difficulties in those instances in which the condition results from an underlying abnormality. Furthermore, the term has connotations with the ageing process and suggests the condition to be an inevitable consequence of growing old.

The two terms in common parlance are osteoarthritis and osteoarthrosis. On occasions some affected joints exhibit obvious inflammatory reactions which may justify the term osteoarthritis. However, the consensus is that inflammation is a secondary response which follows the underlying joint disintegration.

Though perhaps being etymologically confusing the term osteoarthrosis is the preferred nomenclature.

Traditionally, osteoarthrosis is divided into two aetiological groups: primary, implying a condition developing *de novo* and secondary, resulting from the effects of previous injury or other derangement of the joint. Osteoarthrosis may also be categorized clinically into the generalized and erosive types. In the former group the distal interphalangeal joints are characteristically affected together with the carpometacarpal joint of the thumb, the first tarsometatarsal joint, the metatarsophalangeal joint of the hallux, the knee and the interfacetal joints of the cervical and lumbar spine (Kelsey, 1982). A subset of generalized osteoarthrosis, so-called generalized nodal osteoarthrosis, is characterized by bony protuberances on the margins of the distal interphalangeal joints, Heberden's nodes. The proximal interphalangeal joints may also become involved – the Bouchard swelling.

Erosive osteoarthrosis is an aggressive form of the condition which particularly affects the distal interphalangeal joints of the fingers.

A number of crystals may be found in the synovial fluid and synovium of some cases of severe 'osteoarthrosis' but there is doubt that they are the cause of the arthropathy and this is particularly the case in those degenerative joint conditions associated with calcium pyrophosphate (pseudo-gout) and hydroxyapatite. Certainly crystal deposition alone is not a sufficient cause for the arthopathy and many elderly people have crystal deposits in otherwise normal joints. The incidence of crystal deposition seems to rise in an almost linear fashion from less than 1% in the under 50s to more than 40% in those over 90 years old. Similarly, crystal deposition can result from other joint conditions such as previous meniscectomy.

In order to accommodate the above observations a hypothesis has been proposed which suggests that calcium pyrophosphate and other forms of crystal deposition can act as an 'amplification loop' accelerating the joint damage seen in many chronic arthropathies including osteoarthrosis (Dieppe *et al.*, 1985).

Rheumatoid arthritis

Rheumatoid arthritis is a chronic inflammatory disease which has been described both as 'one of the great mysteries of medicine' (Cecil *et al.*, 1930) and 'a baffling enigma' (Buchanan and Boyle, 1971). It involves the connective tissue of all organs and the painful joints display swelling, effusion, deformity and varying degrees of loss of function. There is a sweeping destruction of joint cartilages and ligaments.

In the early stages only one joint may be effected but rapid progress can occur with involvement of multiple joints especially the small joints of the hands and feet. Larger joints become subsequently involved including the elbows, knees, shoulders and hips and this is usually in a symmetrical fashion.

Prevalence

Osteoarthrosis

Mason (1956) found that of those patients attending a physiotherapy department with joint problems the majority suffered from osteoarthrosis. It is the most prevalent chronic joint condition and carries with it severe social, economic and personal implications, especially in the elderly. Felson (1988) reported radiographic evidence of osteoarthrosis in the majority of people by 65 years of age and described

Table 6.1 Prevalence (cases/1000) of moderate to severe osteoarthrosis in different anatomical sites

Joint	Male	Female
Distal interphalangeal	110	170
Proximal interphalangeal	23	121
Metacarpophalangeal	64	15
First carpometacarpal	64	160
Wrist	170	0
Cervical spine	35	30
Lumbar spine	79	73
Hip	84	31
Sacroiliac	12	16
Knee	111	151
Tarsi	12	29
Lateral metatarsophalangeal	0	10
First metatarsophalangeal	87	175
Total	434	69

(*Source*: Kellgren and Lawrence, 1958)

involvement in more than 80% of people over the age of 75 years.

Kellgren and Lawrence (1958) surveyed both moderate and severe osteoarthrosis in a population and reported fingers, hips and knees to be mostly affected but with a marked sexual variation (Table 6.1). Females were more affected in the fingers, knees and feet whereas men dominated in hip involvement. With regard to hips and knees these findings have in part been verified by Allander (1974) but not so in the HANES I survey (Tables 6.2, 6.3).

Lindberg (1985) showed in a study of 4027 normal barium enemas that the prevalence of primary osteoarthrosis of the hip is 2.1% with 3.1% occurring after the age of 55 years. Both sexes were effected equally and bilateral osteoarthrosis of the hip was found in 35%.

In comparing one group examined for osteoarthrosis of the hip with one examined in exactly the same way 20 years later Danielsson, Lindberg and Nilsson, (1984) found that the prevalence had not changed nor was there any change in sex ratio or distribution between bilateral and unilateral cases or between the various types of osteoarthrosis of the hip.

In the Framingham Osteoarthritis Study Felson *et al.* (1987) examined the standing knee radiographs of 1424 individuals from 63 to 94 years. Radiographically there was an increase of osteoarthrosis with age. In individuals younger than 70 years the prevalence was 27% which rose to 44% at 80 years and over.

Osteoarthrosis has approximately the same prevalence in different population groups as well as geographic distribution within the western

Table 6.2 Prevalence (cases/1000) of osteoarthrosis of the hip

Age	Allander (1974) Male	Female	Age	HANES I[a] Male	Female
30–35	0	0	25–34	6	
42–46	10	5	35–44	2	
56–60	35	25	45–54	15	17
70–74	90	75	65–74	62	39

[a] National Health and Nutrition Examination Survey I.
(*Source*: Maurer, 1979)

Table 6.3 Prevalence (cases/1000) of arthrosis of the knee

Age	Allander (1974) Male	Female	Age	HANES I[a] Male	Female
30–35	30	20	25–34	3	1
42–46	70	60	35–44	24	21
56–60	70	160	45–54	37	54
			55–64	83	107
70–74	160	340	65–74	137	249

[a] National Health and Nutrition Examination Survey I.
(*Source*: Maurer, 1979)

hemisphere (Kelsey, 1982; Felson, 1988). The small variations that are sometimes recorded can often be explained by inaccurate readings of radiographs and complexities of the sampling frames.

The prevalence is lower in the Chinese, Jamaicans and South Africans with the exception of some individual joints. Among rural Saudis osteoarthrosis of the hip is less prevalent than in the knee for reasons that are still being debated (Agunwa, 1989).

Rheumatoid arthritis

The prevalence of rheumatoid arthritis is difficult to estimate as diagnostic problems surround the verification of the disease which appears in a number of guises making a 'typical' patient almost a rarity. A distinction is made between classic, definite and probable cases each of which is characterized by a number of diagnostic criteria (Ropes, 1958). Not infrequently these groups merge to become one entity when prevalence calculations are made. The criteria have been revised from time to time and different sets have been created for different purposes. Thus the ARA criteria were created for clinical use while the New York Criteria (Benett and Burch, 1967) were intended for epidemiological investigations. Applied to the same population they give divergent results on the prevalence of the disease (Cathcart and O'Sullivan,

Table 6.4 Prevalence in percent of classic, definite and probable rheumatoid arthritis in persons aged 18–79 years by sex and age, United States 1960–62

Age (years)	Male	Female	Both sexes
18–24	0.2	0.3	0.3
25–34	—	0.6	0.3
35–44	0.5	2.1	1.3
45–54	1.5	4.4	3.0
55–64	4.2	8.3	6.3
65–74	3.1	14.1	9.2
75–79	14.1	23.5	18.8
Total (18–79)	1.7	4.6	3.2

(*Source*: US National Centre for Health Statistics, 1960–1962)

1970) and reported prevalences hence vary from 0.1% (Beighton, Solomin and Valkenburg, 1975) to 6% (Henrad, Benett and Burch, 1975; Harvey *et al.*, 1981). In most European populations the prevalence is about 2–3% (Laine, 1962; Allander, 1970).

In the United States National Center for Health Statistics study (1960–62) 3.2% of the population between 18 and 70 years were found to have classic, definite or probable rheumatoid arthritis including 4.6% females and 1.7% males. In Table 6.4 the distribution of rheumatoid arthritis in different age groups is presented.

Finally, a comparison is made in Table 6.5 of the prevalence of osteoarthrosis and rheumatoid arthritis in different joints.

Table 6.5 Comparison of osteoarthrosis (OA) and rheumatoid arthritis (RA) regarding prevalence of clinical joint involvement ($n = 50$)

Joint	Percentage	
	OA	RA
Temporomandibular	9	23
Cervical spine	22	34
Sternoclavicular	7	5
Acromioclavicular	4	19
Shoulder	35	62
Elbow	7	68
Wrist	17	85
CMCP	36	42
MCP	11	80
PIP	43	63
DIP	66	22
Hip	38	27
Knee	46	79
Ankle	5	39
Talocalcaneal	3	11
Midtarsal	6	24
MTP	49	71
PIP	13	24

(*Source*: Buchanan and Boyle, 1971)

Aetiology

The aetiologies of both osteoarthrosis and rheumatoid arthritis are unknown though many suggestions have been made.

As for osteoarthrosis the ageing process is accepted as an important contributor as are traumatic injury to the articular surfaces, internal joint derangement (principally the knee) and joint hypermobility. The role of obesity has been discussed but not conclusively proved. Is it the weight *per se* or an abnormal metabolism or both which act as the risk factor?

Similarly, the aetiology of rheumatoid arthritis remains unknown. Viral and heredity causes have been suggested but some of those studies which show a genetic predisposition have had serious methodological flaws (O'Brian, 1967). At present, interest is focused on aberrant immunological responses in rheumatoid patients but the specific agents involved have so far not been satisfactorily identified.

Radiography

Osteoarthrosis

The radiographic appearance of osteoarthrosis is characterized by joint space narrowing (Fredensborg and Nilsson, 1978), osteophytes and subchondral sclerosis with cyst formation and if all of these are not present there must be some doubt. If only one is present, the diagnosis cannot be made radiologically.

The joint space narrowing may be irregular with some portions of the joint relatively well maintained. The joint space may appear normal on a single radiograph and special views may therefore be required. In the weight-bearing joints such as the knees, joint narrowing may not be obvious unless the films are obtained with the patient in a weight-bearing stance. Preoperative assessment of osteoarthrosis of the knee should therefore include weight-bearing films (Ahlbäck, 1968) that allow measurement of the hip-knee-ankle angle (HKA) (Figure 6.1). Osteophytes are outgrowths of bone into capsular attachments and will develop with any kind of cartilaginous injury and, by themselves, do not indicate osteoarthrosis.

Subchondral sclerosis tends to be most obvious where the cartilage loss is most advanced which has led some to suggest that the sclerosis is a factor in causing progression by interfering with nutrition of the overlying cartilage. Subchondral cysts are typical and occasionally can be large enough to mimic other conditions and distract one's attention from the true underlying condition.

Osteoporosis is not a feature.

Crystal-associated osteoarthropathy can be frequently diagnosed radiologically in the elderly. Characteristically pyrophosphate crystal deposition disease is seen as osteoarthrosis with chondrocalcinosis and profuse osteophyte production. The cystic and destructive changes in bone are often exaggerated with disproportionate signs in the patellofemoral joints. Conversely, hydroxyapatite arthropathy is usually characterized by the changes of osteoarthrosis but with considerable loss of bone stock, and capsular and ligamentous calcifications. These changes may mimic a neuropathic joint.

Rheumatoid arthritis

Active rheumatoid arthritis is characterized by synovial swelling, osteoporosis, uniform joint narrowing and marginal erosions of the subchondral cortical bone. Bilateral symmetry is the rule and the extent of this symmetry may be remarkable. Periostitis is rare and enthesopathy (inflammation of tendon and ligament insertions into bone) does not occur.

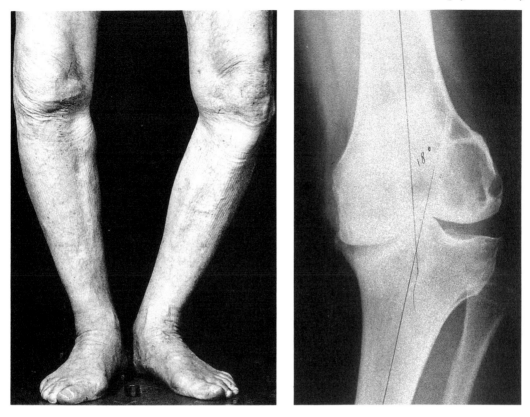

Figure 6.1 Advanced osteoarthrosis predominantly involving the medial compartment. The knees are in varus alignment with a hip-knee-ankle (HKA) angle of 18 degrees

In the late stages deformity due to soft tissue involvement as well as extensive destruction is characteristic. Subluxation/dislocation is common. In the hip, the femoral head may protrude into the acetabulum and in the fingers characteristic deformities described as swan neck, boutonnière and hourglass are seen.

Relationship between radiography and symptoms

When considering osteoarthrosis it is important to emphasize that the correlation between radiographic appearances and symptoms is poor. In two studies Kellgren and Lawrence (1957, 1958) reported in a 1 in 10 sample of an English industrial and mining town that 87% of females and 83% of males displayed radiographic evidence of osteoarthrosis. In this population sample however only 22% of the females and 15% of the males complained of symptoms. The same applies to rheumatoid arthritis. Not all patients with radiographically destroyed joints report symptoms.

Symptoms and signs

Pain is the most disabling symptom of both osteoarthrosis and rheumatoid arthritis. Pain on movement may be relieved by rest but it is not uncommon for a severely destroyed joint to cause sleep disturbance. This is especially so with respect to the hip.

Stiffness is occasional in osteoarthrosis but is typical of rheumatoid arthritis – particularly in the morning.

Swelling is common in both disorders and is due to a combination of a swollen synovial membrane (more so in rheumatoid arthritis) and effusion.

Deformities develop in both conditions. In osteoarthrosis these occur in the distal and proximal interphalangeal joints of the fingers with node formation. In the hip flexion and external rotation contractures are frequent and a varus deformity is commonly seen in the knee (Fig. 6.1).

In rheumatoid arthritis the deformities of the fingers include the swan neck, boutonnière, telescoping of the thumb and ulnar deviation of the fingers at the metacarpophalangeal joints. Traditionally, it has been thought that valgus deformity of the knee is typical for rheumatoid arthritis but Isacson (1987) demonstrated varus to be equally, if not more frequent.

Decreased function due to a combination of pain, stiffness and deformity is a hallmark of both osteoarthrosis and rheumatoid arthritis. Added to this is muscular wasting which is a frequent feature of both conditions. Walking distance may become limited and an antalgic and/or short-limbed limp may develop. Contractures contribute to a restricted range of motion.

Joint instability may develop in the later stages of both conditions and is due to a loss of cartilage and bone resulting in incongruous joint surfaces. Muscle weakness and capsular contracture may also contribute to instability as will collateral ligament attenuation. In the rheumatoid knee it is not uncommon for the problem to be compounded by a rupture of the anterior cruciate ligament.

Medical treatment

Medical (conservative) treatment was recently reviewed by Bird (1990) and must include a full and frank discussion with the patient of the expected course and prognosis of the disease. A medication programme should be outlined and the benefits of physiotherapy advocated. Self activity, self improvement and self reassurance must be encouraged. The aim should be to diminish pain, to increase the range of motion and in so doing to restore the individual's independence.

The prognosis for osteoarthrosis is not as dull as many anticipate and fluctuations of the disease offer relatively long periods of relief of symptoms. As regards the hip joint it has been demonstrated by Nilsson, Danielsson and Hernberg (1982), in a group of patients which they re-examined 10 years after the initial diagnosis, that during this period 12% became completely pain-free and a considerable reduction in pain was experienced by no less than 59%. Similar figures were found in a recent audit of patients waiting for total hip replacement for osteoarthrosis in the Department of Orthopaedics, Karolinska Hospital, Stockholm. In more than 30% of the patients the symptoms had so diminished in the 2–3 year wait to surgery that there was no longer any indication for operation. Furthermore, none of these patients came to surgery in the following 2 years.

As far as the knee is concerned the pattern is somewhat reversed with progressive deterioration, increase in pain and further decreased function almost always being the rule.

In rheumatoid arthritis the prognosis is more gloomy and about half the patients may be expected to develop severe functional incapacity within 10 years of the initial diagnosis. Conversely, 10% will remit completely and some 20–30% will exhibit the disease in a more modest form.

Physiotherapy including transcutaneous nerve stimulation, ultrasound and vibration are recommended for both conditions. Suitable footwear and appropriate aids and appliances should be prescribed and these are fully discussed in chapters 7 and 18.

Pain relief can be achieved in both osteoarthrosis and rheumatoid arthritis by simple analgesics such as paracetamol but non-steroidal anti-inflammatory drugs may be more effective. Disease modifying agents such as gold, penicillamine and anti-malarials may be used in severe and resistant rheumatoid arthritis. Because of side effects they require careful and continuous control by a rheumatologist.

A topic of current debate is the role of intra-articular injection of corticosteroids. In general, this form of treatment cannot be recommended for patients with osteoarthrosis since in most cases the inflammatory reaction is modest. Conversely, in rheumatoid arthritis inflammatory painful effusions and swollen synovial membranes respond well to a steroid injection which can be repeated two or three times at 4–6 week intervals. This form of treatment should not be repeated more frequently as it has been suspected of increasing damage to the already existing destruction of joint cartilage. This has, however, not been supported by conclusive evidence.

Intra-articular injections are relatively easy to place into the knee and the joint usually responds well to this form of treatment. The other site in the body which is also very rewarding to treat by injection therapy is the shoulder. However, it must be borne in mind that the shoulder is composed of at least five functionally inter-related subunits all of which can be effected synchronously or metachronously to varying degrees by rheumatoid arthritis. These are the sternoclavicular joint, the acromioclavicular joint, the subacromial region and bursa, the glenohumeral joint and the scapulothoracic 'functional' joint. It is therefore mandatory that prior to injection treatment being suggested the exact site of the pain, i.e. whether it be extrinsic or intrinsic to the glenohumeral joint should be accurately localized and this is most reliably achieved by selective injection of local anaesthetic (Newman, 1989). Rheumatoid arthritis of the acromioclavicular joint responds well to this form of treatment as does subacromial impingement syndrome.

Failure of medical therapy is the indication to consider surgery.

Surgical treatment

Arthritis surgery in the elderly aims to relieve pain, increase the range of motion and offer an improvement in the quality of life. Before considering surgery it is essential to ascertain that all conservative approaches have been tried and proved to be unsatisfactory.

In order to achieve a gratifying result from surgery it is also necessary to adhere to strict indications. Similarly, an operation on a joint should be considered ill-planned if the operated joint improves but the surrounding joints are allowed to deteriorate such that little or no benefit can be afforded by the local surgical intervention.

It is also necessary to have some insight into the way results of surgery are reported. Scoring systems are popular but not always reliable (Andersson and Möller-Nielsen, 1972) since several physiologically unrelated modalities (radiography, symptoms and range of movement) may be individually measured and then summated. This seldom, if ever, reflects the true result of the surgical procedure being evaluated. The current trend is to break away from such scoring systems and to introduce an approach with greater practical applicability, e.g. a comparison of pre- and postoperative activities. A good example of this technique is seen in a review of the results of total hip arthroplasty (Goldie, 1983). Preoperatively 67% of patients could not perform ordinary household tasks but after surgery only 16% were unable to do so. Before operation 46% could not go out shopping but after surgery only 10% were unable to

do so. Similar measurements were made for tying shoelaces, for putting on and taking off stockings and independently taking care of oneself. Other studies on the postoperative improvement in the quality of life and sexual activity have also been published (Wiklund and Romanus, 1988).

The length of follow-up following a procedure is also critical. According to Morscher (1984) '... five years of follow-up are needed for femoral prostheses and eight to ten years for acetabular components before an assessment can be made as to the superiority of one fixation method over another'.

It is also necessary to have some knowledge of the complications of various procedures in order that the potential risks of an operation can be explained to the patient. Once a patient understands that all operations are not necessarily successful he or she will carry with greater forbearance a result which has turned out unsatisfactorily. It is the patient who really experiences the complication – not the surgeon!

The surgical procedures available may be classified as soft tissue, arthrodesis, osteotomy and arthroplasty.

Soft tissue procedures

Osteoarthrosis

In view of the rapid and successful development of total joint arthroplasty soft tissue procedures such as synovectomy are becoming increasingly less indicated in the elderly. Synovectomy, however, not as a single procedure but performed as part of a joint debridement procedure ('spring clean') may still have a place for the occasional individual who for various reasons objects to the operation of arthroplasty. This procedure includes removal of synovial tissue, osteophytes, softened and fibrillated cartilage, torn or degenerated menisci and loose bodies. Multiple, small holes are also drilled into denuded bone to stimulate the formation of fibrocartilage. Reasonable results have been reported by Insall (1967) and Hirohata (1973).

Rheumatoid arthritis

Synovectomy of the metacarpophalangeal and proximal interphalangeal joints yields very good

Table 6.6 Fourteen-year follow-up study of synovectomy of the knee for rheumatoid arthritis in 51 knees in 44 patients

Year	Stage of disease process				Knees/patients
	I	II	III	IV	
1965	7	21	20	3	51/44
1965		2 dead	2 dead		
		2 art	2 art		
Lost	0	8	10	1 art	19/15
		2 ank	2 ank		
1973		2 arth	4 arth		
1973					
Lost	0	4 arth	6 arth	0	10/10
1977					
1977	7	9	4	2	22/19
1977					
Lost	3 (dead)	3 arth	2 arth		8/8
Total remaining in 1979	4	6	2	2	14/11

ank = ankylosis
art = arthrodesis
arth = arthroplasty
(*Source*: Goldie, 1984)

results when the joints are stable and the cartilage not yet destroyed. In fixed deformities synovectomy has no place.

Synovectomy in the wrist, often combined with excision of the ulna head (Newman, 1987) is a recommended procedure.

In the elbow synovectomy combined with excision of the radial head gives good results in 80% (Laine and Vainio, 1969). The operation is reliable with regard to initial pain relief and the aquisition of good function (Raunio, 1981) but the results with regard to movement are variable, though gains in flexion and extension have been reported in up to 55% (Stein, Dickson and Bentley, 1975). The operation does not appear to arrest radiological deterioration and the recurrence of synovitis is not uncommon. For example, Summers, Webley and Taylor (1987) reviewed 50 patients and whereas 84% were pain-free at 6 months only 54% were within this category 5 years later. Recurrent synovitis occurred in almost 40% of patients and this is also the experience of Souter (1989).

Synovectomy cannot be recommended for the rheumatoid hip but has proved to be a satisfactory procedure for the knee. Goldie (1984) reported a follow-up of over 14 years with initial good results but with deterioration with time depending on the aggressiveness of the disease (Table 6.6). Synovectomy is a worthwhile procedure which, if not permanent in its results, may offer a comparatively long-standing deferral of a more aggressive intervention.

Arthrodesis

A successful arthrodesis relieves local pain, corrects deformity and gives stability. However, in view of the rapid development of successful arthroplasty procedures arthrodesis has become quite outmoded for the treatment of major joints in the elderly. Such individuals, whether victims of degenerative or inflammatory disease, are so anxious to retain whatever mobility is possible that arthrodesis is perceived by them as an abomination. Furthermore, arthrodesis is contraindicated if the joint above or below is also degenerate – something not uncommon in the elderly. Similarly, because of the fear of metachronous disease arthrodesis is contraindicated for most major joints in patients with rheumatoid disease.

In a limited number of joints arthrodesis is still the operation of choice – even in the elderly rheumatoid. These include those joints of the thumb and fingers necessary for a functional grip (Flatt, 1963), the wrist (Mannerfelt and

Malmsten, 1971), the ankle and toes. Arthroplasty alternatives in these sites currently appear superfluous.

Osteotomy

Rehabilitation following osteotomy is time consuming and is just as badly accepted by the elderly as is arthrodesis. The results are unpredictable and certainly not as good as total joint arthroplasty, and therefore the indications for osteotomy around the hip are nowadays increasingly limited in the elderly patient with either osteo- or rheumatoid arthritis.

Tjörnstrand (1981) reviewed the results of high tibial osteotomy for osteoarthrosis and concluded that the procedure conferred inferior results to arthroplasty. Similarly, Odenbring's 10–19 year follow-up study of 314 tibial osteotomies for osteoarthrosis revealed an almost 20% overall revision rate (Odenbring *et al.*, 1990).

There is no place for osteotomy in aged patients with disabling hip and knee problems due to rheumatoid arthritis.

Arthroplasty

It becomes apparent when attempting to assess the results of replacement surgery that a distinction between the observations made on patients with osteoarthrosis and those with rheumatoid arthritis is not always made in the literature. With experience however it has become clear that no major differences separate the results obtained in these two diagnostic groups and many of the conclusions drawn from the treatment of osteoarthrosis may be applied to patients with rheumatoid arthritis and *vice versa*. However, a consideration which does vary between the two groups and which must be emphasized is the necessity to consider the functional capacity of the neighbouring joints when planning a replacement procedure for an elderly rheumatoid patient. Such individuals invariably suffer multiple joint involvement. Consequently, a knee may be replaced with a perfect local result but will never function satisfactorily if the ipsilateral hip is painful and contracted in flexion and adduction. In this situation it is necessary either to replace both joints at the same operative session if the patient's condition so permits (Hoekstra, 1989; Stanley, Stockley and

Getty, 1990) or to decide which joint should be given priority.

Pain usually dictates the order of surgery but, in general, it is preferable to start with the hip before the knee. Furthermore, for practical reasons it is easier to exercise a recently operated hip when the patient has a painful and contracted knee than *vice versa*. The immediately dramatic results of hip surgery tend to motivate the patients with their rehabilitation programmes and encourage them to persist with other – at times more demanding – surgical procedures such as knee replacement.

If both hips and one knee require surgery bilateral total hip replacement will facilitate personal hygiene and sitting. If on the other hand early ambulation is the goal it may be preferrable to replace the hip and ipsilateral knee which will then give the patient one reliable lower extremity before the other one is dealt with.

Generally, arthroplasty of the upper extremities take second place after lower extremity surgery provided that the upper extremities are not more painful (Poss and Sledge, 1981).

Hoekstra (1989) has described 14 patients in whom both hips and knees were replaced with the hip surgery being performed prior to that on the knees. At follow-up (32–92 months postoperatively) five patients were rated as excellent, seven as good and two as fair. Improved performance in daily activities was, however, achieved less consistently.

The hip

Total replacement of the hip has revolutionized orthopaedic surgery in the elderly patient. The satisfactory functional results over a long period of time have made the method immensely popular and more than 400 000 total hip replacements are performed per year worldwide. More than 90% exhibit excellent results as regards pain relief and walking ability at more than 12 years follow-up and similar results have also been reported after 20 years' observation (Wroblewski, 1990). The obvious success of this procedure has made it almost inevitable that the operation has on occasion been used indiscriminately. If consistently good results are to be obtained with this form of treatment it is essential that certain indications are strictly adhered to including the combination of severe pain

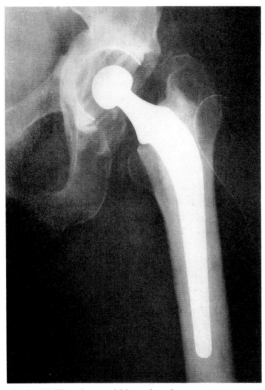

Figure 6.2 Charnley total hip arthroplasty

(especially nocturnal) uncontrolled by conservative means, restricted motion and radiographic evidence of joint destruction.

The procedure which was refined and made almost a routine practice by Sir John Charnley (1979) includes replacement of the femoral head with a metal ball mounted onto a stem which fits into the femoral canal and replacement of the acetabulum by a polyethylene cup. Both components are fixed to bone with polymethylmethacrylate cement (Figure 6.2) which interlocks with the prosthetic irregularities and bony trabeculae. Failure of this mechanical interlock allows micromotion at the interfaces and leads to subsequent implant loosening.

Since the late 1970s fixation without the use of cement has been developed based on the principles of initial stability rendered by intimate bone contact and suitable prosthetic biocompatibility to stimulate biological fixation by osseointegration and/or bony ingrowth (Lord *et al.*, 1979). The former term implies the ability of bone cells to integrate into the surface of appropriate implants (usually titanium) and the nature of this bond is presumed to be chemophysical at the molecular level.

The term 'bony ingrowth' denotes growth of bone close to the surface of a suitable implant. These are generally covered by a porous layer of metallic mesh, net or microspheres and direct contact between living bone and implant surface has been reported (Chen *et al.*, 1983; Memoli *et al.*, 1983).

Because of concern about the osteoblastic response of the elderly as well as the difficulty that such patients have in cooperating with the partial or non-weight bearing postoperative rehabilitation regime necessary for cement-free procedures, 'biologically fixed' prostheses have not been widely offered to elderly arthritic patients and the cemented arthroplasty has become the standard implant type for them. Nonetheless, it is well documented that cemented total hip replacement is associated with a slowly increasing rate of failure. Whether this also applies to the non-cemented procedure is still unknown.

In 1989 Wykman presented his analysis of two randomized groups of patients aged 60 years and over treated by total hip replacement; one group received a cemented Charnley prosthesis and the other a non-cemented Honnart–Patel–Garches prosthesis. Within the follow-up period of 5 years no major advantages were found with the non-cemented prosthesis compared with the cemented prosthesis and the probability of prosthesis survival was 88% for the cemented and 82% for the non-cemented type.

The benefit of a total hip replacement to an elderly, arthritic patient is a medical victory over pain and distress. The functional advantages are obvious with an improvement in social relations, increased activity, improvement in quality of life, return of self respect and, often, prolonged independence. These in combination lessen the burden of the care of the elderly on society. In purely economic terms it has been estimated that for individuals more than 65 years of age the 'profit' of a hip replacement to society is roughly double the costs of the operation and hospitalization.

The procedure is associated with several systemic, short- and long-term complications and Table 6.7 shows that venous thrombosis is the most frequent systemic complication. The reason for this is unknown but an assumption is that venous return becomes compromised during the operative procedure which involves extreme angulation of the hip during insertion

Table 6.7 Non-specific, systemic complications following total hip replacement

Complication	Per cent
Mortality	0.5–2[a]
Urinary retention	20–35
Urinary tract infection	5–18
Thrombosis	20–70
Pulmonary embolism	2–4
Paralytic ileus	0–3
Postoperative psychosis	0–3
Pulmonary complication	0–2
G–I tract haemorrhage	0–1
Cardiac arrythmia	0–1

[a] This figure may rise to 4% at age 80 years (Ling, 1984)
(*Source*: Ahnfelt, 1987)

Table 6.8 Specific early complications after total hip replacement

Complication	Per cent
Infection	0.5–2
Dislocation	0.5–5
Fracture	1 –2
Nerve palsy	0.5–1.7
Ectopic bone formation	20 –70
Trochanteric problems	1.2–8.3

(*Source*: Ahnfelt, 1987)

Table 6.9 Specific late complications after total hip replacement

Complication	Per cent
Loosening	3–7.5
Bone resorption	0–30
Implant complications	0.2–1.0

(*Source*: Ahnfelt, 1987)

of the prostheses. Pre- and postoperative prophylaxis is therefore necessary but recommendations differ. In the Department of Orthopaedics, Karolinska Hospital, Stockholm the routine is 500 ml Macrodex (Dextran 70) peroperatively and then 500 ml on days 1 and 3 postoperatively together with early ambulation. The use of heparin and warfarin remains controversial and the proposed benefits of this treatment must be balanced against the increased risks in the elderly of haemorrhage, haematoma and subsequent wound infection (Sikorski, 1984). Anti-embolism stockings are routinely prescribed.

The specific early and late complications of this operation are listed in Tables 6.8 and 6.9 and infection is clearly a problem. The use of prophylactic antibiotics is mandatory to prevent sepsis with consequent premature implant loosening. In the aforesaid orthopaedic department it has been found that a single preoperative dose (2 g dicloxacillin i.v. 15–30 min preoperatively) is as effective as multiple doses (Al-Dabbagh, Svenberg-Appelgren and Wallensten, in press). Theatre enclosure with a laminar airflow system is recommended for all replacement procedures.

Death is feared even by elderly patients and certainly by their family. It is therefore essential that both are warned of this complication of total hip arthroplasty since the mortality rate of this procedure is approximately 1% in the first postoperative month when all patients irrespective of age are considered. However, the rate rises significantly with age to be 4% in a group of patients with a mean age of 80 years (Ling, 1984). Lindberg *et al.* (1984) calculated the mortality rate after total hip replacement and found that this decreased after the first postoperative year in women over the age of 70 years. There was no such effect in men. Revisions did not affect the mortality rate in women. In men over the age of 70 years the risk was increased after a revision. Patients (men or women) who undergo total hip replacement after hip fracture and/or rheumatoid arthritis had an increased mortality rate after the first postoperative year.

Heterotopic ossification is a frequent radiological finding but does not often significantly limit mobility. The perioperative administration of non-steroidal anti-inflammatory drugs will however reduce its incidence.

The diagnostic criteria for loosening are controversial which may account for the variation in the results presented in Table 6.9. The reported rate of radiographic loosening varies from less than 1% (Paterson, Fulford and Denham, 1986) to 38% (Wejkner and Wiege, 1987) for the acetabular component and from 1% (Harris, McCarthy and O'Neill, 1982) to 47% (Wejkner and Wiege, 1987) for the femoral component.

Contraindications for total hip replacement in the elderly include advanced cardiopulmonary disease, morbid obesity and sepsis. Advanced age in itself is not a contraindication but the risks of complication are somewhat higher, in particular with regard to dislocation, femoral fracture and hospital mortality. This is particularly so for patients aged 80 years or more (Newington, Bannister and Fordyce, 1990). Nevertheless, 75% of such patients have a satisfactory outcome.

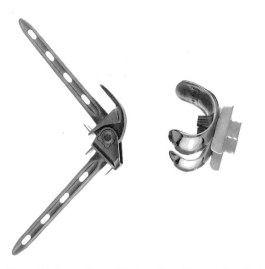

Figure 6.3 Comparison of design of total knee arthroplasty prostheses. (left) A fully constrained all-metal knee prosthesis (Walldius) with a uni-axial hinge and long intra-medullary fixation stems. (right) A non-constrained, two-part, metal on high density polyethylene prosthesis

Total failure of the operation results in revision surgery (Goldie, 1986). The rate for this varies between different series and 10 years postoperatively ranges between 1.5 and 19% (Amstutz *et al.*, 1982; Kavanagh, Ilstrup and Fitzgerald, 1985).

The knee

Knee arthroplasty is an ideal operation for the older individual in whom knee function has been compromised because of uncontrollable pain and/or deformity. Several prosthetic designs are available and these are categorized into the constrained, non-constrained and semi-constrained varieties. The constrained types are fitted with stemmed components (Figure 6.3) linked by a uni-axial hinge though some limited rotatory ability has been incorporated into the designs of late. The stability of the operated knee is then imparted by the prosthesis. The non-constrained types are surface replacements and rely principally for their stability on the integrity of the remaining ligaments (Figure 6.3). The semi-constrained such as the Sheehan are a compromise between the constrained and non-constrained types (Dreghorn *et al.*, 1990).

In all these designs both femoral condylar surfaces are either replaced or recovered. This approach may be excessive when one considers

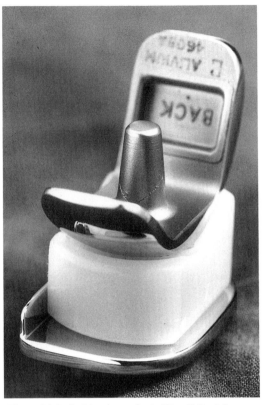

Figure 6.4 Oxford knee prosthesis (Goodfellow) for unicondylar arthroplasty. The design incorporates a high density polyethylene 'meniscus' which articulates between the tibial and femoral resurfacing components

that in many cases osteoarthrosis affects predominantly only the medial tibiofemoral articulation. In some cases, the lateral tibiofemoral joint may be relatively spared and the concept that only one side of the femorotibial joint needs to be replaced – so-called unicondylar arthroplasty – is becoming increasingly accepted. A typical example of this design is the Oxford knee (Figure 6.4) (Goodfellow and O'Connor, 1988; Barrett, Biswas and MacKenney, 1990).

Like total hip prostheses there are cemented and non-cemented knee replacements. Time will show which type is superior but in comparative studies the rate of complications in cementless cases has been higher than in cemented (Insall *et al.*, 1983; Rorabeck, Bourne and Nott, 1988). It is the quality of bone which is decisive for the fate of any prosthetic replacement and this is especially so for the cementless variety.

In 1975 a multicentre study on total knee replacement was introduced in Sweden (Svenska knäartroplastiker) and to date more than 17 000 operations have been registered. In this way detailed follow-up information has been recorded on the quality of arthroplasty techniques. In general, knee arthroplasty has been shown to be a satisfactory procedure in the elderly resulting in decreased pain and increased function. Survivorship analysis of different prostheses after 6 years indicates better survival for surface replacements than for stemmed ones. Within the former group the best survival was observed for a design called total condylar including replacement of the patella with a 'button'. Unicondylar arthoplasties as mentioned above yielded excellent results.

In 1988 Ranawat and Boachie-Adjer reported the 8–11 year results in 72 patients (90 knees) with total condylar knee arthroplasties; 93% were excellent, 3% fair and 4% poor. Radiography revealed well-fixed components in 40% thus leaving 60% with radiolucencies. These radiolucencies were not necessarily associated with symptoms despite being an accepted radiological sign of loosening which does occur in varying degrees. There was a correlation between body weight and the presence or absence of radiolucencies.

Gschwend, Drobny and Radovanovic (1988) using a semi-constrained, low-friction stemmed type of prosthesis with patellar replacement reported 75% overall improvement for pain, range of motion and functional gain after 14 years.

Complications have been similar to those seen with total hip replacement and include infection, wound drainage, thromboembolism, nerve palsy and loosening. Problems specific to the knee have included patellar fracture, subluxation and maltracking. In Gschwend's series re-operations were necessary in almost 8%, of which half were caused by the patella only. In total knee replacement it is essential that the dynamics of the patella are borne in mind since malalignment and aberrations of the extensor mechanism may be secondary to the surgical procedures. Preoperatively a tendency for abnormal patellar function may be present and allowance has to be made for this in the planning of the replacement procedure. No matter whether the patella is subjected to resurfacing or patelloplasty, postoperative patellar abnormalities including subluxation, dislocation and pain are most often the result of inadequate soft-tissue balance or rotational malalignment of the prosthetic components. Nowadays resurfacing the patella with a 'button' is generally advocated but conclusive evidence for its benefit is still awaited (Goldie *et al.*, 1988).

Irrespective of cause, failure may result in removal of the prosthesis with attempted arthrodesis as the salvage procedure. In the nationwide Swedish study 91 patients with attempted arthodesis after failed knee arthoplasty were identified from 6342 arthroplasties (Knutson *et al.*, 1984). There were 43 hinged, 34 bi- or tricompartmental and 14 unicompartmental designs used. Infection was the cause of failure in 75%. Fusion was achieved in only half of the 108 attempts in the 91 knees. The suggested reasons for this poor fusion rate were loss of bone stock, poor bone quality, inadequate technique of fixation and persistent infection.

In summarizing knee arthroplasty it may be well to cite Whiteside (1990): 'Much of the decision making processes in surgery of the arthritic conditions of the knee have changed drastically in the last ten years. With the success of total knee arthroplasty fusion has been limited to infection, multiply-failed arthroplasty and some cases of Charcot arthropathy and the role for osteotomy has been significantly reduced. However, the variety of arthroplasties available and the selection of methods of bone resection and ligament balancing, have added several layers of complexity to this subject. The statement "Do a total knee replacement" is only a beginning to the discussion of how to perform surgery on an arthritic knee with present methods'.

The shoulder

In those cases where the symptoms and disability are demonstrated to be arising in the true glenohumeral joint total shoulder arthroplasty is the procedure of choice. In the most recent review solely dedicated to a cohort of 42 patients with rheumatoid arthritis Kelly, Foster and Fisher (1987) found almost 90% to have no significant pain when treated using the Neer technique (Figure 6.5). Flexion and extension were both improved by approximately 30 degrees and internal and external rotation were improved by a similar amount. Though patients experienced improvement in their functional abilities leading to greater personal independence none could use their hand above shoulder level.

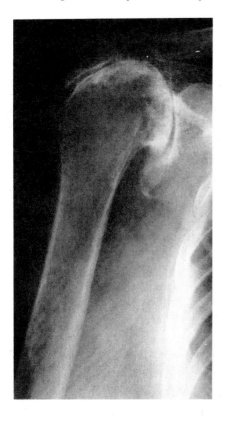

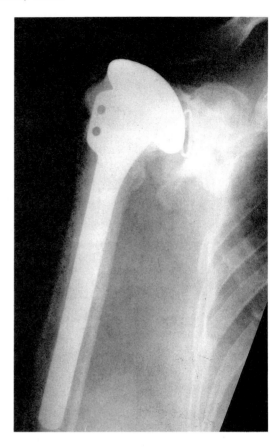

Figure 6.5 (left) Shoulder severely affected with rheumatoid arthritis showing superior subluxation of the humeral head. (right) Neer total shoulder arthroplasty

In the author's series of shoulder arthroplasty the range of motion following surgery did not increase and no patient could raise his arm above 90 degrees in abduction or flexion. However, feeding, personal hygiene and everyday tasks could be carried out without difficulty (Goldie, 1987).

Prostheses currently available can be categorized as constrained and non-constrained and examples of the latter types are the Neer (Figure 6.6), (Neer, Watson and Stanton, 1982) Bechtol (1987), O'Leary-Walker (1982) and DANA (Designed After Natural Anatomy). Examples of the constrained variety are Fenlin (1975), Kessel (Kessel and Bayley, 1979) and Kölbel (Kölbel *et al.*, 1977). The advantage of a non-constrained prosthesis is that it decreases the forces acting at the bone–cement interface and in so doing, theoretically at least, reduces the incidence of loosening. In contrast, a constrained prosthesis has the advantage of inherent stability but the disadvantage of increased stresses at the interface. The static fulcrum will however theoretically allow the deltoid muscle to elevate the arm in the absence of a functioning rotator cuff.

Whereas in the past it was thought that the absence of a rotator cuff should lead a surgeon to use a constrained device it has now become apparent that rotator cuff deficiency should not necessarily be considered to be an absolute contraindication to unconstrained arthroplasty.

Shoulder arthroplasty should be considered as a procedure which gives pain relief rather than necessarily increasing the range of motion. This is particularly so in rheumatoid arthritis when the cuff is diseased and often functionless. When the operation is performed for osteoarthrosis a greater degree of postoperative movement can be expected.

Glenoid bone erosion occurs much more in rheumatoid arthritis than osteoarthrosis and may be marked so prejudicing the sound fixation of a glenoid component. An alternative

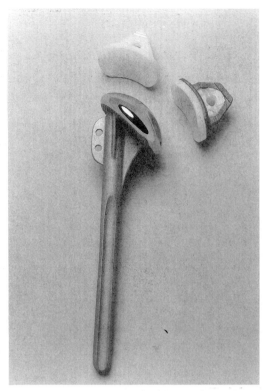

Figure 6.6 Mark II Neer total shoulder prostheses. Two types of glenoid component are shown; both are of high density polyethylene but the one on the right is metal backed. (Photograph kindly provided by 3M Health Care Limited)

approach is to manage these shoulders without using a glenoid component, i.e. by hemiarthroplasty only. Few publications have compared the results of total with hemiarthroplasty in a controlled manner but it has been suggested that total joint replacement fairs slightly better than hemiarthroplasty (Marmor, 1977; Gschwend, 1988).

The elbow

The surgical management of the elbow with advanced rheumatoid or osteoarthrotic disease may be by arthoplasty (Figure 6.7) and the design of prostheses has changed dramatically over the course of the last two decades. From fully constrained implants with long stemmed fixation such as the Dee (1972), Stanmore and Shires designs have changed to semi-constrained models such as the Volz (1984), Coonrad (1982),

Pritchard (1983) and Mayo Clinic and, finally, to unconstrained prostheses such as the Souter–Strathclyde (Figure 6.8) and Liverpool prostheses. Several designs are currently available but a recent 10-year review of the Souter–Strathclyde prothesis has showed that whereas preoperatively 85% of the patients experienced severe elbow pain, 92% had no pain or only the occasional twinge of discomfort 1 year after surgery and this gratifying result was maintained at 5 years. Pronation and supination are improved by this procedure, flexion is usually increased but fixed flexion deformity is almost irremovable (Souter, 1989).

The commonest complication of this procedure is ulnar neuropathy which occurs in approximately 15% (Souter, 1989).

The wrist and hand

A great contribution to prosthetic replacement of the joints of the rheumatoid hand has been made by Swanson who has designed a flexible hinge implant made of silicone elastomer. The importance of the implant is to maintain proper joint alignment and spacing while early movement is started with the implant then acting as a dynamic spacer. Swanson and de Groot Swanson (1981) have expressed this as:

bone resection + implant + fibrous

encapsulation = new joint

'The new joint' concept has been used successfully in the trapeziometacarpal joint, the metacarpophalangeal joints and the interphalangeal joints. On comparing different designs such as those of Flatt (1963), Niebauer (Niebauer and Landry, 1971) and Swanson and de Groot Swanson (1981), Dryer *et al.* (1984) found that patient satisfaction was high and the ability of the patients to perform activities of daily living was acceptable. However, the author concluded that the Swanson spacers must be used cautiously, with a firm knowledge of ancillary soft tissue procedures and a realistic expectation of clinical efficacy.

Arthrodesis is a very successful operation for a chronically painful wrist joint in patients with rheumatoid arthritis (Mannerfelt and Malmsten, 1971). Prostheses have been designed but long-term results are not yet available (Meuli, 1984; Volz, 1984).

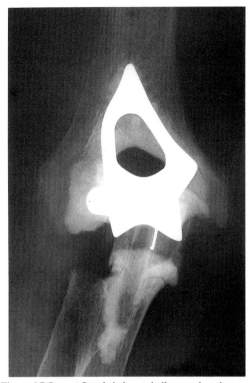

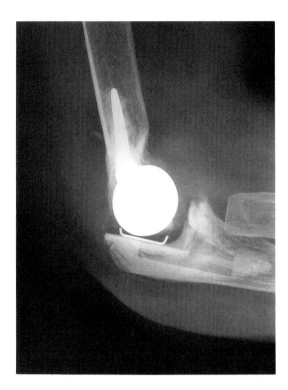

Figure 6.7 Souter–Strathclyde total elbow arthroplasty. The radial head is resected and not replaced with this technique

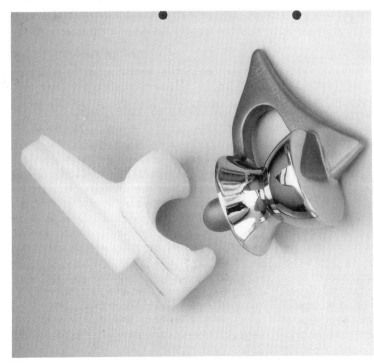

Figure 6.8 Souter–Strathclyde total elbow prosthesis. The use of capitellar and medial epicondylar pegs allows the fixation of the humeral component to span the maximum width of the epicondyles and this is further supplemented by a stirrup cemented into the excavated supracondylar ridges. The high density polyethylene ulnar component is cemented into the medullary cavity of the ulna. (Photograph kindly provided by Howmedica (UK) Ltd)

Summary

The surgical treatment of osteoarthrosis and rheumatoid arthritis is exciting but though the results are good they are not yet good enough to warrant complacency. As for prosthetic replacement, further advances in design and materials are required. It is also clear that there is a positive relationship between the technical expertise with which surgery is performed and the long-term functional results. Nonetheless, the benefits that joint replacement surgery can confer to the severely afflicted patient with regard to pain relief and improved function are such that there should be little hesitation in offering this form of treatment to all such patients who fail conservative treatment. However, it must always be remembered that the results of even the most sophisticated surgery can be improved by an intensive rehabilitation programme including pre- and postoperative occupational therapy and physiotherapy, the prescription of appropriate appliances and the optimization of medical therapy.

As a final comment Charnley (1979) in a summary of joint replacement surgery may be cited, '... only by performing easy operations very well shall we avoid an appalling accumulation of untreatable failures in the next two decades'.

References

Agunwa, W.C.R. (1989) Low incidence of osteoarthritis of the hips in contrast with osteoarthrosis of the knees among rural Saudis: Why? *Ann. Rheum. Dis.*, **48**, 351–352

Ahlbäck, S. (1968) Osteoarthrosis of the knee. *Acta Radiol.* (Suppl.) 277.

Ahnfelt, L. (1987) Reopererade totala höftledsplastiker i Sverige under åren 1979–1983. Thesis, Gothenburg

Al-Dabbagh, Z., Svenberg-Appelgren, P. and Wallensten, R. Single-dose versus multiple dose antibiotic prophylaxis in primary joint replacement surgery. *Acta Orthop. Scand.* (in press)

Allander, E. (1970) A population survey of rheumatoid arthritis. *Acta Rheumat. Scand.* (Suppl.) 15

Allander, E. (1974) Prevalence, incidence and remission rates of some common rheumatic diseases or syndromes. *Scand. J. Rheumatol.*, **3**, 145–153

Amstutz, H.C., Ma, S.M., Jinnah, R.H. and Mai, L. (1982). Revision of aseptic loose total hip arthroplasties. *Clin. Orthop.*, **170**, 21–33

Andersson, G. and Möller-Nielsen, J. (1972) Hip assessment: A comparison of nine different methods. *J. Bone Joint Surg.*, **54B**, 621–625

Barrett, D.S., Biswas, S.P. and MacKenney, R.P. (1990) The Oxford knee replacement. A review from an independent centre. *J. Bone Joint Surg.*, **72B**, 775–778

Bechtol, C.O. (1987) *Recent Advances in Orthopaedics* (ed. A. Catterall), Churchill Livingstone, Edinburgh, p. 102

Beighton, P., Solomin, L. and Valkenburg, H.A. (1975) Rheumatoid arthritis in a rural South African negro population. *Ann. Rheum. Dis.*, **34**, 136–141

Benett, P.H. and Burch, T.A. (1967) New York Symposium on population studies in the rheumatic diseases: New diagnostic criteria. *Bull. Rheum. Dis.*, **17**, 453–458.

Bird, H.A. (1990) Medical treatment for rheumatic diseases. *J. Roy. Soc. Hlth*, **110**, 157–160

Buchanan, W.W. and Boyle, J. (1971) *Clinical Rheumatology*, Blackwell Scientific, Oxford

Cathcart, E.S. and O'Sullivan, J.B. (1970) Rheumatoid arthritis in a New England town. *N. Engl. J. Med.*, **228**, 421–424

Cecil, R.L., Nicholls, E.E. and Stainsby, W.J., (1930). The etiology of rheumatoid arthritis. *Am. J. Med. Sci.*, **181**, 12

Charnley J. (1979) *Low Friction Arthroplasty of the Hip*, Springer Verlag, Berlin, Heidelberg, New York

Chen, P.-Q., Turner, T.M., Ronningen, H., Galante, J., Urban, R. and Rostoker, W. (1983). A canine cementless total hip prosthesis model. *Clin. Orthop.*, **176**, 24–33

Coonrad, R. (1982) History of Total Elbow Arthroplasty. In: *Total Joint Replacement of the Upper Extremity* (ed. A. Inglis), St Louis, CV Mosby, Chapter 8, pp. 75–90.

Danielsson, L.G., Lindberg, H. and Nilsson, B., (1984) Prevalence of coxarthrosis. *Clin. Orthop.*, **191**, 110–115

Dee, R. (1972) Total replacement arthroplasty of the elbow for rheumatoid arthritis. *J. Bone Joint Surg.*, **54**, 88–95.

Dieppe, P.A., Doherty, M., Macfarlane, D. and Maddison, P. (1985) *Rheumatological Medicine*, Churchill Livingstone, London, pp. 157–189

Dreghorn, C.R., Newman, R.J., Shea, W., McBride, D., McCreath, S. and Whitefield, G. (1990) The Sheehan knee arthroplasty. British Orthopaedic Association presentation, Glasgow

Dryer, R., Blair, W., Shurr, D. and Buckwalter, J. (1984) Proximal interphalangeal joint arthroplasty. *Clin. Orthop.*, **185**, 187–194

Felson, D., Naimark, A., Anderson, J., Kazis, L., Castelli, W. and Meenan, R. (1987) The prevalence of knee osteoarthritis in the elderly. The Framingham Osteoarthritis Study. *Arth. Rheum.*, **30**, 914–918

Felson, D. (1988) Epidemiology of hip and knee osteoarthritis. *Epidem. Rev.*, **10**, 1–28

Fenlin, J. (1975) Total glenohumeral replacement. *Orthop. Clin. North Am.*, **6**, 565–583

Flatt, A.E. (1963) *The Care of the Rheumatoid Hand*, CV Mosby, St Louis

Fredensborg, N. and Nilsson, B.E. (1978) The joint space in normal hip radiographs. *Radiology*, **126**, 325–326

Goldie, I. (1983) Nya leder (New Joints). Instructional course, Karolinska Hospital, Stockholm

Goldie, I. (1984). A synopsis of surgery for rheumatoid arthritis. *Clin. Orthop.*, **191**, 185–192

Goldie, I. (1986) Failed joint replacement. *Current Orthop.*, **1**, 3–5

Goldie, I. (1987) Joint replacement in the upper limb. In *Recent Advances in Orthopaedics* (ed. A. Catterall), Churchill Livingstone, Edinburgh No. **5**, pp. 101–121,

Goldie, I., Broström, L.-A., Josefsson, A. and Söderlund, V. (1988) The patella in total knee replacement: a problem or not? In *Total Knee Replacement* (eds Niwa, Paul, Yamamoto), Springer Verlag, Tokyo, p. 277

Goodfellow, J.W. and O'Connor, J. (1988) The Oxford knee: The role of a meniscal bearing arthroplasty. In *Total Knee Replacement* (eds Niwa, Paul, Yamamoto), Springer Verlag, Tokyo, p. 227

Gschwend, N. (1988) Is glenoid component necessary for rheumatoid patients? *Proc. 2nd. Cong. Europ. Shoulder Elbow Soc.*, Berne, Switzerland

Gschwend, N., Drobny, T. and Radovanovic, D.I. (1988) GSB – 14 years experience with total knee arthroplasty. In *Total Knee Replacement* (eds Niwa, Paul, Yamamoto), Springer Verlag, Tokyo, p. 241

Harris, W. H., McCarthy, J.R.J. and O'Neill, D.A. (1982) Femoral component loosening using contemporary techniques of femoral cement fixation. *J. Bone Joint Surg.*, **64 A**, 1063–1067

Harvey, J., Lotze, M., Stevens, M.B., Lambert, G. and Jacobson, D. (1981) Rheumatoid arthritis in a Chipewa band. *Arth. Rheum.*, **24**, 717–721

Henrad, J.-C., Benett, P.H. and Burch, T.A. (1975) Rheumatoid arthritis in the Pima Indians of Arizona: an assessment of the clinical components of the New York criteria. *Int. J. Epidemiol.*, **4**, 119–126

Hirohata, H. (1973). Synovectomy in arthritis of the knee joint. *Int. Congr. Rheumatol.*, Kyoto, Japan

Hoekstra, H. J., (1989) Bilateral total hip and knee replacement in rheumatoid arthritis patients. *Arch. Orthop. Traum. Surg.*, **108**, 291–295.

Insall, J. N. (1967) Intra-articular surgery for degenerative arthritis of the knee. A report of the work of the late P.H. Pridie. *J. Bone Joint Surg.*, **49**, 211–228

Insall, J.N., Hood, R., Flawn, L. and Sullivan, D. (1983) The total condylar knee prosthesis in gonarthrosis. *J. Bone Joint Surg.*, **65 A**, 619–628

Isacson, J.B.I. (1987) *The Knee Joint in Rheumatoid Arthritis. An Epidemiologic, Radiologic and Goniometric Study*, Thesis, Stockholm

Kavanagh, B.F., Ilstrup, D.M. and Fitzgerald, R.H. (1985) Revision total hip arthroplasty. *J. Bone Joint Surg.*, **67 A**, 517–526

Kellgren, J.H. and Lawrence, J.S. (1957) Radiological assessment of osteo-arthrosis. *Ann. Rheum. Dis.*, **16**, 494–502

Kellgren, J.H. and Lawrence, J.S. (1958) Osteo-arthrosis and disk degeneration in an urban population. *Ann. Rheum. Dis.*, **17**, 388–397

Kelly, L.G., Foster, R.S. and Fisher, W.D. (1987) Neer total shoulder replacement in rheumatoid arthritis. *J. Bone Joint Surg.*, **69 B**, 723–726

Kelsey, J.L. (1982) *Epidemiology of Musculoskeletal Disorders*, Oxford University Press, New York, Oxford

Kessel, L. and Bayley, I. (1979) Prosthetic replacement of the shoulder joint. Preliminary communication. *J. Roy. Soc. Med.*, **72**, 748–752

Knutson, K., Hovelius, L., Lindstrand, A. and Lidgren, L. (1984) Arthrodesis after failed knee arthroplasty. A nationwide multicentre investigation of 91 cases. *Clin. Orthop.*, **191**, 202–211

Kölbel, R., Rohlmann, A., Bergmann, G. and Friedebold, G. (1977) Shoulder joint replacement Kölbel–Friedebold method. In *Endoprosthesis and Alternatives for the Arm* (ed. C. Burri), Hans Huber, Bern, Stuttgart, p. 47–61.

Laine, V.A.I. (1962) Rheumatic complaints in an urban population in Finland. *Acta Rheum. Scand.*, **8**, 81–88

Laine, V.A.I. and Vainio, K. (1969). *Elbow in rheumatoid arthritis in early synovectomy*, Excerpta Medica, Amsterdam

Lindberg, H., Carlsson, A., Lanke, J. and Horstmann, V. (1984) The overall mortality rate in patients with total hip arthroplasty with special reference to coxarthrosis. *Clin. Orthop.*, **191**, 116–120

Lindberg, H. (1985). *Epidemiological Studies on Primary Coxarthrosis*, Thesis, Malmö

Ling, R.S.M. (1984) Systemic and miscellaneous complications. In *Complications of Total Hip Replacement* (ed. R.S.M. Ling), Churchill Livingstone, Edinburgh, pp. 201–211

Lord, G., Hardy, J.R. and Kummer, F.J. (1979) An uncemented total hip replacement: Experimental study and review of 300 madreporique arthroplasties. *Clin. Orthop.*, **141**, 2–16

Mannerfelt, L. and Malmsten, M. (1971) Arthrodesis of the wrist in rheumatoid arthritis a technique without external fixation. *Scand. J. Plast. Reconstr. Surg.*, **5**, 124–130

Marmor, L. (1977) Hemi-arthroplasty for the rheumatoid shoulder joint. *Clin. Orthop.*, pp. 122, 201–203

Mason, R.M. (1956) Osteoarthritis. *Ann. Phys. Med.*, **3**, 143–152

Maurer, K. (1979) Basic data on arthritis of knee, hip and sacroiliac joints in adults, ages 25–74 years: United States, 1971–75. (National Health and Nutrition Examination Survey (HANES I, 1971–75)). Vital and Health Statistics, series 11, No. **213**, DHEW publication no. (PHS) 79–1661, National Center For Health Statistics, Hyattsville, MD

Memoli, V.A., Woodman, J.L., Urban, R.M. and Galante, J.O. (1983) Long term biocompatibility of porous titanium fiber metal composites. *Proc 29th ORS Meeting*, Anaheim

Meuli, H. (1984) Meuli total wrist arthroplasty. *Clin. Orthop.*, **187**, 107–111

Morscher, E. (1984) *The Cementless Fixation of Hip Endoprostheses*, Springer Verlag, Berlin

Neer, C., Watson, K. and Stanton, J. (1982). Recent experience in total shoulder replacement. *J. Bone Joint Surg.*, **64 A**, 319–337

Newington, D.P., Bannister, G. C. and Fordyce, M. (1990) Primary total hip replacement in patients over 80 years of age. *J. Bone Joint Surg.*, **72 B**, 450–452

Newman, R.J. (1987) Excision of the distal ulna in patients with rheumatoid arthritis. *J. Bone Joint Surg.*, **69B**, 203–206

Newman, R.J. (1989) Chronic shoulder pain in rheumatoid arthritis. *Br. Med. J.*, **299**, 530.

Niebauer, J. and Landry, R. (1971) Dacron-silicone prosthesis for metacarpophalangeal and interphalangeal joints. *Hand*, **3**, 55–62

Nilsson, B., Danielsson, L.G. and Hernberg, S.A.J. (1982) Management of degenerative joint diseases. *Scand. J. Rheumat.*, (Suppl. 43) 13–21

O'Brian, W.M. (1967) The genetics of rheumatoid arthritis. *Clin. Exp. Immun.*, **2**, 785–802.

Odenbring, S., Egund, N., Knutson, K., Lindstrand, A. and Larsen, S. (1990) Revision after osteotomy for gonarthrosis. A 10–19 year follow-up of 314 cases. *Acta Orthop. Scand.*, **61**, 128–130

O'Leary-Walker, P. (1982.) Some bioengineering considerations of prosthetic replacement for the glenohumeral joint. In *Total Joint Replacement of the Upper Extremity*. (ed. A. Inglis), CV Mosby, St Louis, Chapter 23, pp. 273–288.

Paterson, M., Fulford, P. and Denham, R. (1986) Loosening of the femoral component after total hip replacement. The thin black line and the sinking hip. *J. Bone Joint Surg.*, **68 B**, 392–397

Poss, R. and Sledge, C. (1981). Total hip replacement in rheumatoid arthritis. In *Surgery in Rheumatoid Arthritis* (ed. I. Goldie), Karger, Basel, pp. 139–146

Pritchard, R. (1983) Anatomic surface elbow arthroplasty. *Clin. Orthop.*, **179**, 223–230

Ranawat, C.S. and Boachie-Adjer, O. (1988) Total condylar knee arthroplasty: 8–11 year follow-up. In *Total Knee Replacement* (eds Niwa, Paul, Yamamoto), Springer Verlag, Tokyo, pp. 71–76

Raunio, P. (1981) Synovectomy of the elbow in rheumatoid arthritis. In *Surgery in Rheumatoid Arthritis* (ed. I. Goldie), Karger, Basel, pp. 63–69

Ropes, M.W. (1958) Diagnostic criteria for rheumatoid arthritis. *Ann. Rheum. Dis.*, **18**, 49–53

Rorabeck, C.H., Bourne, R.B. and Nott, L. (1988) The cemented kinematic-II and the non-cemented porous-coated anatomic prostheses for total knee replacement. *J. Bone Joint Surg.*, **70 A**, 483–490

Sikorski, J.M. (1984) Thromboembolic complication. In *Complications of total hip replacement* (ed. R.S.M. Ling), Churchill Livingstone, London, pp. 51–81

Souter, W.A. (1989) Surgery for rheumatoid arthritis: (i) upper limb. Surgery of the elbow. *Curr. Orthop.*, **3**, 9–13

Stanley, D., Stockley, I. and Getty, C.J.M. (1990) Simultaneous or staged bilateral total knee replacements in rheumatoid arthritis. A prospective study *J. Bone Joint Surg.*, **72 B**, 772–774

Stein, H., Dickson, R.A. and Bentley. (1975) Rheumatoid arthritis of the elbow. Pattern of joint involvement results of synovectomy with excision of the radial head. *Ann. Rheum. Dis.*, **34**, 403–408

Summers, G.D., Webley, W. and Taylor. A.R. (1987) Synovectomy excision of the radial head in rheumatoid arthritis: a short term palliative procedure. *Clin. Exp. Rheumatol.*, **5**, (suppl 2) 115 (abst)

Swanson, A.B. and de Groot Swanson, G. (1981) Flexible implant resection arthroplasty for the digits in the hand. In *Surgery in Rheumatoid Arthritis* (ed. I. Goldie), Karger, Basel, pp. 111–138

Tjörnstrand, B. (1981) *Tibial Osteotomy for Medial Gonarthrosis*, Thesis, Lund

United States National Center for Health Statistics 1960–1962. *Rheumatoid Arthritis in Adults*, Series 11, No. **17**

Volz, R. (1984) Total wrist arthroplasty: a clinical and biomechanical analysis. In *Total Joint Replacement of the Upper Extremity* (ed. A. Inglis), CV Mosby, St Louis, chapter 23, pp. 273–288.

Wejkner, B. and Wiege, M. (1987) Correlation between radiologic and clinical findings in Charnley total hip replacement. A ten-year follow-up study. *Acta Radiol. Diagn.*, **28**, 607–613

Whiteside, L.A. (1990) Total knee arthroplasty. *Curr. Orthop.*, **4**, 99–102

Wiklund, I. and Romanus, B. (1988) Bättre livskvalitet efter höftledsartroplastik. *Ortopediskt Magasin*, **3**, 7–9

Wroblewski, B.M. (1990) *20 Years Experience of Charnley Total Hip Replacement*, Golden Jubilee Symposium, Karolinska Hospital, Stockholm

Wykman, A. (1989) *Cemented and Non-cemented Total Hip Arthroplasty*, Thesis, Karolinska Institute, Stockholm

7

Foot surgery in the elderly

Leslie Klenerman

Many people over the age of 65 years have some trouble with their feet – 'for possibly a quarter of elderly people these problems represent a restriction on their activities or cause appreciable pain or discomfort' (Cartwright and Henderson 1986). In this age group many problems that were previously disregarded, when the patient was young and active, in later life become a source of symptoms which require relief. This applies particularly to the forefoot where hallux valgus, hallux rigidus and claw toes can be very troublesome (Barlow, Braid and Jayson, 1990).

Although this chapter is entitled 'foot surgery in the elderly' one should approach these problems from a conservative viewpoint. One must beware of unnecessary or ill-judged operative procedures since the penalty could be loss of a digit or even a more extensive ablation of the limb.

The patient must be assessed with special care to the blood supply of the foot. A good rule is to be able to palpate at least one pedal pulse, preferably the posterior tibial. If there is any doubt a Doppler probe must be used to measure the ankle/brachial ratio, i.e. the blood pressure in the distal leg is compared with that in the antecubital fossa. The normal ratio is approximately 1. The ratio may be falsely raised in patients with arteriosclerosis but any measurement below 0.75 is indicative of peripheral vascular disease. This is usually associated with reduced skin temperature, nail thickening, loss of hair and peripheral cyanosis.

Because of the need for a predominantly non-operative approach the role of footwear is of paramount importance and will be discussed first.

Footwear

Many of the common forefoot problems can be solved by the use of extra-depth footwear (Figure 7.1) and the black felt boot – traditional in many centres – should be considered obsolete. The lasts for these shoes are designed with extra volume to give greater width and depth than a commercially available shop shoe. They are usually supplied as standard depth shoes with one or more insoles which can be removed for up to 12 mm of extra depth. They are useful for toe deformities or when a made-to-measure insole is required. An insole inserted into an ordinary shop shoe is very likely to occupy so much space that the patient will not use it. When toe deformity is combined with the need for an insole then extra depth of 18 mm is required. Extra-depth shoes are not generally available to the public and are usually supplied by orthotists. There is an ever-changing variety of styles and manufacturers which should allow an element of choice. In practice it is usual for a single make to be used depending on the affiliation of the orthotist.

Surgical shoes, i.e. bespoke shoes made specifically for the patient, are required if the foot cannot be comfortably accommodated in an extra-depth shoe. This applies especially for those with hind- and mid-foot deformities. They are made from a last produced by detailed measurements by the orthotist or from a positive plaster-of-Paris cast and consequently cost about four times as much as the extra-depth variety. Virtually any foot deformity can be accommodated provided the foot is placed on a level base and the shoe or boot constructed around it.

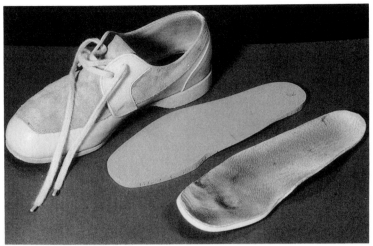

Figure 7.1 Extra-depth shoes

Drewshoes were introduced in 1979 and are made of the moulded thermoplastic material, plastazote. They are suitable for very awkwardly shaped, swollen or ulcerated feet because the plastazote can be spot heated or cut away to make it fit.

For the flat foot valgus supports are needed inside the shoe together with an inside wedge to the heel and sole (the latter can simply be a short inside wedge of the metatarsal bar type). In severe cases prolonged heels or fully elongated heels are necessary to fill in the waist of the shoe for improved medial support.

For hallux rigidus the sole should be as stiff as possible. This may be further reinforced with a steel plate or with an Ortholen support, plus a varus wedge on the outer side of the sole (as patients tend to walk off the area of pain) in conjunction with a rocker bar. The rocker bar should be about 5 cm wide. The object is to produce a rocking motion and reduce the need for dorsiflexion at the metatarsophalangeal joint of the great toe.

Total contact insoles are useful for the management of metatarsalgia due to prolapsed metatarsal heads. The insole is made from a weightbearing cast of the sole of the foot and those areas which bear the highest vertical loads, i.e. the prominent metatarsal heads, are accommodated in depressions in the surface of the insole. Thus, the load is shared with the surrounding normal plantar skin. The insoles are made of a composite of a high density plastazote base which is firm and hard and acts as a cradle,

plus a soft poron surface to cushion the painful areas.

When special shoes are prescribed it is hoped that patients will wear them for all or most of their waking hours. There is a case to be argued for indoor and outdoor shoes to be made available on prescription so that they can be worn alternately.

The foot in diabetes mellitus

The prevalence of known diabetes in the United Kingdom is approximately 1% of the population (Neil, Gatling and Mather, 1986). Diabetics are known to occupy more hospital bed-days per person than non-diabetics (Williams, 1985) and foot problems contribute significantly to these numbers and substantially to the cost. Connor (1986) found that 12% of the admissions to a diabetic unit were for foot problems and these patients accounted for 47% of the total bed-days.

Foot problems occur because of the diabetic complications of neuropathy and peripheral vascular disease. Neuropathy in diabetes may be classified into several different types but essentially it is a symmetrical distal polyneuropathy encompassing motor, sensory and autonomic modalities. Motor involvement leads to a weakness of the intrinsic muscles which is associated with an imbalance between the long flexors, extensors and peronei – leading to a cavus foot and claw toes. Autonomic neuropathy has two effects; first, it reduces sweating leading to dry plantar skin which easily cracks and, second, it alters the normal autoregulation of the microcirculation, leading to capillary basement membrane thickening and arteriovenous shunting. The overall bloodflow through the foot is increased resulting in a warm, dry foot with bounding pulses and distended veins. Sensory neuropathy may be painful or painless depending on which nerve fibres are predominantly affected. Those with painful neuropathy do not seem to develop foot ulcers. Painless neuropathy results in a peripheral sensory loss in a 'stocking' distribution with impairment of pinprick, light touch and vibration senses. The patient may thus injure the foot without being aware of it.

Atherosclerosis appears in the diabetic at a younger age, progresses more quickly and shows less male bias than in non-diabetics. In the lower limb the vessels particularly involved are the distal superficial femoral, tibial and peroneal arteries. This involvement is usually diffuse rather than within a single vessel. It has long been assumed that a microangiopathy similar to that found in diabetic retinopathy existed. This has been challenged by Logerfo and Coffman (1984) who found as many small vessels, i.e. as small as 10 µm, in diabetics as in non-diabetics. They did, however, confirm the presence of capillary basement membrane thickening.

Whether ulceration occurs in a neuropathic or ischaemic foot the fundamental cause is mechanical stress. In the ischaemic foot low pressures maintained for a period of time may lead to necrosis. This can occur with ill-fitting shoes. Common sites affected are the bunion area and the corresponding site over the lateral aspect of the fifth metatarsal head. In the neuropathic foot the patient may precipitate ulceration either by direct high pressure injury (as for example by walking on a drawing pin and being unaware of it) or more gradually through what has been described by Brand (1988) as 'repetitive moderate stress'.

Callosities build up in those areas of the foot subjected to increased pressures, in particular under the metatarsal heads and heel. The subcutaneous tissue is now trapped between bone and thick, unpliable skin and subjected to high shearing forces on walking. These forces eventually lead to tissue breakdown.

In the assessment of a diabetic ulcer it is essential to know whether it is due to ischaemia or neuropathy, or a combination of both. The

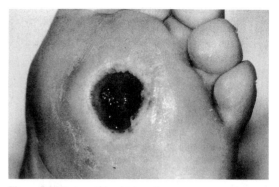

Figure 7.2 Neuropathic plantar ulcer

neuropathic ulcer commonly occurs under a metatarsal head, is surrounded by thick hyperkeratosis, has a pink punched-out base and is painless (Figure 7.2). The foot is warm with dilated veins and palpable pulses. In contrast, the ischaemic ulcer is cool and pulses are absent. The ulcer is not surrounded by hyperkeratosis and is usually painful to touch.

Once the decision has been made on the aetiology of the ulcer it is then necessary to determine whether any active infection is present as this will require antibiotic therapy. Assessment of the vascular status of the foot is performed with a Doppler probe and the opinion of an experienced vascular surgeon is sought on those patients with clear evidence of ischaemia.

Neuropathic ulcers which result from mechanic forces can be healed by removing or reducing these forces. The simplest, but not necessarily the best, method is by strict bed-rest or non-weight-bearing on crutches. However, this is time consuming and tedious for the patient. The use of the total contact cast for the management of neuropathic ulcers is effective and prevents unnecessary admission to hospital. Essentially this is a below-knee walking cast applied with minimal padding over the bony prominences and with a rocker on the sole (Figure 7.3). It needs to be carefully applied and any competent plaster technician can learn the technique in a short time. The great advantage is that the patient is treated as an outpatient and remains ambulant. Before the cast is applied the ulcer is debrided and this can readily be done in the insensitive foot. Casts are changed after the first week and thereafter at 3-week intervals. A 25-

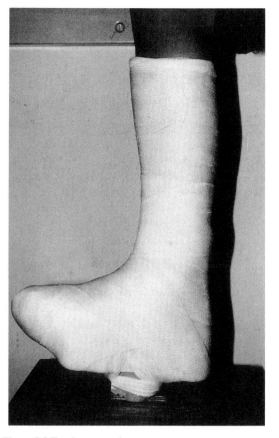

Figure 7.3 Total contact plaster cast

mm diameter ulcer should be healed in about 6 weeks with this technique.

The patient with a healed ulcer, either recent or remote, is at risk of further ulceration unless the foot is protected from excessive forces. It is therefore essential that at the end of a period in a total contact cast the patient is fitted with surgical shoes and appropriate total contact insoles. A 30-degree rocker is added to the sole of the shoe to reduce forefoot loading.

Surgery for the neuropathic foot is required to drain abscesses and to remove sequestra or gangrenous digits. Bony excrescences may sometimes need to be trimmed, as for example on the sole of a patient with a Charcot foot and a rocker-bottom deformity. Where there is extensive infection local amputations of digits or a Syme's procedure can be attempted rather than the mandatory below-knee amputation where vascular disease predominates.

The rheumatoid foot

Because of the nature of the disease many patients carry the sequelae of rheumatoid arthritis into old age. The foot is affected in 89% of long-standing cases (Vainio, 1956) and the commonest site is the forefoot. The least common joint to be affected is the ankle. Hindfoot involvement occurs in about one-third of patients and is rare without the forefoot being affected as well (Vidigal *et al.*, 1975).

The great toe is commonly valgus, rigid or a combination of both. The lesser toes are clawed and frequently dorsally dislocated with large callosities under the adjacent metatarsal heads. Occasionally there is a prominent bunionette or bony prominence on the lateral aspect of the fifth metatarsal head. The patient complains of 'walking on stones' or 'pebbles' because the fat pad normally present beneath the metatarsal heads is drawn up anteriorly to the metatarsal heads.

Subtalar joint involvement is often associated with hindfoot valgus. Ankle joint damage may result in an equinus deformity.

Treatment

As already mentioned surgery is best avoided if possible and many problems can be managed by extra-depth shoes and custom-made insoles of the total contact pattern. Valgus hindfoot deformities may need the support of an outside-iron and inside T-strap and occasionally a double below-knee iron with round ankle sockets might be necessary to control an ankle joint.

Where conservative management has failed and the blood supply to the foot is healthy a forefoot arthroplasty may solve the problem of intractable metatarsalgia. Many different techniques have been described (Newman and Fitton, 1983) but the author favours a modification of the original method described by Hoffmann (1912) who advocated excision of all metatarsal heads via plantar incisions. It is easier to perform this operation through three dorsal incisions, one medial, one between the second and third metatarsal shafts and one between the fourth and fifth metatarsal shafts. It is essential to retain the relative proportions of the length of the metatarsals.

For the hindfoot a triple arthrodesis is effective in the control and correction of hindfoot valgus. In cases of gross valgus deformity extensive mobilization of the calcaneum on the talus will be required in order to reduce the deformity. Alternatively, if this is difficult to achieve bone grafts from the iliac crest may be necessary to hold the calcaneum in a corrected position at the subtalar joint. Ankle deformity and pain are well controlled by arthrodesis and ankle arthroplasty has not been proved to be a better solution so far. Occasionally a combination of ankle and subtalar pathology will require a pantalar fusion.

Hallux valgus, hallux rigidus and hammer toes

Deformities of the great toe are common and may occur in combination with deformities of the lesser toes. Hallux rigidus is always associated with a dorsal exostosis and with hallux valgus it is medially situated. A bunion may be present and can occasionally, if infected, produce local ulceration. Hammer toes (i.e. toes with a fixed flexion deformity at the proximal interphalangeal joint, a straight distal interphalangeal joint and associated corn on the dorsal aspect of the proximal joint) often involve the second toe, but other toes may also be similarly deformed. Because of the piston effect of shoe pressure on the flexed proximal joint the metatarsal head is prolapsed plantarwards and symptoms of metatarsalgia may result.

If possible extra-depth shoes should be used with appropriate insoles to relieve pressure beneath the metatarsal heads. If this fails and the patient will accept operative treatment a number of options are available if the vascular supply to the foot is adequate. For gross hallux valgus the only effective remedy to restore the position of the great toe and reduce the large medial prominence is an arthrodesis of the metatarsophalangeal joint with the toe fixed at an angle of about 10 degrees to the planter surface of the foot. The patient, especially if female, must be warned that she will be permanently restricted to wearing shoes with low heels. For lesser degrees of hallux valgus or hallux rigidus there is a place for Keller's operation, which both weakens and shortens the great toe. It provides good symptomatic relief and since the patient has probably had very poor function from the deformed great toe for many years the functional loss is minimal.

There is little role, if any, for metatarsal osteotomy (Wilson, 1988) in the management of hallux valgus in elderly patients since their joints tend to be slightly degenerate and the foot somewhat stiff.

Hammer toes are best treated by interphalangeal fusion using a Kirshner wire for internal fixation (Newman and Fitton, 1979). At the time of operation the dorsal corn may be excised. A tenotomy of the long extensor and a radical capsulotomy of the metatarsophalangeal joint is performed to avoid the problem of a straight toe pointing upwards. For a hammer deformity of the little toe excision of the proximal phalanx provides a satisfactory solution.

Metatarsalgia

This is not a diagnosis but a symptom to describe pain in the forefoot. It is not surprising that it occurs frequently as the forefoot is loaded for 75% of the stance phase of gait. It is essential to identify the specific cause if possible. It may result from prolapse of a metatarsal head in association with a hammer toe, from rheumatoid arthritis, or as result of a bony irregularity on the under-surface of a metatarsal head. Morton's metatarsalgia which is the result of an entrapment syndrome of the intermetatarsal nerve between either the contiguous surfaces of the second and third, or third and fourth toes is not uncommon in this age group (Guiloff, Scadding and Klenerman 1984). The cleft between the third and fourth toes is most commonly affected and pain, often of a burning nature, is experienced at the tip of the digit. It is aggravated by walking, relieved by removal of the shoe and often there is no pain on walking barefoot. The diagnosis is made on the history and by accurate localization of the pain to the plantar surface of the intemetatarsal space where the nerve is trapped against the intermetatarsal ligament. Occasionally a painful click can be produced by compression of the forefoot ('Mulder's click' – Mulder, 1951) which reproduces the patient's symptoms. The most effective remedy is excision of the affected intermetatarsal nerve through a plantar incision.

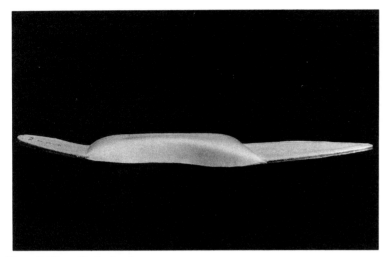

Figure 7.4 Rose–Taylor insole

The painful heel syndrome (policeman's heel, postman's heel)

This is a common condition. The patient complains of pain in the heel which is usually localized to the inner side at a site approximately level with the medial tubercle of the calcaneum. The symptoms are described as worst first thing in the morning on putting the affected foot on the floor. The pain then wears off with increased activity. The patient is usually overweight and often spends a considerable time standing during the course of the day. Physical examination rarely provides very much additional information and radiographs may show a spur in the line of the long plantar ligament. The significance of spurs is unclear. They are common in the general population, increase in frequency with age and have no direct relation to heel pain (Bassiouni, 1965). The pathology is likely to be due to ligamentous traction, and in a series of 45 patients 60% showed an increased bone blood flow in the calcaneum (Williams *et al.*, 1987).

The treatment should always be conservative. The most effective remedy is a steroid injection directly into the most painful part of the heel. Repeat injections may be necessary on one or two occasions. An insole (Rose–Taylor insole as advocated by Rose, 1955) which tilts the heel into varus and relaxes the plantar fascia is also useful (Figure 7.4). The combination of these two treatments and the passage of time will usually result in relief of symptoms.

Ingrown toenails and onychogryphosis

Both these problems affect the great toenail. In the presence of diabetes or ischaemia the infection associated with the ingrown toenail must be regarded as serious. The medial border of the toenail is most commonly affected. The treatment of choice is a wedge resection of a 5-mm segment of nail and the application of phenol BP to the adjacent nail matrix. This method has a 97% success rate (Tait and Tuck, 1987).

The grossly thickened, curved and overgrown nail of onychogryphosis is a result of inadequate nail care. Removal of the nail and application of phenol BP to the entire nail matrix should prevent recurrence. Both these procedures are within the scope of a competent chiropodist and can be performed under local anaesthesia.

References

Barlow, A.M., Braid, S.J. and Jayson, M.I.V. (1990) Foot problems in the elderly. *Clin. Rehab.*, **4**, 217–222

Bassiouni, M. (1965). Incidence of calcaneal spurs in osteoarthritis and rheumatoid arthritis. *Am. Rheum. Dis.*, **24**, 490

Brand, P.W. (1988) Repetitive stress in the development of the diabetic foot. In *The Diabetic Foot* (eds M.E. Levin and L.W. O'Neil), CV Mosby, St Louis, pp. 83–90

Cartwright, A. and Henderson, G. (1986) *More trouble with feet: a survey of the foot problems and chiropody needs of the elderly*, HMSO, London

Connor, H. (1986) The economic impact of diabetic foot disease. In *The Foot in Diabetes* (eds H. Connor, A.J.M. Boulton and J.D. Ward), John Wiley, Chichester, pp. 145–149

Guiloff, R.J., Scadding, J.W. and Klenerman, L. (1984) Morton's metatarsalgia: clinical, electrical and histological investigations. *J. Bone Joint Surg.*, **66B**, 586–591

Hoffmann, P. (1912) An operation for severe grades of contracted or clawed toes. *Am. J. Orthop. Surg.*, **9**, 441

Logerfo, F.W. and Coffman, J.D. (1984) Vascular and microvascular disease of the foot in diabetes. *N. Engl. J. Med.*, **311**, 1615–1619

Mulder, J.D. (1951) The causative mechanism of Morton's metatarsalgia. *J. Bone Joint Surg.*, **33B**, 94–95

Neil, H.A.W., Gatling, G. and Mather, H.M. (1986) A reassessment of the prevalence of known diabetes in England and Wales. *Diab. Med.*, **3**, 360A

Newman, R.J. and Fitton, J.M. (1979) An evaluation of operative procedures in the treatment of hammer toe. *Acta Orthop. Scand.*, **50**, 709–712

Newman, R.J. and Fitton, J.M. (1983) Conservation of metatarsal heads in surgery of rheumatoid arthritis of the forefoot. *Acta Orthop. Scand.*, **54**, 417–421

Rose, G.K. (1955) The painful heel. *Br. Med. J.*, **ii**, 831

Tait, G.R. and Tuck, J.S. (1987) Surgical or phenol ablation of the nail bed for ingrowing toenails: a randomised controlled trial. *J. Roy. Coll. Surg. Edin.*, **32**, 358–360

Vainio, K. (1956) The rheumatoid foot: a clinical study with pathological and roentgenological comments. *Am. Chir. Gynaec.*, **45**, Suppl. 1

Vidigal, E., Jacoby, R.K., Dixon, A. St J., Ratcliff, A.H. and Kirkup, J. (1975) The foot in rheumatic disease. *Ann. Rheum. Dis.*, **34**, 292–297

Williams, D.R.R. (1985) Hospital admissions of diabetic patients: information from hospital activity analysis. *Diabet. Med.*, **2**, 27–32

Williams, P.L., Smibert, J.G., Cox, R., Mitchell, R. and Klenerman, L. (1987) Imaging study of the painful heel syndrome. *Foot Ankle*, **7**, 345–349

Wilson, D.W. (1988) Hallux valgus and rigidus. In *The Foot* (eds B. Helal and D. W. Wilson), Churchill Livingstone, London, Chap. 21, pp. 411–483

8

The ageing spine

Robert A. Dickson and Peter A. Millner

Introduction

Many of the conditions which afflict the ageing spine are not pathognomonic of longevity but are simply states encountered with increased frequency with advancing years and those mechanical derangements of the spinal column secondary to degenerative processes of bone, joint and soft tissues typify this. Metabolic disorders such as osteomalacia and osteoporosis, inflammatory arthropathies, infection and neoplastic involvement are again not unique to the elderly patient but are more commonly associated with old age. The range of disease processes affecting the geriatric spine reflects the more generalized senescence of the body as a whole, from a cellular level upwards and expressed as macroscopic disease entities in clinical practice.

In terms of applying scientific knowledge of the pathophysiology of such conditions to therapeutics, our options are often limited by socio-economical considerations as well as the effects of ageing on other vital body systems. The principle of holistic medicine is applicable in orthogeriatric spinal practice as it is anywhere else in the body and this has an important bearing on our attitude to the elderly 'back patient'. Whilst an aggressive, investigational and interventional approach may be indicated in the younger patient with motion segment instability it is often inappropriate to the geriatric patient who may neither physically tolerate nor rehabilitate from complex spinal surgery. This has to be balanced with the very real benefits to be gained in, for example, combined two-stage anterior and posterior decompression with instrumented stabilization for impending paraplegia and pain in a case of metastatic spinal disease. The 'risks and rewards' equation is a common problem to be solved in clinical practice and never more so than in spinal surgery of the aged patient.

Lumbar disc degeneration

From maturity through to old age intervertebral discs and cartilaginous end-plates undergo a natural and constitutional process of biochemical degeneration with loss of nuclear protein and water and collagen fibrillation (Markolf and Morris, 1974; Roberts, Menage and Urban, 1989; Naylor, 1990). *Pari-passu* biomechanical changes also occur with loss of disc elasticity and height, annular tears and bulging, end-plate sclerosis, facet joint osteoarthrosis with irregularity, loss of joint cartilage and thickening of joint capsules (Frymoyer and Stokes, 1990; Goel and Weinstein, 1990). The degenerative process leads to subluxation of the posterior facet joints with the superior facets of the inferior vertebra progressively approximating the local exiting nerve root. Loss of vertical height of the functional spinal unit leads to progressive ligamentous redundancy and local instability with traction spurs forming 1 mm or so above and below the end-plates together with translation forwards (degenerative spondylolisthesis) or backwards (retrolisthesis) (Farfan, 1980).

Unlike the spondylolisthesis of youth associated with a pars interarticularis defect (spondylolysis), degenerative translation does not dissociate the front and back of the spine and thus only a few millimetres of slip may give rise to serious neurological consequences (Figure 8.1). Nonetheless, the spine is a capricious structure and some of the worst looking spines radiologically can perplexingly be symptom-free and *vice versa*. Moreover, these degenerative processes occur over many years and thus the fourth dimension, time, has a crucial effect; the clinical sequelae of such processes reflect this rate-dependency. A complete block at one disc level on a myelogram may have no clinical consequences whatever in the patient with degenerative spinal stenosis while a fraction of that degree of neural compression occurring acutely due to a prolapsed intervertebral disc may rapidly result in irreversible neurological loss. Moreover, a degree of pathology producing significant problems in one patient leaves many others unharmed and this varying clinical response makes objectivity difficult to achieve. The process of degeneration itself is almost certainly asymptomatic in that epidemiological surveys have clearly demonstrated its presence radiologically more frequently in older individuals regardless of symptoms (Jeffrey and Ball, 1963; Lawrence, 1987). The two processes which appear to be important with regard to symptoms are motion segment instability and neurological compromise.

Motion segment instability

Intervertebral disc degeneration leads to disc space narrowing and abnormal mobility of the segment and this may or may not be symptomatic. There may be irritable low back pain provoked by the stresses of bending, twisting, lifting or extending the back. There may also be referred pain to the buttocks and proximal thighs (not beyond the knees) but no radicular pain or neurological features in the lower limbs (Frymoyer and Stokes, 1990).

Radiologically, disc space narrowing is easily visible together with traction spurs and tends to be more obvious in the lower lumbar spine. Rotational deformities or degenerative retrolisthesis or spondylolisthesis may also be evident. Facet joint osteoarthrosis develops within a few years of the onset of segmental degeneration. Pain on provocative discography and its relief with local anaesthetic indicates a symptomatic segment derangement.

Frank clinical instability is associated with lumbar spine dysrhythmia, the normal smooth arc of flexion and extension being interrupted by

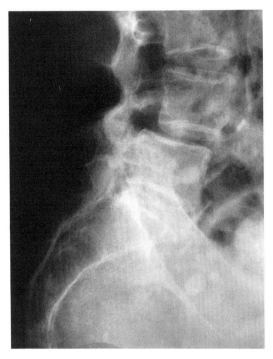

Figure 8.1 Anterior translation of L4 on L5 in degenerative spondylolisthesis

'catching' or 'giving way', particularly on resuming the erect position. There is little to find on physical examination and if straight leg raising is reduced it is because of back and not leg pain. Signs of translational, angular and rotational instability may be seen on both erect and bending X-ray films. If the traction spurs seen 2 or 3 mm above and below the end-plate are unduly large it suggests that the segment has regained stability and is now asymptomatic, while traction spurs seen on both AP and lateral films indicate circumferential spurring and rotational instability. Bending films require to show an approximately 10° change in angulation or 5 mm in translation before instability should be regarded as significant (Figure 8.2). Additional pain on prolonged sitting when the lumbar lordosis is obliterated suggests symptomatic facet joint degeneration.

Much can be achieved non-operatively in patients with clinical instability or facet joint involvement. Lumbosacral orthoses (corsets), facet joint and epidural injections, facet rhizotomy and back school programmes will produce symptomatic relief in the majority especially when combined with anti-inflammatory medication. The mood of the elderly can be appreciably

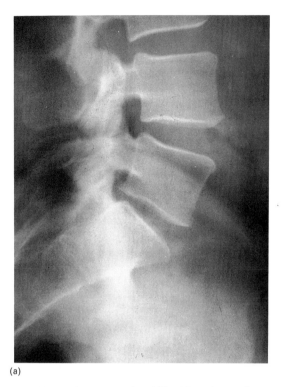

(a)

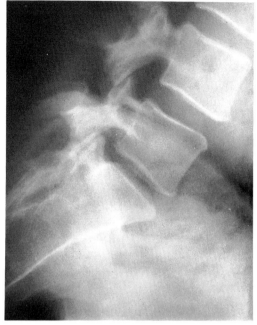

(b)

Figure 8.2 Motion segment instability. Note the retrolisthesis (backwards translation and angulation) of L5 on S1 on backwards bending (a) compared with forwards bending (b) indicating significant instability

affected by prolonged lumbar disability and anti-depressant preparations can be very beneficial. Spinal fusion may be necessary in a minority although it is often difficult to localize accurately the site of symptoms. These patients should therefore 'earn' their operation but if the offending motion segment can be identified in the patient with intractable painful instability by provocative discography or facet joint injection, then localized spinal fusion performed posterolaterally at the intertransverse level should produce a sound bony fusion in 80–90% of cases (Frymoyer and Stokes, 1990). However, for reasons that are not abundantly clear, a substantially smaller percentage will actually achieve symptomatic relief. Multiple level fusion should be avoided and therefore normality in adjacent segments should be demonstrated preoperatively. The addition of metalwork to a one-level fusion is probably unnecessary although increasingly fashionable. The advantage of earlier and more aggressive mobilization of the elderly patient which instrumentation allows has to be balanced against the increased operative time and the presence of a foreign body implant – a good example of the 'risks and rewards' dilemma.

Neurological compromise

The degenerative process can compress the cauda equina, the emerging nerve roots or both. Root entrapment is typically the result of gross narrowing of the disc space and consequent subluxation of the facet joint with the superior articular process of the vertebra below moving upwards and forwards, so narrowing the lateral part of the root canal and foramen. This foraminal encroachment is compounded by osteophyte formation of the facet joint itself and posterolateral vertebral body. Oblique films and CT scanning demonstrate this process particularly well (Figure 8.3). Symptomatically, in addition to back pain there are radicular symptoms down the leg in the form of dysaesthesiae and a claudication-type of pain not relieved by standing still for a few minutes. These patients are not

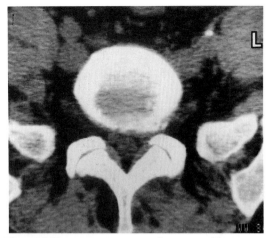

Figure 8.3 Nerve root entrapment demonstrated by transverse section computed tomography. The lateral part of the left root canal is narrowed by osteophytes on the posterolateral vertebral body and facet joint, compressing the emerging nerve root

helped by fusion and require root decompression to achieve symptomatic relief.

Degenerative spondylolisthesis can produce both root and central canal compression. It is typically a condition of ageing females with primary generalized osteoarthrosis and osteoporosis. The L4/5 level is most commonly affected and there is a lower than normal intercristal line, often with sacralization of the L5 vertebra; the L4/5 level thus becomes the first mobile motion segment. Although the lateral X-ray films appear to show anterior translation, the deformity is chiefly rotational with degenerative change in the disc permitting abnormal rotational stresses with distraction of one facet joint and subluxation of the other. Compression fractures may produce laminar shortening and facet subluxation may lead to the inferior articular processes contacting the laminae below.

With degenerative spondylolisthesis there is low back pain with either symptoms of central canal stenosis or root pain which may be bilateral, although usually on the side of the more stenosed lateral recess. Both central and root canals require decompression with partial facetectomy. Fusion is generally added but is probably unnecessary in the elderly with end-stage degeneration which reconfers stability.

To most medical personnel the term lumbar spinal stenosis tends to focus attention on the central canal although concomitant root canal narrowing is also important (Verbiest, 1954;

Kirkaldy-Willis, 1976). Interestingly, although the development of a trefoil-shaped canal is most obvious in the lower lumbar region spinal stenosis is most evident at the L4/5 level followed by the L3/4 level. Although patients typically present with evidence of severe degenerative changes at these motion segments, the majority probably start with a canal that was constitutionally too narrow, i.e. developmental stenosis. There is a reduced anteroposterior diameter with hypertrophic, medially placed facet joints and short thick laminae with overlapping inferior facets. The lateral recesses are proportionately narrowed and there is little if any epidural fat. Facet capsular thickening, disc herniation and end-plate hypertrophy further compromise nerve tissue and its vascularity. Myelography, computed tomography scanning and magnetic resonance imaging are all important in defining more precisely the relevant stenotic levels.

Elderly males are particularly affected and symptoms are more important than signs in making the diagnosis. There is generally a combination of both backache and leg symptoms, the latter being of tiredness, cramps, aching, paraesthesiae and dysaesthesiae, not of a radicular type. The stenotic lumbar spine does not tolerate lordosis which induces further stenosis from posterior facet joint capsular bulging, laminar shingling and ligamentum flavum infolding. Accordingly, walking in the erect position readily produces symptoms which are in turn not relieved by merely stopping walking. Affected patients require to lean forward or sit in order to reduce the lumbar lordosis and thus gain symptomatic relief. Walking up hill or upstairs is easier than walking downwards while cycling may be unaffected. Symptoms can, however, be much less specific in the form of difficulty with balance and increasing dependency on a walking stick.

The nerve supply to the lower urinary system is frequently involved and while incontinence is the most dramatic feature, urgency, frequency and recurrent infection all indicate incomplete bladder emptying. Such features are often wrongly diagnosed as being prostatic or gynaecological in origin. The condition is differentiated from vascular claudication by having a less regular temporal relationship with exercise, a lack of relief by simply standing still for a few minutes and by the presence of normal peripheral pulses. There is often little to find on physical examination with good spinal movements, normal straight leg raising and a normal neurological examination of the limbs though reflex changes may be identified by examination after exercise.

Conservative treatment is generally much less beneficial than with instability problems but facet joint and epidural injections may be useful in those patients deemed unfit to undergo the necessary decompressive surgery. This is better performed earlier rather than later by which time irreversible nerve root changes may have occurred. It is important to decompress both central and lateral canals and undercutting facetectomies should obviate postoperative instability. It should therefore be unnecessary to have to proceed to a localized spinal fusion and in any event the elderly, very degenerate, stenotic segment is not unduly unstable. As with most types of back surgery, it is the peripheral expression of the problem in the lower extremities that best responds to surgical decompression rather than the backache itself, some 60–70% of patients benefiting from operative treatment (Dickson, 1987).

Evidence of Paget's disease is occasionally identified on plain X-ray films of patients with spinal stenosis and the condition may have both mechanical and vascular effects. Paget's disease is a cause of vertebra magna with increasing size of all components of the vertebra thus narrowing both central and lateral canals. There may also be a mechanical component from spondylotic changes. In addition, a local diminution of blood supply to the spinal cord or cauda equina may occur due to diversion by the hypervascular Pagetic tissue (steal syndrome). Should imaging fail to reveal impressive mechanical stenosis a trial of calcitonin or diphosphonates may obviate the need for surgery (Douglas *et al.*, 1981; Smith and Houghton, 1990).

Cervical disc degeneration

The same constitutional processes of degeneration that occur in the lumbar spine also occur in the cervical spine with the additional problem of hypertrophy of the joints of Luschka causing anterolateral foraminal stenosis. Again, it is degenerative new bone formation in association with hypertrophy of joint capsules and ligamentum flavum which narrows the available space for nerve tissue. There is usually a long history

of increasing symptoms often with more acute exacerbations induced by incidents such as mild head injury or neck sprains. The clinical picture is very variable and may involve nerve roots on one or both sides, the spinal cord, or both (Cameron, 1990). There is typically brachial neuralgia with root compression in association with lower motor neuron signs in the upper extremities. Concomitant myelopathy produces increasing difficulty in walking and upper motor neuron signs in the lower extremities. There may also be urinary frequency and intermittent retention while encroachment into the foramina transversaria produces symptoms of vertebrobasilar insufficiency including dizziness, vertigo and intermittent loss of consciousness. The presence of lower motor neuron signs in the lower extremities suggests co-existent lumbar canal stenosis and this area should always be investigated carefully in addition to the cervical region.

Plain X-ray films indicate the likely involved segments with disc space narrowing and marginal syndesmophytes while osteophytes of the joints of Luschka narrow the forminae. Cervical myelography confirms the diagnosis and indicates more precisely the sites of nerve compression that require to be addressed surgically (Figure 8.4). Root or foraminal compression should be dealt with by anterior Cloward-type excision of disc and all compressing bone with concomitant fusion (Cloward, 1962). Myelopathy is treated by posterior decompressive laminectomy stopping short of the joints of Luschka in order not to endanger the integrity of the vertebral arteries. Intervertebral fusion is usually unnecessary.

Despite meticulous intraoperative care and the use of the microscope the results of this surgery are often good only in the short to medium term. Established myelopathy is recalcitrant to what appears to be satisfactory decompression. Temporary urinary retention is common but intraoperative nerve damage should occur in substantially less than 1% of cases (Cameron, 1990).

Rheumatoid arthritis

In addition to intervertebral synovial joint involvement by rheumatoid synovitis the bursae are susceptible, particularly those surrounding the odontoid process of the axis within the dens ligament. The cervical spine bears the brunt of

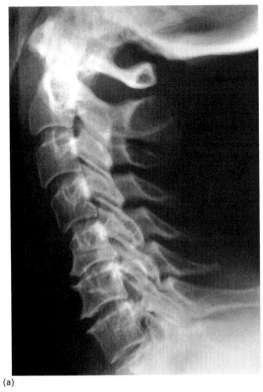

(a)

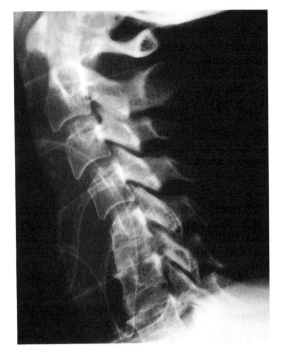

(c)

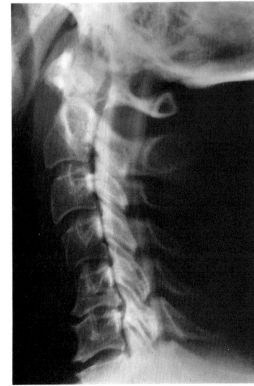

(b)

Figure 8.4 Cervical disc degeneration. A plain lateral radiograph (a) reveals degenerative changes at C5–C6 and C6–C7. Anterior thecal indentation by osteophytes is shown on the lateral cervical myelogram (b). Postoperatively, a plain lateral radiograph (c) clearly shows the anterior inter-body fusion at two levels after excision of compressing disc material and bone

the rheumatoid disease and is involved in a third of cases within 2 years of onset (Winfield *et al.*, 1981). Thoracolumbar spine involvement is more difficult to diagnose in the elderly where degenerative conditions prevail, but is probably more common than is thought.

In the cervical spine, bone and soft tissue erosion from synovial proliferation produce four clinicopathological conditions (Lipson, 1984; Bossingham and Dickson, 1990) each with the potential for producing cervical cord and root compression. Atlantoaxial impaction (AAI) with upward migration of the odontoid peg towards or through the foramen magnum occurs in up to 30% of rheumatoid patients. Atlantoaxial subluxation (AAS) with forward displacement of C1 on C2 is even more prevalent, occurring in up to 71% of patients and 46% of rheumatoid patients at post mortem. Both AAI and AAS are more likely to occur in patients receiving steroid therapy and with long-standing disease (Lipson, 1984; Pellici *et al.*, 1981). Subaxial subluxation (SAS) is present in up to 20% of patients, often at more than one level. The co-existence of all three types of instability is not an infrequent finding and all may play a part in producing the clinical picture of neurological deficit and pain. Extradural rheumatoid granulation tissue can further compromise the cervical cord, particularly if combined with often apparently minor SAS, tipping the neurological balance unfavourably (Kudo, Iwano and Yoshizawa, 1984).

Erosive discitis, paravertebral joint erosions, motion segment instability, vertebral collapse and lumbar root compression are among the range of pathologies seen in the rheumatoid lumbar spine and with an incidence greater than in non-rheumatoid patients (Bywaters, 1974; Heywood and Meyers, 1986). As in the cervical spine, subluxation can result and may proceed to a true spondylolisthesis with neurological deficit. Similarly, a minor degree of subluxation can result in severe or even complete cord compression in the presence of extradural granulation tissue (Bossingham and Dickson, 1990).

Pain, stiffness and neurological deficit are the major presenting features of spine involvement, although radiographic disease may be present without symptoms in as many as 50% of patients (Pellici *et al.*, 1981). The concomitant involvement of the extremities with muscle atrophy, peripheral neuropathies and joint deformities may make accurate assessment well nigh impossible. Furthermore, the insidious, progressive nature of the systemic disease often masks the development of neurological dysfunction and this problem is compounded in the elderly by the increased frequency of features unrelated to the disease such as urinary incontinence. Beware of the elderly rheumatoid patient who 'goes off his legs'.

A variety of neurological features are found depending on disease site, severity and progression rate. Vertebrobasilar disturbances, pyramidal tract involvement, sensory deficits, sphincter dysfunction and bulbar palsies may occur from cervical spine disease, giving rise to a plethora of clinical findings. As previously stated, such diverse combinations of symptomatology may not be readily attributable to rheumatoid cervical spine disease.

The clinical features of lumbar discitis with often confusing radiographic changes can

Table 8.1 Ranawat classification

Class 1: no neurological deficit

Class 2: subjective weakness with hyper-reflexia and dysaesthesia

Class 3: objective findings of weakness with long tract signs; subdivided into:
a: ambulatory
b: quadriparetic, non-ambulatory

suggest an infective discitis, subsequently disproved on biopsy. In cases of lumbar spine subluxation or florid spondylolisthesis, lower motor neuron signs may be produced although upper motor neuron signs occasionally result. Finally, mechanical low back pain secondary to motion segment instability and vertebral collapse pose as much of a problem as they do in the non-rheumatoid patient.

Despite the multitude of difficulties obstructing thorough and accurate neurological assessment, in order to judge response to treatment an attempt should be made to classify pain and neurological deficit. A variety of grading systems exist though the classification proposed by Ranawat (Table 8.1) is in common usage (Ranawat *et al.*, 1979).

Most would agree that neurological deficit is an indication for operative intervention although the presence of intractable pain from symptomatic instability may warrant surgical intervention (Zoma *et al.*, 1987). No investigation of a rheumatoid spine patient is complete without accurate radiographic localization of the pathology, though it should be recognized that radiographic changes may not correlate with the severity of the clinical picture (Rana *et al.*, 1973). Ideally, a triad of orthopaedic spinal specialist, neurologist and a radiologist experienced in musculoskeletal imaging should bring their combined expertise to bear on the patient. Plain radiographs, tomography and, latterly, computed tomography and magnetic resonance imaging are invaluable adjuncts to quantifying instability and therapeutic planning; each modality has its specific indication.

Conservative treatment using collars and splints has little effect in stabilizing the spine (Althoff and Goldie, 1980; Pellici *et al.*, 1981). The operative treatment of the rheumatoid spine is a subject of controversy with a variety of approaches and techniques proposed (Bossingham and Dickson, 1990). Forwards subluxation at the atlantoaxial joint (AAS) is by far the commonest problem encountered and is almost always reducible with a short period of halo-traction and extension of the cervical spine. This alone often produces a substantial improvement in neurological signs. The reduced position is maintained by posterior C1-C2 fusion with wire support. Irreducible AAS requires preliminary transoral excision of the odontoid but in practice this is an unusual circumstance. Although AAI is radiologically common it is seldom the cause of neurological problems unless the degree of impaction is extreme, in which case it should be treated as a space-occupying lesion of the posterior fossa and dealt with by neurosurgical means. Reducible SAS needs stabilization with a posterior fusion and wire fixation supplemented by a metal rectangle if multiple levels are involved. Irreducible SAS is best dealt with by anterior dural decompression followed by posterior instrumentation and fusion at a second stage. Extradural granulation tissue is excised from whichever approach – anterior or posterior – is appropriate.

Anterior cervical fusion has had a variable press, and may give disappointing results (Ranawat *et al.*, 1979). The results of posterior fusion for all types of subluxation are similarly diverse; Lipson (1984) quotes non-union rates of 20–33%, postoperative mortalities of 8–20% and neurological improvement in 42–92% of cases reported. Following a pragmatic treatment protocol as outlined above, the authors have personal experience of more than 40 cases of rheumatoid cervical spine disease. The results suggest that the figures quoted in the literature are unduly depressing; we have seen no cases of non-union or postoperative mortality and all patients improved by at least one grade in the Ranawat classification (Dickson and Dreghorn, 1989). A commonsense approach to management is the critical factor rather than a surgical *tour de force*.

Lumbar spine disease without neurological deficit is often amenable to a conservative approach. Discitis without abnormal neurology or subluxation often proceeds to spontaneous interbody fusion and can be treated symptomatically. Significant subluxations with neurological dysfunction require anterior decompression and iliac crest strut grafting supplemented by posterior instrumented stabilization. It goes without saying that the pathological level should be identified accurately by preliminary myelography, computed tomography or magnetic resonance imaging.

Osteoporosis

The term osteoporosis is applied to the process of ossified bone mass reduction without any change in its true chemical composition. It is due to either decreased bone formation, increased bone resorption or both. Bone mass reaches a maximum in early adult life and at this time males have more bone mass than females. Thereafter, bone is lost, often rapidly in the post-menopausal phase in females. The condition is generally multifactorial in its aetiology and a lower bone mass to start with combined with less efficient osteoblastic new bone formation in old age, together with relative immobility of the elderly, all contribute to clinical recognition (Smith and Houghton, 1990).

The clinical importance of osteoporosis is solely in its ability to produce structural skeletal failure and it tends to do so in wrists, femoral necks and vertebrae. Asymmetric vertebral biconcavity or anterior wedge compression produces foreshortening of stature and increase in kyphosis with episodes of local pain when acute vertebral failure occurs and this may be associated with minor physical or traumatic events. Radiographs may appear to show less dense vertebral bodies although at least half the normal bone mass needs to be lost before this visual impression is really valid (Waddell, 1982). It is then end-plate biconcavity and vertebral compression which enables the diagnosis to be made. Bone biochemistry (serum calcium, phosphorus and alkaline phosphatase) is not abnormal. While in the younger adult the differential diagnosis includes the secondary osteoporosis of thyrotoxicosis or Cushing's syndrome, in the elderly the differential diagnosis includes secondary malignancy and myeloma. In most patients the natural history favours gradual stabilization with subsequent loss of pain, albeit with the spine shorter and more kyphotic.

Conservative treatment is of very limited value and braces sufficiently strong to prevent the progression of kyphosis are extensive and not well tolerated. In the established case prevention of further bone loss by calcium, fluoride or hormone replacement is only marginal. Prevention of bone loss at an earlier stage appears to be a more promising therapeutic avenue. Exercise to promote a maximal bone mass, the cessation of smoking and hormone replacement therapy starting about the menopause are the most important considerations (Woolf and Dixon, 1988; Smith and Houghton, 1990).

The introduction of segmental spinal instrumentation more than a decade ago led to a rash of instrumentation of the osteoporotic elderly spine but the complication rate is relatively high due to the weakness of the bone. However, intractable pain can be particularly distressing and internal metallic splintage can be effective on rare occasions when all else fails.

Osteomalacia

Unlike osteoporosis in this condition there is normal or even increased bone mass and the problem is one of defective mineralization of the matrix such that biopsy reveals wide bands of unmineralized osteoid. The typical skeletal lesion is the Looser's zone, usually found in the pelvis, scapulae and ribs but also in the long bones, interestingly on the compression side, in contrast to the fissure fractures of Paget's disease which occur on the tension side. The spine is commonly affected with symmetrical biconcavity of many vertebrae and this vertebral collapse can be painful over and above the proximal muscle weakness and generalized bone pain and tenderness that typifies its clinical presentation.

Dietary vitamin D deficiency, malabsorption and renal disease (both tubular and glomerular) are the main causes and the condition is frequently seen in both the elderly and Asian immigrants (Smith and Houghton, 1990). Staying indoors shields them from sunlight and inhibits the natural synthesis of vitamin D in the skin. In the Asian immigrant a dietary intake of Asian bread (chapatis and the like) can compound the issue by favouring intestinal malabsorption via chelation of dietary calcium by the phytates found in certain types of Asian flour (Thomas and Gillham, 1985). Bone biochemistry reveals lower than normal values of both serum calcium and phosphorus with the alkaline phosphatase level being raised. This provokes secondary hyperparathyroidism which enhances osteoclastic resorption of bone. The condition is very probably much more common than is generally recognized.

Medical treatment is much more rewarding than with osteoporosis and vitamin D replacement is rapidly beneficial. For painful increasing thoracolumbar kyphosis spinal orthoses are frequently prescribed but are generally ineffective or ill-tolerated, but occasional patients can benefit from internal support using segmental instrumentation.

Spinal infection

Two-thirds of spinal infections are pyogenic and one-third tuberculous and, although there are certain clinical characteristics peculiar to each, the majority of cases present with an initial common pathway that is indistinguishable (Wedge and Kirkaldy-Willis, 1990). Metastatic spread from a septic focus results in spinal infection aided by Batson's plexus and the valveless venous network throughout the spine. Most infections settle primarily in the highly vascular end-plate region and cause destruction of local bone and disc by way of toxin-induced arterial spasm or pressure infarction, leading to septic necrosis and sequestration of both bone and disc. Thus, infection can be differentiated from tumour on plain radiographs by disc narrowing with involvement of the adjacent vertebrae, while tumour causes vertebral collapse with preservation of the discs on each side (Figure 8.5). In addition to a systemic upset and local pain, progressive paralysis can occur by way of angular kyphosis, pressure from necrotic disc or bone, local abscess formation or vascular compromise of the cord.

More than half of all cases of pyogenic infection are due to *Staphylococcus aureus* but many other organisms, including *Streptococcus, Pseudomonas, E. coli, Salmonella, Brucella* and *Meningococcus* can be the causative agent. There is a more rapid onset with pyogenic than with tuberculous infection and the lumbar spine is the most common site. A recent history of urinary tract infection or catheterization, debilitation from malignancy, alcoholism, diabetes mellitus and drug addiction or steroid medication are all predisposing factors. Spinal tenderness with back pain and pyrexia constitute the essential

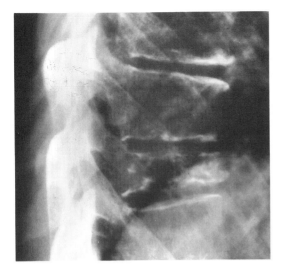

(a)

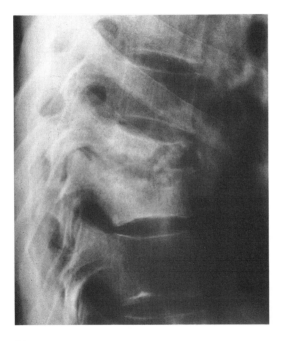

(b)

Figure 8.5 Infection or tumour? Vertebral body collapse with disc space preservation (a) is typical of malignant disease. Pyogenic and tuberculous infections initially invade the disc and end-plates leading to loss of disc space and contiguous vertebral body involvement (b). In either case, a paraspinal soft-tissue mass may be visible

clinical triad and laboratory investigations indicate a raised white cell count and a high plasma viscosity.

Tuberculous spinal infection has a more insidious onset, tends to affect the thoracolumbar junction, less significantly raises the white cell count and plasma viscosity and tends to present with more kyphosis and more evidence of neurological loss (Wedge and Kirkaldy-Willis, 1990). The Mantoux test is usually but not always positive. The situation is frequently confused by previous antibiotic therapy and percutaneous needle biopsy has a central role in providing material for both pathological and bacteriological analysis (Newman, Butt and Dickson, 1991). Should bacteriological assessment yield no growth a histological report of chronic inflammatory tissue with Langerhans' giant cells and caseation establishes the diagnosis of tubercle but does not of course indicate the particular type of organism or its sensitivity.

Treatment of spinal infection may be both medical and surgical. For pyogenic infection the appropriate antibiotic is prescribed for a minimum of 6 weeks. For tuberculous infection rifampicin and isoniazid are given in daily divided doses orally for a period of 9 months, with some specialists adding 3 months of streptomycin (Wedge and Kirkaldy-Willis, 1990).

The indications for surgery are not generally agreed and the Medical Research Council research groups still favour a non-surgical approach even for the tuberculous patient with abscess formation and complete paralysis (Eighth Report of the MRC Working Party on tuberculosis of the spine, 1982). They claim that the results of anti-tuberculous chemotherapy equal those following surgical treatment. Some spinal authorities disagree and state that significant abscess formation, progressive neurological loss and progressive spinal deformity with instability constitute indications for immediate surgery (Wedge and Kirkaldy-Willis, 1990). As with tumour the problem exists in front of the dura and laminectomy is not only futile but positively harmful. Effective surgical treatment should comprise anterior dural decompression with anterior strut grafting. Thereafter, additional posterior instrumented support is advisable (Figure 8.6). Unlike patients with terminal spinal malignant disease those with spinal infection can, by combined medical and surgical treatment, expect to be cured even when paralysis has been complete for some time.

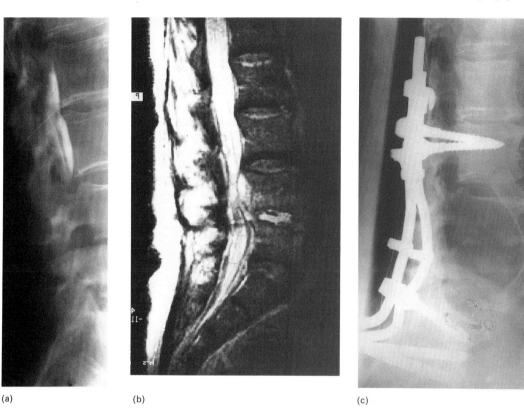

(a)   (b)   (c)

Figure 8.6 In (a), lumbar myelography shows a block to contrast flow at L4 in this patient who had a progressive neurological deficit and clinical features suggestive of infection at the L4/L5 level. Magnetic resonance imaging (b) confirmed anterior dural compression and involvement of L4, L5 and the intervening disc. The appearance after anterior decompression, strut grafting and posterior stabilization with Cotrel-Dubousset instrumentation is shown in the plain lateral radiograph (c)

Malignant disease of the spine

Primary tumours of the spine are rare while metastatic malignant disease has a marked propensity to involve the spine (Dreghorn *et al.*, 1990). The spine is third following the lungs and liver as the site of predilection for metastatic malignant deposits. Indeed, one in 20 patients with metastatic disease will develop some spinal cord compression. The thoracic region is the most common site followed by the lumbosacral and cervical regions. Breast, bronchus, prostate and renal primaries account for the great majority of deposits and while much is talked about thyroid tumours, vertebral secondaries are practically never encountered from this source. Whether multiple myeloma is primary or secondary is a matter of semantics but along with lymphoma, it is not that uncommon (Leatherman and Dickson, 1988). It is thought that Batson's plexus provides relatively free access from breast and prostate to the spine.

The important symptoms are local pain (especially nocturnal) and neurological embarrassment and the former can be intractable and disabling while the latter can progress to total neurological loss long before the underlying disease calls a merciful halt to the proceedings. In many patients the presence of vertebral secondaries is the first sign of malignancy and thus the spinal surgeon frequently makes the initial diagnosis. If no clues are provided by the history and physical examination (including rectal examination) then a full blood count and a chest radiograph should be performed. Moderate elevation of plasma viscosity is characteristic of disseminated cancer while the value is much higher in cases of multiple myeloma. Radioisotope scanning will indicate the extent of skeletal spread and also defines suitable sites for needle biopsy should the diagnosis have not yet been confirmed (Newman, Butt and Dickson, 1991). In patients with neurological compromise, particularly of breast origin, full length spinal myelography is essential before embarking upon surgical treatment as multiple sites of dural compression are commonly encountered despite the presenting problem being localized to one level.

Surgery is indicated for intractable pain, neurological loss or both and in almost all cases the problem exists in front of the dura as an anterior space occupying lesion or a local angular kyphosis causing neural tension. The literature is replete with the disappointing results of posterior decompressive laminectomy (Hall and Mackay, 1973) although every few years

another group attempts to justify it (Galasko, 1991). As with trauma and infection the latter approach is illogical – one cannot adequately decompress from the back something that is occurring at the front nor can one replace the anterior and middle columns from the back in any satisfactory way. Moreover, there is no muscle attached to the anterior spinal column from the first thoracic vertebra to the sacrum and an anterior approach (transthoracic, combined thoracic and lumbar or lumbar retroperitoneal) is straight forward. Myeloma and renal secondaries can be extremely vascular but in practical terms little is gained by preliminary angiography or embolization. The essence of treatment is thorough anterior dural decompression followed by anterior and middle column

(a)

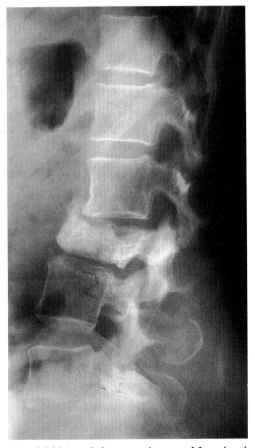

(b)

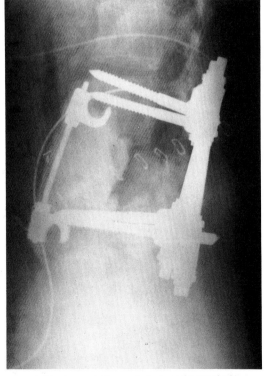

Figure 8.7 Metastatic breast carcinoma at L3 produced a painful kyphosis with neurological loss (a). Anterior decompression, methylmethacrylate cement support and segmental instrumentation anteriorly and posteriorly resulted in a complete resolution of both pain and neurological disturbance (b)

support which can be either by tricortical iliac crest bone graft if the defect is short and the pelvis amenable or methylmethacrylate cement (Harrington, 1981). Anterior segmental instrumentation provides more definitive stability and if necessary the back of the spine can be supported with metalwork too (Figure 8.7).

Relief of pain and neurological loss is the rule rather than the exception although the longer nerve tissue has been totally functionless the less good the result. There are very few areas of spinal surgery which are as rewarding as those which mitigate the distressing terminal state of painful paralysis.

Summary

The axial skeleton comprises a series of complex articulations but as with joints anywhere in the body ageing is coupled with degeneration and this process involves both bone and joint. Bone ages with a progressive loss of ossified matrix (osteoporosis), particularly in the post-menopausal female, while the ability to mineralize osteoid frequently becomes substandard (osteomalacia). The degenerative process is equally obvious in the interverebral areas (functional spinal units or motion segments) and both the anterior interbody syndesmoses as well as the posterior synovial articulations all degenerate with the passage of time producing spondylosis with increasing age. The spinal column can be regarded as a glorified cylinder conducting nervous tissue to relevant target areas while providing central mechanical support to the host. As the mechanically protective effect of disc or cartilage is progressively lost from the functional spinal unit the underlying more labile bone responds to increased stress by thickening and thus the central canal and its peripheral ramifications become progressively narrowed to produce a variety of neurological abnormalities (spinal stenosis). The relatively rich blood supply to the cancellous bodies and the valveless communications to adjacent vascular plexuses favours the local seeding of both infection and tumour. The ageing spine can therefore be disadvantaged by a number of different pathologies – some are best treated medically, some surgically and some by a combination of therapies. In all cases however the risks and rewards equation

must be carefully considered and the most appropriate treatment tailored for the elderly, and often frail, patient.

References

Althoff, B. and Goldie, I.F. (1980) Cervical collars in rheumatoid atlanto-axial subluxation; a radiographic comparison. *Ann. Rheum. Dis.*, **39**, 485–489

Bossingham, D.H. and Dickson, R.A. (1990) Inflammatory arthritis. In *Spinal Surgery; Science and Practice* (ed. R.A. Dickson), Butterworths, London, Chapter 14,

Bywaters, E.G.L. (1974) Rheumatoid arthritis in the thoracic region due to spread from costo-vertebral joints. *Ann. Rheum. Dis.*, **33**, 408–409

Cameron, M.M. (1990) Cervical disc and degenerative disease. In *Spinal Surgery: Science and Practice* (ed. R.A. Dickson), Butterworths, London, Chapter 12

Cloward, R. (1962) New methods of diagnosis and treatment of cervical disc disease. *Clin. Neurosurg.*, **8**, 93–102

Dickson, R.A. (1987) The surgical treatment of low back pain. *Curr. Orthop.*, **1**, 387–390

Dickson, R.A. and Dreghorn, C.R. (1989) The unstable rheumatoid neck: management protocol. Br. Orthop. Ass., Rhodes,

Douglas, D.L., Duckworth, T., Kanis, J.A., Jefferson, A.A., Martin, T.J. and Russell, R.G.G. (1981) Spinal cord dysfunction in Paget's disease of bone. *J. Bone Joint Surg.*, **63B**, 495–503

Dreghorn, C.R., Newman, R.J., Hardy, G.J. and Dickson, R.A. (1990) Primary tumours of the axial skeleton. Experience of the Leeds Regional Bone Tumour Registry. *Spine*, **15**, 137–139

Eighth report of the Medical Research Council Working Party on tuberculosis of the spine (1982). A ten year assessment of a controlled trial comparing debridement and anterior spinal fusion in the management of tuberculosis of the spine in patients on standard chemotherapy in Hong Kong. *J. Bone Joint Surg.*, **64B**, 393–398

Farfan, H.F. (1980) The pathological anatomy of degenerative spondylolisthesis – a cadaveric study. *Spine*, **5**, 412–418

Frymoyer, J.W. and Stokes, I.A. (1990) Biomechanics of the motion segment. In *Spinal Surgery: Science and Practice* (ed. R.A. Dickson), Butterworths, London, Chapter 6

Galasko, C.S.B. (1991) Spinal instability secondary to metastatic cancer. *J. Bone Joint Surg.*, **73B**, 104–108

Goel, V.K. and Weinstein, J.N. (1990) *Biomechanics of the Spine: Clinical and Surgical Perspective*, CRC Press Inc., Boca Raton, FL

Hall, A.J. and Mackay, N.N.S. (1973) The results of laminectomy for compression of the cord or cauda equina by extradural malignant tumour. *J. Bone Joint Surg.*, **55B**, 497–505

Harrington, K.D. (1981) The use of methylmethacrylate cement for vertebral body replacement and anterior stabilisation of pathological fracture dislocation of the spine due to metastatic malignant disease. *J. Bone Joint Surg.*, **63A**, 36–46

Heywood, A.W.B. and Meyers, O.L. (1986) Rheumatoid arthritis of the thoracic and lumbar spine. *J. Bone Joint Surg.*, **68B**, 362–368

Jeffrey, M.R. and Ball, J. (1963) *Atlas of standard radiographs of arthritis. The epidemiology of chronic rheumatism II*, Blackwell Scientific, Oxford, pp. 22–23

Kirkaldy-Willis, W.H. (1976) Lumbar spinal stenosis and nerve root entrapment syndromes; definition and classification. *Clin. Orthop.*, **115**, 4

Kudo, H., Iwano, K. and Yoshizawa, H. (1984) Cervical cord compression due to extradural granulation tissue in rheumatoid arthritis. *J. Bone Joint Surg.*, **66B**, 426–430

Lawrence, J.S. (1987) The epidemiology of low back pain. *Curr. Orthop.*, **1**, 361–365

Leatherman, K.D. and Dickson, R.A. (1988) *The management of spinal deformities*, Wright, London

Lipson, S.J. (1984) Rheumatoid arthritis of the cervical spine. *Clin. Orthop.*, **182**, 143–149

Markolf, K.L. and Morris, M.W. (1974) Structural components of the intervertebral disc. *J. Bone Joint Surg.*, **56A**, 675–687

Naylor, A. (1990) Lumbar disc disorders. In *Spinal Surgery: Science and Practice* (ed. R.A. Dickson), Butterworths, London, Chapter 9

Newman, R.J., Butt, W.P. and Dickson, R.A. (1991) An audit of percutaneous needle biopsy of the axial skeleton. *Br. Orthop. Ass.*, Cambridge

Pellici, P.M., Ranawat, C.S., Tsairis, P. and Bryan, W.J. (1981) A prospective study of the progression of rheumatoid arthritis of the cervical spine. *J. Bone Joint Surg.*, **63A** 342–350

Rana, N.A., Hancock, D.O., Taylor, A.R. and Hill, A.G.S. (1973) Atlanto-axial subluxation in rheumatoid arthritis. *J. Bone Joint Surg.*, **55B**, 458–470

Ranawat, C.S., O'Leary, P., Pellici, P., Tsairis, P., Marchisello, P. and Dorr, L. (1979) Cervical spine fusion in rheumatoid arthritis. *J. Bone Joint Surg.*, **61A**, 1003–1010

Roberts, S., Menage, J. and Urban, J.P.G. (1989) Biochemical and structural properties of the cartilage end-plate and its relationship to the intervertebral disc. *Spine*, **14**, 166–174

Smith, R. and Houghton, G. (1990) Metabolic and inherited disorders of the spine. In *Spinal Surgery: Science and Practice* (ed. R.A. Dickson), Butterworths, London, Chapter 24

Thomas, J.H. and Gillham, B. (1985) Nutrition: general aspects. In *Wills' Biochemical Basis of Medicine* (2nd edn), Wright, London, Chapter 10

Verbiest, H. (1954) A radicular syndrome from developmental narrowing of the lumbar vertebral canal. *J. Bone Joint Surg.*, **36B**, 230–237

Waddell, G. (1982) An approach to backache. *Br. J. Hosp. Med.*, **28**, 187–219

Wedge, J.H. and Kirkaldy-Willis, W.H. (1990) Infections of the spine. In *Spinal Surgery: Science and Practice* (ed. R.A. Dickson), Butterworths, London, Chapter 25

Winfield, J., Cooke, D., Brooke, A.S. and Corbett, M. (1981) A prospective study of the radiological changes in the cervical spine in early rheumatoid arthritis. *Ann. Rheum. Dis.*, **40**, 109–114

Woolf, A.D. and Dixon, A. St J. (1988) *Osteoporosis: a clinical guide*, Martin Dunitz, London

Zoma, A., Sturrock, R.D., Fisher, W.D., Freeman, P.A. and Hamblen, D.L. (1987) Surgical stabilisation of the rheumatoid cervical spine. *J. Bone Joint Surg.*, **69B**, 8–12

9

Lower limb amputation surgery

David I. Rowley and Amar S. Jain

Amputation is an ancient surgical procedure and evidence exists of its practice among prehistoric man. Early amputation was a crude affair in which the patient was not anaesthetized, the limb was rapidly removed and boiling oil or a burning branch applied to the bleeding cut surface. This left a stump which was unsuitable even for the primitive prostheses then available. With the development of refined anaesthesia and appropriate surgical techniques stumps can now be fashioned which confer good postoperative function. The relatively new science of prosthetics is based upon sound bioengineering principles allowing amputees to be fitted with prostheses which fit and function satisfactorily.

The destructive nature of amputation can give rise to a defeatist attitude in which the operation is considered undesirable though necessary. Amputation of a diseased limb however should be thought of as the first step towards returning the patient to a normal place in society.

In general the younger, more active amputee will learn to use his prosthesis without too much difficulty and usually is able to return to an acceptable lifestyle fairly soon after surgery. His problems are likely to be prosthetic rather than physical and are often encountered when the function of the artificial limb fails to match that of the 'real' limb during sporting or recreational activities. Conversely, the elderly amputee often has problems in adapting to even limited prosthetic use. Therefore a skilled and accurate assessment of the elderly patient's capabilities is vital to establish a realistic rehabilitation goal. All too often aged, infirm patients are referred for prosthetic fitting regardless of their general physical condition including exercise tolerance, mental attitude towards the loss of a limb and their appreciation of the hard work required in learning to use a prosthesis.

It is particularly important that the patient displays enthusiasm for the proposed rehabilitation programme. Even the most skilled and energetic rehabilitation team will be unable to train an amputee to achieve independent gait using a prosthesis if the patient is uncooperative. For some elderly people, especially those with chronic disability or disease processes, walking and leading a functionally independent life even with normal legs is an extremely difficult affair. It is therefore unreasonable to expect such patients to become independent artificial limb users. It also makes little sense to commit expensive therapy, time and expertise in attempting to restore walking ability to such patients who will inevitably spend most of the day in a chair.

Close collaboration between all members of the clinical team is vital if satisfactory and appropriate rehabilitation is to be achieved. The patient's immediate family and of course the patient himself must be involved in discussions on his future lifestyle. The decision to abandon any attempt at prosthetic fitting and subsequent gait training should only come after careful evaluation of the patient – though experience shows that the suggestion will often come first from the amputee himself. If ambulation on a prosthesis is not considered possible then a cosmetic non-weight bearing prosthesis can be prescribed which may make the patient's self-image more acceptable.

Once a person becomes an amputee his lifestyle changes dramatically and in the elderly this often means loss of independence with its associated psychological consequences. It is therefore important at the outset that those concerned

Table 9.1 New amputees attending British Artificial Limb and Appliance Centres for the first time, 1984

Lower limb	
Single	4552
Double	165
Double, previously single	328
Total	5045
Upper limb	
Single	155
Double	3
Double, previously single	0
Total	158
Multiple amputation (upper and lower)	15
Without amputation (mainly due to congenital deformities)	152
Overall total	5370

Source: Review of Artificial Limb and Appliance Centre services (1986)
For 1985 and 1986 data see Gregory-Dean (1991)

with the management of these patients make every effort to make their lives both comfortable and worthwhile. It must be recognized that all amputees require total care by a multidisciplinary team. In specialized centres with ideal facilities an identified group of qualified and appropriately experienced medical and paramedical staff may be justified both in terms of individual care and in cost benefits to the community. Such a team would include not only the surgeon but also physiotherapists, occupational therapists, prosthetists and, of course, nursing staff. Unfortunately, the majority of hospitals do not possess these resources and in these instances someone must take a special interest in the management of the amputee and plan the pre- and postoperative rehabilitation programme. Simply to perform an amputation on an elderly patient and refer that person to a limb-fitting centre at some unspecified time following discharge allows the opportunity to be lost for achieving optimal rehabilitation.

Amputation can be performed on either the upper or lower limb but that on the lower limb outnumbers that on the upper limb by an overall ratio of more than 30:1 (Table 9.1). Amputations performed in the elderly are nearly always in the lower limb and for these reasons this chapter will only discuss those problems associated with lower limb amputation in this age group. For comparative purposes the tables will contain equivalent upper limb data and the reader is referred to Atkins and Meier (1989), for details regarding the comprehensive management of the upper limb amputee.

Incidence

The total number of amputees in Britain has been reported to be about 60 000 (Table 9.2) with more than 5000 new cases of lower limb amputations performed per year (Table 9.1). The prevalence is 1.05 per 1000 population in the UK and in the United States is 1.7 per 1000 (Malinon, 1981). The incidence of amputation in the Dundee area has remained fairly constant for the past 19 years (Murdoch *et al.*, 1988) at 0.26 per 1000 per year. This apparent discrepancy can only be explained by assuming that this specialized unit, serving a defined population, has collected more accurate figures than elsewhere.

A recent report produced by the Scottish Home and Health Department in 1989 shows a prevalence of 0.13 per 1000 population (Scottish Health Service, 1989).

The aged account for approximately 70% of the total lower limb amputee population (Table 9.2) and a similar proportion of new lower limb cases that attend limb-fitting centres (Table 9.3). The mean age of the 1200 primary amputees seen in the Dundee Limb Fitting Centre between 1966 and 1981 has remained remarkably steady at approximately 70 years with 70% of these patients being over the age of 60 years (Murdoch *et al.*, 1988).

The general physical condition of the elderly amputee is often poor, his adaptability limited and his life expectancy short. For example, the life expectancy of a Dundee vascular amputee is 3 years and 1 month which contrasts markedly with that of approximately 10 years for a 70-year-old peer. Some 80% of amputees are alive 2 years after amputation, 40% alive at 4 years and only 10% by 10 years (Murdoch *et al.*, 1988).

Causal conditions

In general, the medical conditions leading to amputation have not changed over the years but their relative incidence pattern has changed and varies from country to country. The reasons for amputation in Britain are presented in Table 9.4 in which it can be seen that more than 85% of lower limb amputations are performed for peripheral vascular disease secondary to atherosclerosis and/or diabetes mellitus. These data are representative for causes of amputation in the Western world but in Asia, Africa and the

Table 9.2 Total amputee population in Britain, 1984[a]

Age distribution	Male	Female	Total	Percentage of total
Lower limb patients				
0–9	190	123	313	0.6
10–19	473	286	759	1.5
20–39	3711	1202	4913	9.6
40–59	7361	1992	9353	18.3
60–79[b]	22 370	6887	29 257	57.2 ⎫ 70
Over 80[b]	3587	2984	6535	12.8 ⎭
Total	37 692	13 438	51 130	100
Upper limb patients				
0–9	293	317	610	5.2
10–19	490	400	890	7.5
20–39	2040	766	2806	23.7
40–59	2247	617	2864	24.2
60–79[b]	3320	834	4154	35.2 ⎫ 40
Over 80[b]	327	162	489	4.2 ⎭
Total	8717	3096	11 813	100

[a] At the end of 1984 there were 51 130 lower limb and 11 813 upper limb users in Britain. Although the majority were elderly, the total amputee populations included many people in a stable physical condition.
[b] There are 9347 cases where no date of birth is recorded on the computer. The majority of these cases are known to be in the older age groups (i.e. over 60) and have therefore been apportioned accordingly.
Source: Review of Artificial Limb and Appliance Centre services (1986)
For 1986 data see Gregory-Dean, 1991

Table 9.3 Age distribution of amputees attending British Artificial Limb and Appliance Centres for the first time, 1984

Age distribution	Male	Female	Total	Percentage of total
Lower limb				
amputees				
0–9	16	11	27	0.5
10–19	68	23	91	1.8
20–39	172	42	214	4.2
40–59	594	171	765	15.2
60–79	2192	1027	3219	63.8 ⎫ 78
Over 80	346	383	739	14.5 ⎭
Total	3388	1657	5045	100
Upper limb				
amputees				
0–9	2	4	6	3.8
10–19	11	3	14	8.9
20–39	34	14	48	30.4
40–59	34	13	47	29.7
60–79	23	4	5	24.0 ⎫ 27
Over 80	1	4	5	3.2 ⎭
Total	105	53	158	100

Source: Review of Artificial Limb and Appliance Centre services (1986)
For 1986 data see Gregory-Dean, 1991

developing countries the common causes are trauma and infection.

General conclusions about the aetiology of peripheral vascular disease may be drawn from cross-sectional surveys but longitudinal studies are necessary to provide conclusive results. The most important risk factor is probably smoking and this may also be responsible for the abnormalities in haematocrit, blood viscosity and plasma fibrinogen identified in patients with peripheral vascular occlusive disease. High blood pressure, especially systolic hypertension,

Table 9.4 Reasons for amputation in new amputees attending British Artificial Limb Appliance Centres, 1984

	Male	*Female*	*Total*	*Percentage of total*
Lower limb				
Vascular	2292	1020	3312	65.7 ⎤ 88
Diabetes	664	462	1126	22.3 ⎦
Trauma	241	67	308	6.1
Malignancy	96	57	153	3.0
Infection	59	31	90	1.8
Deformity	36	20	56	1.1
Total	3388	1657	5045	100
Upper limb				
Vascular	5	7	12	7.6
Diabetes	—	—	—	—
Trauma	82	23	105	66.4
Malignancy	13	19	32	20.3
Infection	4	1	5	3.2
Deformity	1	3	4	2.5
Total	105	53	158	100

Source: Review of Artificial Limb and Appliance Centre services (1986)
For 1986 data see Gregory-Dean, 1991

may have a significant independent effect. In cross-sectional and case-control studies hyper-triglyceridaemia is univariately associated with peripheral arterial disease but total serum cholesterol and glucose intolerance do not show consistent associations (Leng and Fowkes, 1991).

Selection of level of amputation

It is essential to recognize that the salvage of the knee joint in elderly patients is of prime importance if rehabilitation is to be successful (Pedersen, 1968). However, there is still a disappointingly high ratio of above-knee amputations performed in some parts of the world though the trend is now changing. For example, between 1971 and 1982 the total number of amputations in England and Wales remained virtually static with a ratio of above-knee to below-knee surgery of approximately 2:1. In Dundee in 1966 the ratio was comparable at just under 2:1 but an aggressive policy commenced in 1967 of salvaging the knee joint wherever possible. This had the effect of reducing this ratio almost immediately to 1:1. By 1971 the ratio had been reversed at 1:1.5 and by 1973 the ratio had become 1:3. This was accompanied by a successful rate of healing of 90% for below-knee surgery (Murdoch *et al.*, 1988).

The other advantages of below-knee amputation over the above-knee procedure are well described. Waters *et al.* (1976) assessed the energy consumption of amputees and stated that they used more energy to walk than normal subjects, possibly accounting for the fact that on average non-amputees walk 8366 steps per day while amputees only achieve 2498 (Murdoch *et al.*, 1988). In addition, this increased energy expenditure was found to be directly related to the level of amputation accounting for the observation of Anderson *et al.* (1967) that below-knee amputees are generally more active than above-knee amputees. Fisher and Gullickson (1978) estimated that the above-knee amputee expended 89% more energy than the normal person.

The energy expenditure of the bilateral above-knee amputee is extremely high and it should be apparent and, indeed it is the case, that all elderly bilateral above-knee amputees resort to a highly dependent wheelchair existence.

The other advantages of below-knee amputation over above-knee surgery include improved balance due to proprioception being retained with the salvaged joint, increased ease of 'donning' and 'doffing' the prosthesis and the fact that the bony contours of the stump allow more accurate fitting. These, however, are all secondary to the problems of a very inefficient gait in an already disadvantaged patient. It cannot be overemphasized how important it is to avoid amputation above the knee whenever possible. Liaison with surgeons is therefore pivotal to the success of a rehabilitation programme and their role must start with accurate assessment of both the patient and the limb.

Clinical assessment

The clinical assessment for amputation is, in general, no different from other preoperative clinical assessments but in this instance extra consideration must be given to several particular facets of the case including the patient's skin condition, joint contractures, the general medical condition, mental state and intellectual ability (Hanspal and Fisher, 1991) as well as occupation and hobbies. These criteria are used to determine the optimal level of amputation.

If a patient is clearly mentally and physically incapable of walking with a prosthesis then a decision may be taken in favour of above-knee amputation more readily than in a more able-bodied subject. Such essentially wheelchair bound candidates may indeed be done a disservice by a below-knee amputation which in these circumstances may allow the development of flexion contractures of an unused knee. Such an inconvenient and unnecessary appendage may impede wheelchair sitting and transfers.

Skin conditions, i.e. ulceration, eczematous rashes, previous scars and skin grafts may dictate the level of amputation for successful prosthetic management in spite of a good circulation.

Systolic blood pressure measurements

The use of the Doppler technique for estimating systolic blood pressure has become widely accepted as a standard method for the non-invasive evaluation of the patient with peripheral vascular disease. This is a less than precise method but is undoubtedly useful if taken within the context of a sound clinical assessment in the selection procedure (Clyne, 1991).

Skin blood flow measurement

A quantitative measurement of skin blood flow at the precise level of operation is an added asset to predict wound healing. ^{125}I-4-iodoantipyrine has been used for this purpose and it has been shown to provide a good indication of tissue viability especially below the knee (Spence and Walker, 1984).

Infrared thermography

Infrared thermography has been used in the assessment of peripheral vascular disease for the last 25 years and was suggested as a possible means of selecting amputation levels by Lloyd-Williams (1964). Recently, high resolution digital systems became available and when linked to a microcomputer the outcome from these systems can be quantified. It is now possible to obtain an accurate calibrated thermal map of the limb which provides a highly acceptable assessment of an ischaemic limb. The great advantage of the thermographic mapping of the skin is the ability to adjust the orientation of the skin flaps accordingly and thus obtain good healing in a stump which is longer than it would otherwise be using conventional flaps. In Dundee this technique has, above all others, contributed to the improvement of the ratio of above-knee to below-knee amputation. Indeed, it is strongly suggested that in those centres where thermography of a high order is available, then it should become an integral part of the assessment procedure. Its use, however, is heavily dependent on the concomitant adaptation of the surgical technique in fashioning skin flaps in order to optimize healing.

Concurrent medical problems

The majority of elderly patients requiring amputation have associated medical conditions such as diabetes mellitus, hypertension, chest infection and urinary tract problems which need accurate preoperative assessment and management. It is vitally important that these conditions should be looked after by an experienced physician since they play an important part in the morbidity and mortality of the amputee following surgery.

Preoperative physiotherapy should be instituted to maintain and improve the strength and mobility of the patient in general and of the limb to be operated on in particular. Attention needs to be given to the prevention or reduction of any flexion contractures and the opportunity can be taken to inform the patient and his family of the proposed rehabilitation plans following surgery.

Antibiotic prophylaxis with penicillin should be given. This is most easily performed intravenously for the first 2 days and orally thereafter. A 5-day course of low-dose heparin should also be administered for the prevention of deep venous thrombosis.

The operation

All lower limb amputations in patients with peripheral vascular disease should preferably be performed under spinal anaesthesia unless otherwise contraindicated as this reduces post-operative morbidity and mortality (Mann and Bisset, 1983). A tourniquet should not be used.

Meticulous surgery plays an important part in wound healing, especially in the elderly dysvascular patient. The surgeon's principal objective is to produce a stump which will proceed to primary and uncomplicated wound healing. The stump should be capable of good muscular control and be able to withstand the pressures experienced at the socket/stump interface. To achieve this the techniques of myoplasty and myodesis are employed.

Myoplasty is the suture of the divided muscle ends taking care that the agonist and antagonist muscles are stitched over the divided bone end. This is the most frequent technique used in the patient with peripheral vascular disease.

Myodesis is the reattachment of the muscles to the bone in an anatomical situation and is normally performed through drill holes into the bone. It is not recommended for the patient with peripheral vascular disease.

The Dundee experience showed that amputation surgery failed in approximately 20% at the below-knee level. In these cases the stump could be revised by a below-knee wedge resection (Hadden *et al.* 1987) in 12% with only 8% requiring amputation at a more proximal level. Prostheses were fitted to almost 90% of patients and those considered unsuitable were supplied with a wheelchair. Some received both a limb and a wheelchair.

Contralateral amputation at a later date may be necessary and 97% of cases have vascular-related causes (peripheral vascular disease 62% and diabetes mellitus 35%). Below-knee amputation is, of course, the level of choice and

following the second amputation 68% were fitted with prostheses. Despite the second amputation 80% were fit enough to return either home or to sheltered accommodation.

Sites of amputation

The general principles outlined below are applied to all levels of amputation.

Partial foot amputation

Timely performed limited amputations in the foot are often indicated in the infected diabetic patient. These procedures range from excision of gangrenous or infected toes to resection of rays. It is important that all ischaemic, necrotic and infected tissue is removed. Wounds should be irrigated and left to heal by secondary intention.

Transmetatarsal amputation has some limited application but it is only useful in diabetic gangrene with no major vessel disease. The technique described by McKittrick, McKittrick and Risley (1949) is most favoured. Lisfranc and Chopart amputations have virtually no role to play in peripheral vascular disease in elderly patients.

Syme's amputation

The Syme's amputation is one of the best lower limb amputations from a functional point of view but in vascular disease this is not a favoured level as the healing rate is well below 50% (Sarmiento and Warren, 1969). Indications for this amputation still exist in diabetic foot infections. As suggested by Wagner (1977) this can be performed in two stages.

Below-knee amputation

This is the most favoured level of amputation in elderly dysvascular patients and has gained popularity over the last decade. The best technique is that described by Burgess (1969) using a long posterior flap and a stump measuring 11–12 cm from the medial joint line of the knee. This method is well documented and has been supported by excellent results from various centres (Robinson, 1972; Murdoch, 1975; Cumming *et al.*, 1987, 1988). Since the preservation of the knee joint is of immense importance in walking, every effort should be made to perform this operation as meticulously as possible. The skew flap technique made possible by thermography is a variation on this theme (Robinson, 1991).

Through-knee amputation

There are considerable advantages in an amputation at this level because of the long lever arm and end-bearing properties of the stump. The disadvantage at this level is the poor cosmesis following prosthetic fitting. To obtain adequate cover for the femoral condyles, the technique recently described by Steen Jensen (1988) with side flaps appears to offer a chance of secure wound healing. If possible both menisci should be preserved to ensure a rich proprioceptive supply to the stump.

Above-knee amputation

Amputation above the knee should be performed with as long a stump as possible bearing in mind that space of 10 cm is required to accommodate an artificial knee mechanism between the distal end of the stump and the normal knee joint axis. The amputation should therefore be carried out 10 cm above the knee joint line if the pathology permits. Amputation any more distally leads to prosthetic problems because of the shape of the femoral condyles.

Hip disarticulation and hindquarter amputation

There are no indications for these procedures in the elderly patient (Taylor and Monro, 1952).

Postoperative management

Following surgery the elderly patient's general medical condition requires monitoring and treating as appropriate. Adequate analgesics must be administered and good stump management will result in a sound, comfortable and functional stump.

Following above-knee surgery rigid dressings have been advocated (Mooney *et al.*, 1971) but suspension and maintenance of this form of dressing is difficult. Conversely, if no dressing is applied then the wound is unprotected causing pain and oedema formation which will delay wound healing.

A simple elastoplast adhesive dressing is feasible but the strips must be applied longitudinally and not circumferentially. It protects the wound, offers some support and avoids any adverse pressure gradient.

For through-knee and below-knee amputations a rigid dressing with a plaster-of-Paris cast is an ideal one but care is essential in its application. This type of dressing has been advocated by Burgess, Romano and Zettie (1969) and has subsequently been evaluated by Mooney *et al.* (1971). An alternative form of treatment developed by Redhead and Snowden (1978) is a controlled environment treatment in which the stump is enclosed in a sterile transparent plastic container within which is an 'ideal environment'. This is applied for 5–7 days and thereafter a rigid dressing is applied.

For the Syme's amputation a rigid dressing is an ideal one.

Once the stump has healed regular bandaging should be instituted to control oedema. However, the bandage must be properly applied and the pressure created by the bandage must not exceed intravascular hydrostatic pressure and should not produce an adverse pressure gradient along the stump. The application of this bandage should be supervised by an experienced member of staff who should instruct the patient how to undertake his or her own bandaging once the stump is stable.

An alternative method of reducing stump volume, maintaining a good stump shape and controlling stump oedema is the use of the two-way stretch amputation stump shrinkers. It is important however to use the appropriate size both in terms of length and girth to avoid distal congestion. Similarly, as swelling resolves and the stump reduces in volume the size of the shrinker should be changed accordingly.

Physiotherapy

Those elderly patients who have lost one or both legs rely considerably on their upper limbs and the importance of regular and coordinated exercises to improve the muscle tone, power and stamina in the arms cannot be overemphasized. Such treatment also has subsidiary benefits such as improved respiratory function and overall circulation. Early ambulation not only requires good upper limb function but clearly good control and strength of the stump. In order to

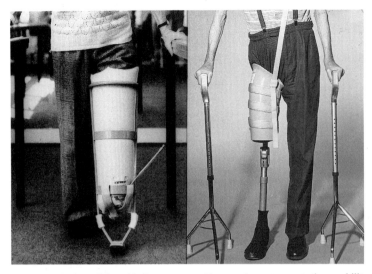

Figure 9.1 Early walking aids for amputees. Pneumatic post-amputation mobility aid (PPAM-aid) (left), Femoret (right)

facilitate postoperative rehabilitation the therapist will have commenced this exercise programme in the preoperative phase and will continue his or her work starting on the first postoperative day. The therapist also instructs the amputee in functional activities including sitting and rising from a chair, rising from a floor, climbing and descending stairs as well as techniques of taking off and putting on the artificial leg.

Prosthetic fitting

In patients with through-knee, below-knee and Syme's amputations the use of the rigid plaster dressing allied to an extension tube and prosthetic foot provides mobility and constitutes immediate postoperative fitting though gait training may usefully be delayed 5–7 days. Most above-knee amputees are able to use one of the early walking aids such as the pneumatic post-amputation mobility aid (PPAM-aid), Tulip or Femoret (Figure 9.1). This enables suitable cases to mobilize within a few days of operation though again this is usually delayed for some 7–10 days. Walking training is part of an intensive rehabilitation programme performed as an inpatient. Unfortunately, even in the best centres, there is an inevitable wait for the delivery of a definitive prosthesis. In order that mobilization

and gait training should not be delayed some sort of temporary prosthesis is used. Such a prosthesis has a socket made out of plaster of Paris or similar material attached to a prosthetic foot by a pylon.

The benefit of using an early walking aid is that early training in standing, balance and gait is allowed. Stump oedema is also controlled and the patient can be assessed as a potential user of a definitive prosthesis. The PPAM-aid is not suitable for a very short stump as the latter tends to slide out of the pneumatic bag when the patient flexes the hip to initiate the swing phase of walking. In these cases additional suspension by means of a shoulder strap or harness should be incorporated. The value of the early walking aid in the assessment of the patient's capabilities is enormous and it is at this stage of the rehabilitation programme that the decision should be made to proceed with prosthetic manufacture and training or to aim for as much independence as possible from a wheelchair. The judgement of an experienced physiotherapist whose patient fails to regain adequate standing balance, weight transference and walking using early walking aids will enable a realistic rehabilitation goal to be set for that patient. This is especially so when her views are considered together with assessments from other members of the rehabilitation team. Even if it is decided that the patient should spend most of his day seated in a chair he should be encouraged to make independent transfers from chair to chair, from bed to chair and from chair to toilet and to make use of a walking frame for one-legged gait if at all possible.

Training begins with the patient seated between parallel bars and he is instructed how to stand and sit safely. Subsequently balance training is given prior to walking being allowed. Ideally, the patient should eventually discard one walking stick and retain the remaining stick in the contralateral hand. This allows one hand to be free for other purposes such as carrying objects, opening doors, etc. The amputee should be instructed in climbing stairs, walking on uneven or soft surfaces such as carpets and in how to negotiate objects in a confined space. It is also important that he is shown how to rise from the floor if a fall occurs. This is best done by 'bumping' along the floor to the nearest piece of stable furniture and then pulling up on to it (Condie, 1988).

It is unlikely that most elderly above-knee amputees will walk great distances. For them stability and the ability to transfer safely from chair to chair and walk with comfort around the house is more important than having the stamina to walk for miles in a straight line.

The definitive prosthesis should have a socket which fits well and which is correctly aligned with the point of ground contact by the artificial foot. Cosmesis should not be underrated and will be of considerable importance to all patients no matter their age. Function is the key factor but even where ambulation is contemplated the device must be perceived as being socially acceptable by the patient. Even when a wheelchair is the inevitable future for the patient it should be remembered that non-functional cosmetic legs are available and many amputees derive a great deal of comfort from such devices.

For the above-knee prosthesis the socket can be made in various shapes and though metal and wood have been used in the past these materials have gradually been replaced by a variety of plastics in both laminated and shell forms. Suspension is obtained by means of a pelvic band often supplemented by a shoulder strap (Figure 9.2). In the more able patient with a strong stump a self-suspending suction socket may be prescribed but this is uncommon in older patients.

The prosthesis for a typical below-knee stump is the patellar tendon bearing (PTB) prosthesis. Almost all such prostheses are fabricated either in sheet or laminated plastic. Suspension is achieved by a cuff situated just above the patella (Figure 9.2).

Modern, so-called 'modular' prostheses made from prefabricated components are tending to replace the more traditionally constructed prostheses in many centres. In recent years the limitation of commercial methods of supply of artifical limbs has also been recognized. The inherent limitation of alignment potential, delaying production and supply has led to advances in the modular assembly system. Essentially this system consists of 'off the shelf' components which can be added to custom-made sockets so allowing alignment and interchange of component as required by clinical prescription. These components form the permanent skeleton of the artificial limb and simply require a suitable covering for good cosmetic appearance (James, 1991).

Rehabilitation

As already indicated the amputee requires total care but the provision of this is complex and requires the participation of all members of the rehabilitation team.

The nursing staff provide day-to-day care and also give continuity to that care mixed with the necessary understanding and compassion needed by their patient. Occupational therapists integrate with the nursing staff and coordinate with the community services. The role of the physiotherapist has already been described.

A suitable home environment is essential if the elderly amputee is to return there from hospital. A home visit should therefore be made by the appropriate staff (usually the occupational and physiotherapist) at an early stage during the patient's rehabilitation. Problems, for example, in the kitchen and bathroom can be identified and appropriate modifications made while the patient is still in hospital. Ease of access to the home should be ensured and this may mean fitting hand rails, stair ramps, etc.

A further home visit by the amputee and therapists prior to final discharge is recommended in order that any remaining areas of difficulty can be clearly established. Appropriate training can be given and/or adaptions made to overcome the difficulties, including the fitting of ramps and rails (Travers, 1991).

The health visitor and social work department also play an important role in arranging the

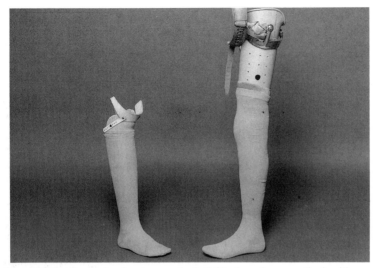

Figure 9.2 Patellar tendon-bearing prosthesis (left), above-knee prosthesis with metal socket and pelvic band (right)

placement of the patient in the community and any extra help that may be needed for the activities of everyday living.

A period of outpatient physiotherapy will be necessary but if possible, a period of domiciliary physiotherapy may be even better for the elderly amputee.

Amputees require regular review at limb fitting centres to monitor the changing stump volume, the effect of a new stump/socket environment and regular appraisal of a prosthetic prescription. Once the stump matures satisfactorily less frequent reviews are required.

'Special cases'

There are some elderly patients who have disabilities in addition to their amputation. These are the 'special cases' whose co-existing conditions include epilepsy, blindness, deafness, obesity, hemiplegia and amputation of the upper limb. The rehabilitation of these individuals requires additional consideration to make them independently safe on their limbs and is fully discussed by Humm (1977).

Complications of amputation surgery

The three important signs which indicate a developing complication in an amputation stump are pain, skin problems and a reduction in the stump volume.

Pain

Pain is always an early warning signal for anything untoward happening in the stump. It can be caused by many factors including infection, neuroma, phantom pain or skin irritation.

Persistent pain is difficult to relieve and usually occurs 24–72 h after operation. This may indicate the formation of a haematoma. This is a serious complication since if not recognized and evacuated immediately it will lead to devitalization of tissue and breakdown of the stump.

Pain due to infection usually occurs during or towards the end of the first week. It is usually throbbing in character and is associated with pyrexia and increases in pulse and respiration rate. When infection is suspected it is necessary to inspect the wound and treat accordingly by antibiotics and drainage.

Pain due to neuroma occurs much later but is less likely where the nerve has been severed under slight traction. This type of pain may be felt during the third postoperative week or at some time later. Repeated continuous percussion of the painful area gives a clue to the diagnosis. The pain can be relieved by infiltration of local anaesthetic and hydrocortisone but if it proves intractable then surgery is required.

Perception of a phantom limb is strongest immediately following operation and it is considered normal for the majority of amputees to experience this phenomenon. Firm bandaging of the amputation stump tends to lessen this sensation and give some degree of comfort, as does the wearing of a prosthesis.

Phantom pain occurs within the phantom limb not in the stump itself. It is an abnormal sensation ranging from a slight tingling or numbness to a severe tearing or crushing pain. Analgesics may give some relief but there may be no satisfactory solution to the problem. There is some evidence that vigilance in relieving pain postoperatively prevents the problem becoming chronic. Spinal anaesthesia also may reduce the frequency of this problem but referral to the pain clinic is sometimes required.

Skin problems

The stump tissues are subjected to a completely new environment in a prosthetic socket. They are compressed and are expected to bear high loads. Air is unable to circulate and perspiration can cause problems with excoriation, contact dermatitis and eczema. Venous and lymphatic stasis may lead to terminal oedema, capillary haemorrhage and blister formation. These conditions may alter the shape of the stump and make the socket of the artificial limb ill-fitting.

Callosities may occur when pressure is taken on the ischial tuberosity in the above-knee amputee and over the patellar tendon on the lateral aspect of the stump in the below-knee amputee. This is, in fact, a protective response of the skin enabling the amputee to bear weight more comfortably, but occasionally proliferation of the tissues occurs resulting in a painful callosity.

Occasional contact dermatitis may arise after months of wearing a prosthesis. The cause may be traced to one of the materials used in the fabrication of the socket which should therefore be altered appropriately.

Epidermoid cysts develop usually in an established above-knee amputee. The commonly affected areas are the inguinal, adductor and ischial bearing areas and infection of the cysts may supervene.

Reduction in stump volume

Owing to muscle inactivity the stump volume reduces, often markedly in the first few months. This can be most easily appreciated by taking note of the number of socks needed by the patient to fit the socket adequately. Should the patient begin to require three or more woollen socks this usually means that the stump volume has reduced to the point where a new socket may be required. If this is not performed expeditiously skin breakdown with ulceration can occur. Regular review at the artificial limb centre prevents such socket/stump interface problems.

Conclusions

The vast majority of patients requiring lower limb amputation surgery are elderly and disadvantaged by peripheral vascular disease due to arteriosclerosis, diabetes mellitus or a combination of the two. The achievement of a well-healed stump and a speedy rehabilitation requires accurate selection of the optimal level of amputation, sound preoperative preparation, meticulous surgery and an intensive rehabilitation programme provided by the various professionals who have but one goal – the restoration of an independent and mobile patient to his community.

References

Anderson, A.D., Cummings, V., Levine, S.L. and Kraus, A. (1967) The use of lower extremity prosthetic limbs by elderly patients. *Arch. Phys. Med. Rehab.*, **48**, 533

Atkins, D.J. and Meier, R.H. III (1989) *Comprehensive Management of the Upper-Limb Amputee*, Springer-Verlag, London

Burgess, E.M., Romano, R.L. and Zettie, J. (1969) *Management of lower extremity amputations: TR10–6*, US Government Printing Office, Washington, DC

Burgess, E.M. (1969) The below-knee amputation. *Inter-Clinic Inform. Bull.*, **VII**, No. 4

Clyne, C.A.C. (1991) Selection of level for lower limb amputation in patients with severe peripheral vascular disease. *Ann. Roy. Coll. Surg. Eng.*, **73**, 155–157

Condie, M.E. (1988), Physiotherapy and the elderly above knee amputee. In *Amputation Surgery and Lower Limb Prosthetics* (eds G. Murdoch and R.G. Donovan), Blackwell Scientific, Edinburgh, pp. 172–177

Cumming, J.G.R., Spence, V.A., Jain, A.S., Stewart, C., Walker, W.F. and Murdoch, G. (1987) Fate of the vascular patient after below-knee amputation. *Lancet*, **ii**, 613–615

Cumming, J.G.R., Spence, V.A., Jain, A.S., McCollum, P.T., Stewart, C., Walker, W.F. and Murdoch, G. (1988) Further experience in the healing rate of lower limb amputations. *Eur. J. Vasc. Surg.*, **2**, 383–385

Fisher, S.V. and Gullickson, G. (1978) Energy cost of ambulation in health and disability: a literature review. *Arch. Phys. Med. Rehab.*, **59**, 124–133

Gregory-Dean, A. (1991) Amputations: statistics and trends. *Ann. Roy. Coll. Surg. Eng.*, **73**, 137–142

Hadden, W., Marks, R., Murdoch, G. and Stewart, C. (1987) Wedge resection of amputation stumps: a valuable salvage procedure. *J. Bone Joint Surg.*, **69**, 306–308

Hanspal, R.S. and Fisher, K. (1991) Assessment of cognitive and psychomotor function and rehabilitation of elderly people with prostheses. *Br. Med. J.*, **302**, 940

Humm W. (1977) *Rehabilitation of the Lower Limb Amputee*, 3rd edn, Bailliere Tindall, London

Leng, G.C. and Fowkes, F.G.R. (1991) Epidemiology of peripheral vascular disease. In *Current Medical Literature. Thrombosis, Scientific and Clinical Perspectives* (ed. C.D. Forbes), Royal Society of Medicine, London, pp. 35–43

James, W.V. (1991) Principles of limb fitting and prostheses. *Ann. Roy. Coll. Surg. Eng.*, **73**, 158–162

Lloyd-Williams, K. (1964) Pictorial heat scanning. *Phys. Med. Biol.*, **9**, 433–456

McKittrick, L.S., McKittrick, J.B. and Risley, T.S. (1949) Transmetatarsal amputation for infection or gangrene in patients with diabetes mellitus. *Ann. Surg.*, **130**, 826–842

Mann, R.M. and Bisset, W.K. (1983) Anaesthesia for lower limb amputations: a comparison of spinal analgesia and general anaesthesia in the elderly. *Anaesthesia*, **38**, 1185–1191

Malinon, M.R. (1981) Regression of atherosclerosis in humans: fact or myth? *Circulation*, **64**, 1–3

Mooney, V., Harvey, J.P., McBride, E. and Snelson, R. (1971) Comparison of post-operative stump management: Plaster v soft dressings. *J. Bone Joint Surg.*, **53A**, 241–249

Murdoch, G. (1975) Below-knee amputation and its use in vascular disease and the elderly. 'Immediate' prosthetic fitting and early walking. *Recent Adv. Orthop.*, **2**, 152–172

Murdoch, G. (1984) Amputation revisited. *Prosth. Orthot. Int.*, **8**, 8–15

Murdoch, G., Condie, D.N., Gardner, D., Ramsay, E., Smith, A., Stewart, C.P.U., Swanson, A.J.G. and Troup I.M. (1988) The Dundee experience. In *Amputation Surgery and Lower Limb Prosthetics* (eds G. Murdoch and R.G. Donovan), Blackwell Scientific, Edinburgh, pp. 440–457

Pedersen, H.E. (1968) The problems of the geriatric amputee. *Artif. Limbs*, **12**, (part 2), i–iii

Redhead, R.G. and Snowdon, C. (1978) A new approach to the management of wounds of the extremities: controlled environment and its derivatives. *Prosthet. Orthot. Int.*, **2**, 148–156

Review of Artificial Limb and Appliance Centre Services (1986) Vol II – *Annexes to the report of an independent working party* (Chairman: McColl). DHSS, London, 1

Robinson, K.P. (1972) Long posterior flap amputation in geriatric patients with ischaemic disease. Review of experience in 1967–71. *Lancet*, **i**, 193–195

Sarmiento, A. and Warren, W.D. (1969) A re-evaluation of lower extremity amputations. *Surg. Gynec. Obstet.*, **140**, 800–802

Scottish Health Service (1989) *Outcomes of artificial lower limb fitting in Scotland*, Health Service Research Reports, ISD Publications, Edinburgh

Spence, V.A. and Walker, W.F. (1984) The relationship between temperature isotherms and skin blood flow in the ischaemic limb. *J. Surg. Res.*, **36**, 278–281

Steen Jensen, J. (1988) Surgery, including transcondylar and supracondylar procedures. In *Amputation Surgery and Lower Limb Prosthetics* (eds G. Murdoch and R.G. Donovan), Blackwell Scientific, Edinburgh, pp. 181–186

Taylor, G.G and Monro, R. (1952) The technique and management of the 'hindquarter' amputation. *Br. J. Surg.*, **39**, 536–541

Travers, A.F. (1991) Ramps and rails. *Br. Med. J.*, **302**, 951–954

Wagner, F.W. (1977) Amputation of the foot and ankle: current status. *Clin. Orthop.*, **122**, 62–69

Waters, R.L. Perry, J., Antonelli, D. and Hislop, H. (1976) Energy cost of walking amputees: the influence of level of amputation. *J. Bone Joint Surg.*, **58A**, 42–46

10

Metabolic bone disease

David L. Douglas

Metabolic bone disease is a major problem in the elderly and may be associated with a significant morbidity. This chapter will concentrate on the three commonest types of this condition namely, osteoporosis, Paget's disease of bone and osteomalacia. These disorders of skeletal metabolism often cause pain, deformity or fracture and many patients present to an orthopaedic surgeon at the point of skeletal failure. Treatment is then aimed at addressing the immediate problem. In osteoporosis the underlying skeletal loss may be irreversible but medical treatments for Paget's disease and osteomalacia are very beneficial.

Composition of bone

Bone consists of cells, mineral and the organic matrix. The marrow cavity contains blood vessels and nerves and cells of the haemopoietic system.

Bone cells

There are at least three main types of bone cells – osteoblasts, osteoclasts and osteocytes – and there is a complex relationship between these and other marrow cells.

Osteoblasts and osteoclasts are responsible for bone formation and resorption respectively. Since bone mass changes little in comparison with the turnover of bone these processes must be very closely interrelated. The serum activity of alkaline phosphatase reflects in part the functional activity of osteoblasts. Osteoclasts produce lysosomal enzymes, e.g. acid phosphatase,

which release hydroxyproline as the bone collagen is resorbed. The urinary excretion of hydroxyproline thus partly reflects the rate of bone resorption. Recent advances allow for the measurement of deoxypyridine derived from the cross-links in the collagen molecule which is a more accurate indicator of bone resorption than hydroxyproline.

The extracellular matrix

The extracellular matrix of bone consists of mineral, collagen, water and non-collagenous proteins. Bone mineral is a crystalline analogue of the naturally occurring mineral hydroxyapatite.

The osteoid, the unmineralized part of the bone matrix consists of 90% collagen and 10% non-collagenous proteins.

Calcium homoeostasis

The skeleton contains 98% of the body's calcium and serum calcium is maintained within a range of 2.2–2.6 mmol/l. The serum concentration is normally controlled by regulation of calcium transport in the gut and kidneys. In health, the fluxes of calcium into and out of the skeleton are equal at skeletal maturity. The three hormones principally involved in calcium homoeostasis are parathyroid hormone (PTH). calcitriol (1,25-dihydroxycholecalciferol or 1,25 $(OH)_2D_3$) and to a lesser extent calcitonin.

Other hormones such as oestrogen, growth hormone, cortisol and thyroxine also affect calcium metabolism but their secretion is not regulated by changes in serum calcium.

Table 10.1   Causes of osteoporosis

Primary (idiopathic)
  Elderly
  Post-menopausal

Secondary
  Immobilization or paralysis
  Oophorectomy and/or hysterectomy
  Thyrotoxicosis
  Drugs (long-term corticosteroids or thyroxine)
  Cushing's syndrome
  Rheumatoid arthritis
  Malabsorption (post-gastrectomy or coeliac disease)
  Primary biliary cirrhosis (often associated with some osteomalacia)
  Alcoholic liver disease

Parathyroid hormone is secreted by the parathyroid glands in response to hypocalcaemia. It acts directly on the kidney to increase renal tubular resorption of calcium, increase skeletal turnover and may increase serum calcium. Parathyroid hormone also stimulates renal 1-hydroxylase which converts 25-hydroxycholecalciferol (25-OH D_3) to 1,25 $(OH)_2D_3$, the active metabolite of vitamin D. Thus, parathyroid hormone indirectly increases active transport of calcium across the small intestine.

Cholecalciferol (the natural form of vitamin D in man) is made from precursors produced by the action of sunlight on the skin. Ergocalciferol, the natural form in plants and fortified foods may also be taken. In the liver it is converted to 25-OH D_3 and in the kidney it is further converted to 1,25 $(OH)_2D_3$ under the control of parathyroid hormone and other factors. 1,25 $(OH)_2D_3$ should be regarded as a hormone rather than a vitamin.

Calcitonin is produced in the thyroid gland by the 'C' cells. Its exact role is not defined, but in pharmacological doses it inhibits bone resorption. Medullary carcinoma of the thyroid may secrete large amounts of calcitonin but causes little change in skeletal metabolism.

Specific examples of metabolic bone diseases

Osteoporosis

Osteoporosis is characterized by a decrease in bone mass per anatomical unit of bone and is associated with an increased risk of fracture principally in sites of cancellous bone such as the wrist, spine and hip. As described in chapter 1 the incidence of hip fracture has doubled over the last 30 years in the United Kingdom and may reach 71 000 per year in 1996 and 117 000 per year by 2016. Hip fractures are increasing not just in the elderly but in all age groups and represent a major cause of morbidity. Their mortality rate is 20–30% within 6 months and they have been estimated to cost the UK approximately £500 million per annum. Causes of osteoporosis are listed in Table 10.1 with the commonest being old age and post-menopausal osteoporosis. Bone mass peaks at about the age of 30 years and thereafter it gradually reduces. This loss is slow at first and more rapid later until a man of 80 years may have only half the bone mineral he had when aged 30 years. Additionally, women have a lower peak bone mass and experience an acceleration of bone loss starting as oestrogen levels decline before the menopause and continuing for about 10 years after it (Figure 10.1). This places women at a much greater risk of fracture due to osteoporosis than men.

Aetiology

The aetiology of osteoporosis is complex. It may be due to increased bone resorption with a failure of bone formation to keep up due to impaired osteoblast function. One model for age-related bone loss is shown in Figure 10.2.

Impaired calcium absorption may result from decreased renal 1α-hydroxylase activity and intestinal resistance to 1,25 $(OH)_2D_3$. The decreased serum calcium then stimulates release of parathyroid hormone resulting in increased bone resorption. However, impaired osteoblast function fails to redress the balance and the net result is a decrease in bone mass.

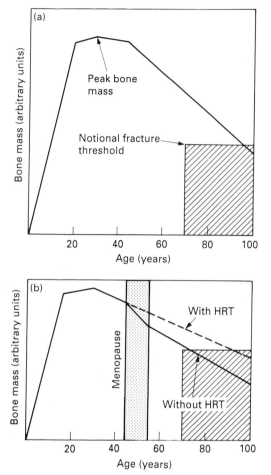

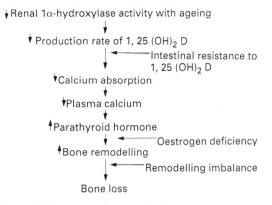

Figure 10.2 A suggested mechanism for age-related bone loss. (Eastell and Riggs, 1987 with permission of the publishers)

Figure 10.1 Total bone mass in men (a) and women (b). Males develop a bigger skeleton during their years of growth, have a higher peak bone mass and usually only cross the notional fracture threshold in old age. Females have a smaller skeleton, lower peak bone mass, suffer accelerated bone loss around the menopause and tend to cross the fracture threshold usually in their 70s.
HRT = hormone replacement therapy (from Dixon, 1991)

Prevalence and clinical presentation

In the absence of a single specific marker for osteoporosis, prevalence has to be measured by the number of osteoporosis-related fractures. Crush fractures of the spine are generally recognized as osteoporotic and other fractures in this category include those in the distal radius, proximal humerus and hip.

Males are affected in the ratio of one man to every 10 women. Osteoporosis in females is post-menopausal or idiopathic in all but 20%. In contrast, in men an underlying cause is present in more than 50% and should be sought.

Spinal osteoporosis

The first vertebrae to collapse are usually those of the lower dorsal or upper lumbar regions. One wedged vertebra is a not uncommon finding in routine radiographs performed on elderly individuals who do not necessarily volunteer a history of either pain or a fall. Two or more wedged vertebrae suggests osteoporosis. When the collapse is acute, there is marked tenderness localized to the fracture site but pain may be more diffuse and symmetrical and may radiate to the front of the body or lower limbs depending on the vertebral level. All movements including coughing may be painful. There is no neurological impairment although testing for straight leg raising may exacerbate the pain. The physical signs may mimic in part a prolapsed intervertebral disc and the differential diagnosis includes other causes of acute spinal collapse, chiefly metastatic disease and myeloma.

Untreated spinal osteoporosis leads to a series of crushed and wedged vertebral bodies with spinal shrinkage and kyphosis. Up to 25 cm of height may be lost. The classic picture is of an elderly woman with a smooth thoracic kyphosis, difficulty in holding her head up, a relatively short trunk compared to her legs or arm span, 'concertina creases' around a protruding abdomen and loss of space between the lower rib margin and the pelvic brim. Breathlessness and symptoms of hiatus hernia reflect the cramping of the viscera in the reduced thoracic and abdominal cavities. Spinal pain although not always a feature is usually dominant. It may arise from continued vertebral microfractures and collapse, from strains on ligaments and posterior spinal joints caused by the altered body shape and possibly from obstruction and congestion of spinal and nerve root venous plexi (Dixon, 1991). Pain can also arise from impingement of the ribs against the pelvic brim. On occasion osteoporosis may be associated with an element of osteomalacia.

Osteoporosis at other skeletal sites

Other important locations for osteoporosis include the hip, shoulder and wrist, and further details can be found in chapters 12–14.

Radiographs

These will show a loss of bone trabeculae and cortical thinning but provide only a subjective estimate of bone density. This can be assessed objectively with single photon absorptiometry, dual photon absorptiometry and quantitative computed tomography scans. The recent development of dual energy X-ray absorptiometry (DEXA) is promising, particularly as a screening procedure as it gives a more reproducible and quicker measurement (Wahner, 1989).

Biochemistry

Serum calcium (which should be corrected for serum albumin) may be normal or low and serum alkaline phosphatase may be normal or slightly raised especially in the event of a recent fracture. In elderly patients the alkaline phosphatase may be elevated for no obvious reason. Serum phosphate is usually normal (Wilton *et al.*, 1987b).

Bone biopsy

This will show reduced trabecular bone mass and signs of a decreased rate of bone formation.

Treatment

The best form of treatment is prevention, i.e. to prevent bone mass decreasing to such an extent that fractures ensue. This option is not usually available in the elderly when the bone mass has already fallen below the fracture threshold. There is evidence in younger patients that hormone replacement therapy (HRT) with combined low dose oestrogen and progesterone decreases the rate of post-menopausal bone loss (Riggs and Melton, 1986; Lindsay, 1988). In

elderly women with an intact uterus cyclical hormone therapy is unacceptable. Furthermore, these elderly women only first present to a physician or surgeon when they are symptomatic with fractures, by which time their bone density has fallen so low that measures simply aimed at decreasing bone loss will be inadequate. Therefore, apart from treatment aimed at their presenting complaint (femoral neck fracture, Colles' fracture, vertebral collapse, etc.) they would also benefit from treatment to increase bone mass. In a recent article the available medical treatments have been discussed (Smith, 1990). Unfortunately there is no treatment which has been shown in the long term to reverse this age-related bone loss. Initial results of fluoride treatment were encouraging (Mamelle *et al.*, 1988) but recent results are disappointing (Riggs *et al.*, 1990). Anabolic steroids such as stanozolol may be effective but have a high incidence of unwanted side effects (Chestnut *et al.*, 1983). More recently etidronate, the original bisphosphonate, has shown early promise (Storm *et al.*, 1990; Watts *et al.*, 1990). However, it must be stated that there there is no conclusive evidence that these therapeutic regimens significantly decrease the fracture rate.

Treatment of fractures is based on prompt internal fixation to facilitate early mobilization and so obviate the complications associated with prolonged bed-rest in the elderly. Because osteoporotic bone is weak the internal fixation devices may cut out (Mainds and Newman, 1989) and several implants have been specially developed for stabilizing fractures through porotic bone. These include Partridge plates and bands and Gallanough plates applied to the side of a long bone to accept the tips of screws. The addition of methylmethacrylate cement to augment fixation is a useful technique and is described in detail in Chapter 11. In general, however, intramedullary devices are preferable to screws and plates for fractures of osteoporotic long bones.

The management of established osteoporosis also includes advice regarding smoking and alcohol consumption as well as the importance of the elderly walking outside in the sunshine. Regular corticosteroids should be reduced to the lowest effective dose or completely withdrawn if possible and all patients on thyroid supplementation should undergo regular blood checks to see if the dose can be reduced. Weight bearing exercises are beneficial at any age but because of the other accompaniments of old age may not always be appropriate or possible in the elderly. Adaptations to the home may improve independence and the National Osteoporosis Society can provide appropriate advice to affected individuals.

Osteomalacia

In the United Kingdom the individuals most at risk from osteomalacia are the elderly and Asian immigrants. This is due to a combination of factors including poor diet and lack of sunshine leading to reduced levels of 25-hydroxycholecalciferol. Malabsorption, renal failure and long-term anticonvulsant therapy are also associated with an increased risk.

Diagnosis

In the adult the features of osteomalacia are those of bone pain, bone tenderness and proximal myopathy. Fractures either in the form of pseudofractures or complete fractures are common.

Radiographs

There may be a generalized reduction in bone density and a chest X-ray may show pathological rib fractures. Deformities of the spine and pelvis may occur due to softening but this happens only in long-standing cases.

Defects in the cortical bone

Transverse translucent bands up to 1 cm in width and often symmetrical (Looser's zones) are characteristically seen in the medial femoral cortex, the pubic ramus, the ribs, the scapula or ulna (Figure 10.3).

Technetium bone scan may show multiple areas of increased uptake which can be confused with metastases.

Biochemistry

This depends on the underlying cause of the condition.

In nutritional vitamin D deficiency, the serum calcium and phosphate are usually low and the serum alkaline phosphatase is raised. Serum 25-OH D_3 levels are low.

The value of screening elderly patients with femoral neck fractures for osteomalacia has

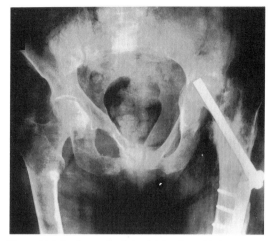

Figure 10.3 Radiograph of the pelvis of an elderly woman with osteomalacia. The diagnosis was missed when she underwent internal fixation for a fractured left femoral neck several years earlier. Looser's zones can be seen in the right subtrochanteric region and right superior pubic ramus

been studied (Wilton *et al.*, 1987a and b). Serum alkaline phosphatase was found to be raised on presentation in up to 23% of normal patients but was normal in those cases of only mild osteomalacia. Serum calcium corrected for albumin was low in 25% of normal patients and was normal in mild cases of osteomalacia. Similarly, serum phosphate was a poor pointer for the condition. The authors concluded that bone biopsy should be performed in those patients who have both low serum calcium (corrected) and raised alkaline phosphatase since this would detect 43% of all osteomalacia (the more severe cases in whom difficulties might arise) and would reduce the need for bone biopsy to 9.5% of the elderly fracture population. Frozen section technique (Wilton *et al.*, 1987a) enables treatment to be started immediately post-operatively.

Early reports of elderly patients presenting with hip fractures suggested an incidence of osteomalacia as high as 30% (Jenkins *et al.*, 1973; Aaron *et al.*, 1974), but in a recent unselected study of more than 1000 patients the true incidence was only 2% (Wilton *et al.*, 1987a). Hip fractures associated with osteomalacia seem therefore to be uncommon but they are associated with a higher risk of surgical complications and mortality than those associated with osteoporosis alone (Chalmers, 1967).

Bone biopsy

Bone biopsy which shows greatly increased amounts of unmineralized osteoid confirms the diagnosis. Undecalcified specimens which display seams with five or more osteoid lamellae or an osteoid area above 5% and a surface extent of osteoid greater than 25% are considered diagnostic of osteomalacia (Wilton *et al.*, 1987a).

Management

MEDICAL TREATMENT

This depends on the underlying cause. In dietary osteomalacia, the stores of vitamin D can be replenished using physiological amounts of ergocalciferol given orally. In malabsorption much higher doses are required and are not always effective. $1,25 (OH)_2D_3$ (calcitriol) or 1α-hydroxycholecalciferol should be prescribed daily with regular checks made of serum calcium and alkaline phosphatase. The calcium often remains low for several weeks but an increase in alkaline phosphatase is seen (the 'flare') which heralds the healing of osteomalacia. Iatrogenic hypercalcaemia is a risk to be avoided and at that stage the dose should be reduced until the serum calcium is normal.

In the confused patient, ergocalciferol may be given as a single intramuscular injection.

SURGICAL TREATMENT

Fractures associated with osteomalacia are often difficult and fixation devices are apt to cut out (Figure 10.4). Additional external support may be necessary in the form of splints while the underlying biochemical abnormality is treated. In the case of long bone fractures intramedullary devices are preferable to plates and screws.

Paget's disease of bone

Paget's disease of bone takes its name from Sir James Paget who in 1877 described a focal disease of bone which he termed 'osteitis deformans'. Increased bone resorption and formation result in characteristic histological, radiological and biochemical changes.

The aetiology of the disease is unknown but the recent detection of inclusion particles in the osteoclast nuclei led to the implication of a slow viral infective process related to measles, paramyxovirus or respiratory syncytial virus. The

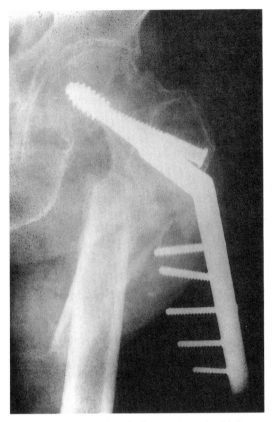

Figure 10.4 Radiographs of a fractured proximal left femur which began as a subcapital fracture treated by Garden screws and which progressed to fracture through the lower screw hole. This has been treated by a Richard's screw and plate which also failed. The patient subsequently died

disease affects the right lower limb twice as often as the left leading to the suggestion that trauma is a possible contributory factor.

Histological features

The osteoclasts are enlarged and the nuclei more numerous than usual. Increased resorption and formation of bone leads to a characteristic mosaic pattern of lamellar bone with increased vascular markings. Three phases have been described – osteolytic, mixed and sclerotic (fibrotic) – and these may overlap.

Radiology and scintigraphy

Osteolytic phase A flame-shaped osteolytic front may be seen advancing along a long bone at approximately 10–30 mm per year or radiating outwards as osteoporosis circumscripta in the skull. Softening may produce bowing, platybasia, protrusio acetabuli and greenstick or avulsion fractures. Bone scans using technetium-99 labelled diphosphonates are usually positive at an earlier stage and show more Pagetoid foci than radiographs.

Mixed phase The skull may assume a 'cotton wool' appearance and the vertebrae appear like 'window frames'. Enlargement of bone is a useful diagnostic feature of Paget's disease.

Sclerotic phase Radiographs show increased bone density and trabecular and cortical thickening. Bone scans may be normal in this stage.

Biochemical features

Common biochemical markers of increased bone turnover are increased serum alkaline phosphatase, which reflects osteoblastic activity and urinary peptide-bound hydroxyproline, which largely reflects osteoclastic resorption.

Other enzymes derived from bone cells such as acid phosphatase may also be increased.

Calcium metabolism Despite increased bone turnover (up to 40–50 times normal) serum calcium and phosphate remain in the normal range indicating a fine homoeostatic control. However, this control may fail in the immobilized patient especially after a fracture when hypercalciuria and hypercalcaemia occur because of the imbalance between bone resorption and formation.

Parathyroid hormone A few reports have suggested that there may be an increased incidence of hypercalcaemia due to hyperparathyroidism in Paget's disease though this could be coincidental.

Uric acid Serum uric acid is elevated in 30% of patients possibly reflecting increased nucleic acid breakdown.

Clinical features

Deformity This is common and may be seen as enlargement of the skull and bowing of the long bones.

Fracture Fracture is the most frequent presenting orthopaedic complication.

Incomplete or fissure fractures are often seen arising perpendicular to the convex side of long bones. The defect may progress to a complete fracture though more often fissure fractures remain asymptomatic. Increasing pain may herald progression to a complete fracture. Fissure fractures probably arise as a result of the bowing (rather than the cause of it) and 50% of the complete fractures occur after little or no trauma. The femur is affected twice as often as the tibia with the commonest site being the subtrochanteric region followed by the middle third of the shaft. Radiographs show a characteristic sharp edge to the fracture which is often transverse. There is an increased risk of delayed or non-union especially in subcapital femoral fractures where the non-union rate is 75%. Refracture may occur in 10% of fractures after apparent healing and avulsion fractures may occur at tendon insertions, usually during the osteolytic phase.

NEUROLOGICAL COMPLICATIONS

These are usually due to nerve compression though other factors may be contributory. Paget's disease of the skull may give rise to lesions of any of the cranial nerves but deafness is the most common neurological disturbance affecting up to 50% of patients with skull involvement. It is commonly of the mixed sensori-neural type and is produced by a combination of temporal bone distortion, invasion of the peri-lymphatic space by inflammatory cells, distortion of the bony wall by Pagetic osteoid and, occasionally, by fixation of the stapes and compression of the eighth cranial nerve in the internal auditory meatus.

Other cranial nerve lesions are uncommon. Blindness may be due to narrowing of the optic foramen giving rise to papilloedema and optic atrophy. Loss of vision may also be due to retinal artery occlusion, retinal haemorrhage and choreoretinal changes (e.g. angioid streaks).

Platybasia and invagination of the base of the skull by the cervical vertebrae are not always associated with neurological complications, but when they occur they may be serious causing vertebrobasilar insufficiency, hydrocephalus, cerebellar herniation, ataxia or lower cranial nerve lesions. The spine is commonly affected by Paget's disease with one or more vertebrae affected. A paraspinal mass of partially calcified osteoid may produce a soft tissue shadow on

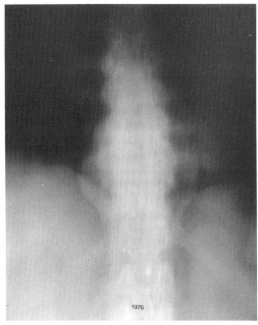

Figure 10.5 A paraspinal mass due to unmineralized osteoid in Paget's disease of the 9th, 10th and 11th thoracic vertebrae associated with paraparesis

radiographs though most patients with disease affecting the spine are symptomless (Figure 10.5). Occasionally, changes in bone lead to spinal cord or nerve root dysfunction and very occasionally quadriplegia occurs. More usually, disease of the thoracic or lumbar spine gives rise to paraparesis, cauda equina syndrome or radiculopathy. Although compression of the cord by the expanded vertebrae can usually be demonstrated by myelography, occasionally paraparesis may present with a normal myelogram. It has been suggested that spinal cord dysfunction is due to a vascular steal syndromes – blood being diverted from the cord to the highly vascular adjacent vertebrae (Douglas *et al.*, 1981). The usual history is that of slowly progressive numbness and weakness over many years finally leading to loss of sphincter control and spasticity in the lower limbs.

OSTEOARTHROSIS

Whether Paget's disease leads to osteoarthritic changes in adjacent joints or not is controversial. Certainly in elderly patients osteoarthrosis of the hip and the knee is commonly seen in association with Paget's disease.

PAGET'S SARCOMA

Most osteosarcomas which develop in later life are associated with Paget's disease but malignant change occurs in less than 1% of all patients with the disease. Fifty percent of the tumours are osteosarcomas, 25% fibrosarcomas and 25% giant cell sarcomas and other unspecified types of tumours. The commonest site is the femur followed by the humerus. The tumour may present as a swelling (especially of the skull), as increasing bone pain or as fracture.

The prognosis of Paget's sarcoma is poor, worse than that for osteosarcoma or fibrosarcoma not associated with Paget's disease. The mean survival is approximately 1 year with only 5% of patients alive after 5 years.

HYPERCALCAEMIA

This may occur if a patient with very active or extensive Paget's disease is immobilized as may occur after a fracture.

High output cardiac failure is also a recognized complicating clinical feature of this condition.

Differential diagnosis

When the classic clinical, radiological and biochemical abnormalities are present the diagnosis is usually not in doubt. Histological difficulty arises in some cases in differentiating Pagetoid bone from hyperthyroidism or fibrous dysplasia. The demonstration of inclusion particles in the osteoclast by electron microscopy is virtually pathognomonic of Paget's disease.

Clinically and radiologically it may be difficult to differentiate Paget's disease from prostatic metatases or tuberculosis of the spine and in doubtful cases X-ray guided biopsy is essential. In those cases where the pelvis is involved a suitable transiliac sample can be obtained under local anaesthesia using as Meunier-type trephine.

Management

MEDICAL TREATMENT

Non-steroidal anti-inflammatory drugs and simple analgesics are important for pain relief.

Human, porcine and salmon calcitonin have been used to treat Paget's disease successfully but side effects include nausea and flushing.

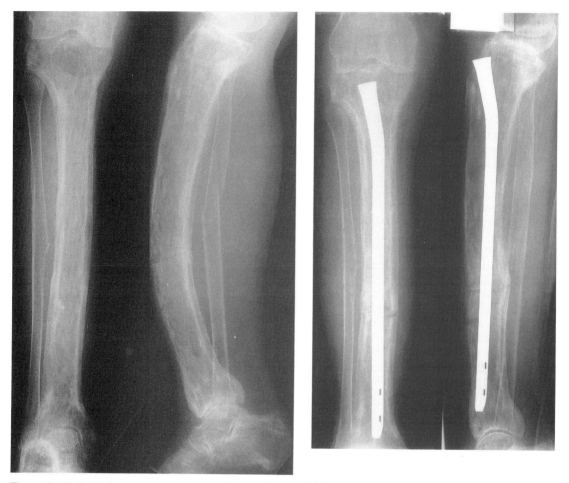

Figure 10.6 (Left) Radiographs showing marked bowing of the tibia in Paget's disease with stress fractures. (Right) Osteosynthesis by means of a closing anteriorly-based wedge osteotomy was subsequently performed with intramedullary internal fixation to correct the deformity and relieve the pain

Diphosphonates or bisphosphonates decrease bone resorption by a direct inhibition of osteoclast function and may suppress bone turnover for months or years. A complication of etidronate, the most commercially available diphosphonate, is that it may cause a mineralization defect. This has not been seen in the subsequent and more potent generations of diphosphonates.

SURGICAL TREATMENT

At operation Pagetoid bone may be hard, soft or normal. Soft bone may not engage screws requiring a Gallannaugh plate to be applied to the opposite cortex to engage the screw tips. Sclerotic bone may be so hard that it is almost impossible to drill or ream or so brittle that it explodes on hammering or reaming. Excessive haemorrhage from active Pagetoid bone may also occur.

Correction of deformity Correction may be required because the deformity is gross and unsightly or because there is severe bone pain. Osteotomy and osteosynthesis can reduce the deformity and also relieve the pain (Figure 10.6). When tibial bowing is associated with osteoarthrosis of the medial compartment of the knee, the pain can be relieved by proximal tibial osteotomy which also corrects the varus deformity.

Surgery for correction of facial bone deformity is rarely indicated and treatment with bisphosphates produces bony remodelling (Bickerstaff *et al.*, 1990).

Management of fractures Initially, the pain from incomplete or fissure fractures (pseudo-fractures) should be treated by a trial of medical management. This can be supplemented, particularly in the management of tibial fractures, with a cast brace or if long-term treatment is considered, weight relieving calipers. If these conservative measures fail or there is progression of the pseudofracture on serial radiographs, consideration should be given to internal fixation by intramedullary nailing.

Complete fractures Treatment of a complete fracture presents the surgeon with an opportunity to correct any pre-existing deformity so reducing the risk of subsequent fracture recurrence. Conservative treatment may be satisfactory but, in elderly patients, prolonged immobilization may lead to hypercalcaemia, bronchopneumonia, deep venous thrombosis, confusion, pressure sores and joint stiffness. Delayed internal fixation is associated with a greater risk of non-union than early internal fixation. In general, the same indications for internal fixation of fractures not associated with Paget's disease apply to patients with the condition.

Subcapital fractures of the femur are a special case because non-union rates are 75% when internal fixation is used. Primary prosthetic replacement of the femoral head is therefore recommended.

Insertion of a nail-plate for trochanteric or subtrochanteric fractures can produce an intra-operative subcapital fracture on hammering in the nail and therefore the use of a dynamic hip screw and plate of the Richard's or AO type is preferable.

Neurological complications Surgical treatment of spinal cord compression reverses neurological changes in 80% of cases. Decompressive laminectomy may need to be extensive and signs and symptoms may recur postoperatively. Occasionally the paraparesis may extend to complete paraplegia following operation. Sudden paraparesis or paraplegia suggest collapse of a vertebra and represents a surgical emergency. In most cases the neurological signs are slowly progressive and medical treatment is preferable – the results are at least as good as those obtained by surgery. Improvement is usually seen within days or weeks of starting

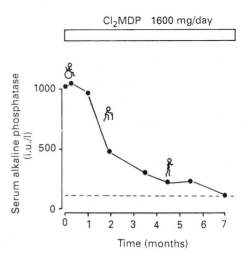

Figure 10.7 The biochemical response to oral dichloro-methylene bisphosphonate in a patient with paraparesis due to Paget's disease of the spine. The muscle power returned to the lower limbs within 2 weeks of starting treatment

treatment. Complete or almost complete recovery can be expected in most patients (Figure 10.7). Long-term follow-up is required with immediate retreatment at the first sign of relapse. A rise in serum alkaline phosphatase or urinary hydroxyproline precedes the clinical deterioration.

Complications of Paget's disease of the skull are amenable to neurosurgery such as relief of hydrocephalus or acute brain stem compression.

Osteoarthrosis Treatment of this condition is along established lines. Occasionally it may be difficult to differentiate between bone pain and joint pain and a 3-month course of medical treatment may determine the source of the pain. If surgery becomes necessary excessive bleeding may be avoided if the patient undergoes prior medical treatment.

Osteoarthrosis of the hip can be treated by total joint arthroplasty though there may be technical difficulties if the femoral shaft is deformed. With the increased bone turnover in Paget's disease there is a theoretical risk of loosening or migration of the prosthesis, though this has not been reported.

Patients with osteoarthrosis of the knee and varus deformity may be helped by proximal tibial osteotomy or total knee replacement if the arthritic changes are extensive.

References

Aaron, J.E., Gallagher, J.C., Anderson, J. *et al.* (1974) Frequency of osteomalacia and osteoporosis in fractures of the proximal femur. *Lancet*, **i**, 229–233

Bickerstaff, D.R., Douglas, D.L., Burke, P.H., O'Doherty, D.P. and Kanis J.A. (1990) Improvement in the deformity of the face in Paget's disease treated with diphosphonates. *J. Bone Joint Surg.*, **72B**, 132–1336

Chalmers, J., Conacher, W.D.H., Gardner, D.L. and Scott P.J. (1967) Osteomalacia: a common disease in elderly women. *J. Bone Joint Surg.*, **49B**, 403–423

Chestnut, C.H. III, Ivey, J.L., Gruber, H.E. *et al.* (1983) Stanozolol in postmenopausal osteoporosis: therapeutic efficiency and possible mechanisms of action. *Metabolism*, **32**, 571–580

Dixon, A. St J. (1991) Osteoporosis and the family doctor. *Reports on rheumatic diseases* (*series 2*). Arthritis and Rheumatism Council, 41 Eagle St, London, No. 17

Douglas, D.L., Duckworth, T., Kanis, J.A., Jefferson, A.A., Martin T.J. and Russell, R.G.G. (1981) Spinal cord dysfunction in Paget's disease of bone. Has medical treatment a vascular basis? *J. Bone Joint Surg.*, **63B**, 495–503

Eastell, R. and Riggs, B.L. (1987) Calcium homeostasis and osteoporosis. In *Endocrinology and Metabolism Clinics of North America*, W.B. Saunders, London, Philadelphia, Toronto, **16**, 829–842.

Jenkins, D.M.R., Roberts, J.G., Webster, D. and Williams E.O. (1973) Osteomalacia in elderly patients with fracture of the surgical neck: a clinico-pathological study. *J. Bone Joint Surg.*, **55B**, 575–580

Lindsay, R. (1988) Management of osteoporosis. *Baillière's Clin. Endocrinol Metab.*, **2**, 103–104

Mainds, C.C. and Newman, R.J. (1989) Implant failures in patients with proximal femoral fractures treated with a sliding screw device. *Injury*, **20**, 98–100

Mamelle, N., Meunier, P.J., Dusan, R. *et al.* (1988) Risk-benefit ratio of sodium fluoride treatment in primary vertebral osteoporosis. *Lancet*, **ii**, 361–365

Riggs, B.L. and Melton, L.J. (1986) Involutional osteoporosis. *N. Engl. J. Med.*, 1676–1686

Riggs, B.L., Hodgson, S.F., O'Fallon, W.M., *et al.* (1990) Effect of fluoride treatment on the fracture rate in postmenopausal women with osteoporosis. *N. Engl. J. Med.*, **322**, 802–809

Smith, R. (1990) Osteoporosis after 60. Advice needs to be individual. *Br. Med. J.*, **301**, 452–453

Storm, T., Thamsborg, G., Steiniche, T., Genant, H.K. and Sorensen, O.H. (1990) Effect of intermittent cyclical etidromate therapy on bone mass and fracture rate in women with postmenopausal osteoporosis. *N. Engl. J. Med.*, **322**, 1265–1271

Wahner, H.W. (1989) Measurements of bone mass and bone density. *Endocrinol Metabol. Clin. N. Am.*, **18**, 995–1012.

Watts, N.B., Harris, S.T., Gerant, H.K. *et al.* (1990) Intermittent cyclinal etidronate treatment of postmenopausal osteoporosis. *N. Engl. J. Med.*, **323**, 73–79.

Wilton, T.J., Hosking, D.J., Pawley, E., Stevens, A. and Harvey, L. (1987a) Osteomalacia and femoral neck fractures in the elderly patient. *J. Bone Joint Surg.*, **69B**, 388–390

Wilton, T.J., Hosking, D.J., Pawley, E., Stevens, A. and Harvey, L. (1987b) Screening for osteomalacia in elderly patients with femoral neck fractures. *J. Bone Joint Surg.*, **69B**, 765–768.

11

Principles of fracture management in elderly patients

Dietmar Pennig

Introduction

Fractures of the skeleton occur in childhood, adolescence, adult life and old age and the principles of treatment differ radically in each age group.

It is a common observation that elderly people today assume a more active role in life and maintain a higher level of activity than their parents and grandparents. This in turn must lead to an increased exposure to conditions in which accidents and bony injuries may occur. Furthermore, the current demands on our trauma services are increasing by the decade. For example, demographic data in Germany reveal that whereas in 1880 only 5% of the population were 65 years or older, only 100 years later it is now more than 15% (Friedel, 1985). These observations when taken together explain why fewer than 60% of adult males aged 60–69 years held a driving licence in 1976 and a recent estimate indicates that this figure will rise to more than 80% by the year 2000. Similarly, more than 50% of all pedestrians killed in road traffic accidents are aged 65 years or more (Friedel, 1985). In Sweden the elderly account for only 16% of the population but they account for 27% of fatal injuries (Voigt and Ottosson, 1985). Similar statistics have been produced in the United States (Oreskowich et al., 1984). The more common isolated injuries in the elderly seem to affect the femoral neck, the distal radius, the proximal humerus but the pattern in multiple injuries involves the head, tibia, chest and pelvis (Oreskowich et al., 1984; Friedel, 1985).

The fact that bones of elderly patients fracture more readily when compared with those of their younger counterparts is explained by the age-related development of osteoporosis. The endosteal bone cylinder decreases in volume and though some periosteal bone apposition occurs the overall balance is negative (Heuck, 1979; Lane and Vigorita, 1983). This can be observed in all long bones and is particularly obvious in the femur. In the metaphyseal area rarefication of the cancellous trabeculae leads to a reduced resistance to strain. The grading of osteoporosis in the proximal femur can be assisted by the classification suggested by Singh, Nagrath and Maini (1970). In cases of severe osteoporosis (Grades 1–3) in the proximal femur difficulties of implant anchorage can be expected to occur in the metaphyseal region of other bones as well.

Fractures in elderly patients unite in the same time as they do in a 30-year-old person (Devas, 1977; Moran, Gibson and Cross, 1990). The healing process per se does not therefore require any special treatment and good fracture alignment and the speedy restoration of mobility are the prime objectives of good fracture management in the elderly. When choosing an operative procedure the osteoporotic changes described have to be taken into account since the purchase of implants is affected by the thinning of the cortices and the rarefication of the trabeculae (Lane and Vigorita, 1983; Davis et al., 1990). These obvious and well-known difficulties however should not lead to a reluctance to employ operative methods when they are otherwise indicated in the patient's best interests. The aim is always to select a technique that is suitable for or adaptable to osteoporotic bone and also to take into account the possibility of reduced compliance in a certain proportion of elderly and sometimes confused patients.

120

General principles

Isolated injuries

Though sometimes difficult to obtain, a detailed history of the injury is necessary including the cause of the accident. It is obviously crucial for the calculation of the prognosis to establish whether it was a 'normal' fall or trip or one secondary to a medical condition such as postural hypotension or myocardial infarction. The overall prognosis obviously is poorer in the latter case. The management has to take this into account since the fall can be a sign of the impending dissolution of the patient. The clinical and radiological examination of the patient should consider that there may be more than one injury in an osteoporotic skeleton and the most likely sites have to be specifically looked at. In the management of long bone fractures it is mandatory that the two adjacent joints are X-rayed in all cases. Local factors including peripheral vascular disease or skin ulcers have to be noted since these will have a significant impact on surgical procedures in that anatomical area.

After establishing the cause and site of the fracture the next issue to address is the prognosis. For this the patient's domestic circumstances have to be known in order that appropriate arrangements can be made to facilitate the patient's subsequent discharge from hospital. A Colles' type fracture of the dominant wrist can temporarily preclude an early return to the normal life style of that individual and a painful though stable fracture of the neck of the humerus will make dressing and undressing impossible for the elderly patient. Similarly, the prescription of a non-weight bearing lower limb cast will render the patient immobile (Nankhonya, Turnbull and Newton, 1991). The routines of daily living are the 'key' to an older person's life and they have to be assessed very carefully in order to institute the most appropriate treatment. In general old people are used to and depend on their environment and can become easily lost and disoriented in any other place. An independent life at home is important when it comes to the quality of remaining life in these patients.

It is now generally accepted that the mortality of a fractured neck of femur is significantly reduced by operative treatment and chapter 12 describes this. The same principles can be advocated for those fractures of the lower extremity that if treated conservatively would require prolonged immobilization of the patient (the femoral shaft fracture being a prime example). Isolated fractures of long bones can be a life-threatening event to an elderly patient and should be appropriately treated.

The skeleton of an adolescent will remodel certain deformities in a number of years and axial malalignment – though obviously not desirable – can be at least partially compensated for. The joints of an elderly patient have been positioned in a certain way for perhaps 70 or more years and will have enormous difficulties in adjusting to axial malalignment secondary to imperfect fracture reduction.

Multiple trauma

The physiological response to major blunt trauma is less favourable in elderly patients (Oreskowich *et al.*, 1984; Voigt and Ottosson, 1985; Haeske–Seeberg, 1988) with the age-induced decrease in organ function with dehydration, the inadequate compensation for blood loss and the reduced immune response seemingly the key factors (Rehn, 1979; Pannike *et al.*, 1981; Albrecht, 1985; Kolbow *et al.*, 1985). Pre-existing illness demands a multi-disciplinary approach on the day of injury and during the postoperative phase. The complications most frequently encountered are pneumonia, pulmonary embolism, urinary tract infection and pressure sores (Friedebold and Wolff, 1986). The mortality may be as high as 46% in these patients (Waydhas, Nast-Kolb and Betz, 1985). Our own data show that patients aged 66 years and older account for 12% of a series of 755 multiple trauma victims and for 21% of the fatalities. In the 75 year and older age group three out of four patients died. The cause of death at autopsy was a head injury in 34% and haemorrhagic shock in 32%. In 24% late pulmonary complications led to a fatal outcome. Further analysis of the figures indicates that an increased likelihood of a fatal outcome after major blunt trauma can be identified in patients aged 56 years and above. This indicates that the high risk group starts at a younger age than previously anticipated (Haeske–Seeberg, 1988).

Skeletal injuries have a considerable impact on the possibility of a fatal outcome (Voigt and Ottosson, 1985). In 145 deaths in hospital in two groups of patients (younger and older than 65 years), the likelihood of a fatal outcome in cases with skeletal trauma as the main injury was considerably higher in patients aged 65 years and older. This indicates the significantly life-threatening element of skeletal injury. To only concentrate on head, chest and abdominal injuries will not assure survival in these patients.

Osteoporotic changes occur in the ribs as well as the long bones (Heuck, 1979), and the decreased elasticity of the rib cage more readily leads to rib fractures. The spectrum varies from simple cracks to an unstable chest with bilateral serial rib fractures and the focus of attention should be on the underlying pulmonary injury and the necessity to turn the patient frequently in bed for effective drainage and ventilation. Internal fixation of the rib fractures is controversial and there is no statistical evidence to support this aggressive surgical approach (Pennig *et al.*, 1990). The stabilization of spinal and long bone fractures in a way that allows movement and positioning of the patient in any desired way must be the surgical aim in treating chest injuries. It is unlikely that poor gas exchange is a function of rib fractures in a ventilated patient. In cases of non-ventilated patients with rib fractures pain-free breathing can be assisted by intercostal nerve blocks and the epidural or intrapleural installation of local anaesthetic agents (Knottenbelt *et al.*, 1991). This may avoid the development of pneumonia as a consequence of impaired breathing.

Since major blunt trauma is unlikely to occur in immobile patients one can therefore assume that a certain minimum activity level was present at the time of injury. It is also obvious that these patients possess their maximum physiological resources on day 1 and will benefit from early treatment (preferably on day 1) of their major injuries such as unstable pelvic and femoral fractures, open joints and compound fractures (Brug *et al.*, 1988; Pennig and Brug, 1989; Waydhas, Nast-Kolb and Betz, 1985). It is important that the stabilization of such injuries is performed using the most effective but least invasive procedures. In the later phase of the treatment after survival has been established, (day 6 and onwards), the main objective is rehabilitation. The odds for a full restoration of normal function have to be evaluated and bearing this and the necessity for rapid mobilization of the patient in mind, operative management of the associated but less severe injuries has to be considered. While a humeral shaft fracture as an isolated injury may be treated conservatively,

there is little sense in handling it this way in a patient who has to use a walking frame or crutches because of associated lower limb injuries (Figure 11.1).

In managing this type of patient both expertise in judgement and surgical skills are required. This generally makes involvement by a senior member of staff necessary if optimal outcome is to be achieved and the number and length of operative sessions are to be minimized. The speed of skeletal stabilization is important for patient survival and the quality of the surgery is the key for early and successful rehabilitation.

Injury patterns

Isolated fractures

The development of osteoporosis predisposes the distal radius, the proximal humerus, the olecranon, the supracondylar femur, the proximal and the distal tibia and the os calcis to fracture. A similar development leads to fractures of the spine. Depending on the forces involved most fractures show mild to moderate displacement with the exception of the olecranon where the triceps tends to pull the fragment apart. Shortening due to crushing of the cancellous bone is common and if the bone is subsequently distracted to its original length, a defect will usually occur. As a general principle, shortening can be tolerated when stabilizing the fracture provided axial alignment is maintained. A limb length discrepancy in the upper extremity is irrelevant. In the lower extremity it is easier to treat this with a shoe raise rather than performing a bone graft with a delay in weight bearing and possible non-union. However, this is not justified in intra-articular fractures with depression resulting in axial malalignment in the lower extremity (Schatzker and Tile, 1987). In the diaphyseal area, fractures tend to be spiral or long oblique thus creating large surfaces which tend to unite readily (Brug and Pennig, 1988). Compound injuries mainly occur in the tibial region and like most high velocity injuries may show marked comminution (Haeske-Seeberg, 1988). Table 11.1 displays the frequency of operative procedures in patients aged 70 years and over (Zimmermann, 1984). Fractures of the proximal femur account for more than 70% of all operations and the femur (distal to the lesser trochanter) is second with 16%. In the upper

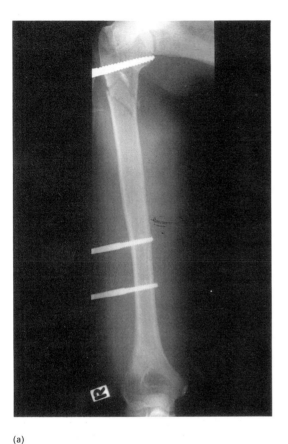
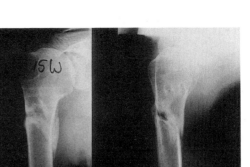

(a)   (b)

Figure 11.1 Closed unilateral external fixation in a displaced fracture of the proximal humerus allowing the use of crutches in a 66-year-old multiple trauma victim (a); periosteal bone healing with medial callus formation 15 weeks after the injury (b)

limb 57% involve the humerus (excluding supracondylar fractures) and the olecranon is second with 30%. More than 90% of the operations affect the lower extremity and in treating these fractures the main objective is the restoration of early mobility.

Multiple trauma

The majority of elderly multiple trauma victims are pedestrians knocked down by motor vehicles (Friedel, 1985; Haeske-Seeberg, 1988) and the head, chest and tibia are the most frequently affected regions (Friedel, 1985). Oreskovich *et al.* (1984) recorded surviving patient injuries of the central nervous system in 11% (non-survivors 20%), of the thorax/abdomen in 31% (non-survivors 33%) and of the extremities in 78% (non-survivors 75%). Only 6% of the surviving

patients were in shock compared with all of the non-survivors. Using the Injury Severity Score (ISS) (Baker *et al.*, 1974) elderly patients were found to die with lower ISS scores compared with the rest of the population (Oreskowich *et al.*, 1984; Friedel, 1985). The aged patient at risk is the one that is or goes into shock as well as those with head injuries. An unstable pelvis or more commonly an unstable femur plays a major role in the development of shock due to the massive blood loss caused by these injuries. Since the pelvis and extremities are injured most often in multiple trauma victims, treatment of these fractures in particular is an essential part of their resuscitation. This is of utmost importance with regard to the unstable pelvis. Every time the patient is moved, e.g. from the bed to an X-ray-table, the bleeding into the retroperitoneum may start again (Pennig and Brug, 1989). With an inadequate capacity for compensation

Table 11.1 Operative procedures in patients older than 70 years

Lower extremity (n = 275)	%
Femoral neck fracture	37.4
Pertrochanteric fracture	36.4
Subtrochanteric fracture	7.2
Femoral shaft fracture	5.5
Supracondylar fracture	3.3
Patellar fracture	2.9
Tibial plateau fracture	1.5
Tibial shaft fracture	2.5
Tibial pilon fracture	1.1
Ankle fracture	0.7
Others	1.5
Upper extremity (n = 30)	
Humeral fracture	56.6
Percondylar fracture	6.7
Fracture of the olecranon	30.0
Forearm fracture	6.7

Source: Zimmermann (1984)

for blood loss, the elderly patient might pass into shock and the chances for a fatal outcome thereby increase. The initial stages in the management must therefore focus on the stabilization of pelvis, femur, open joints and compound fractures. This subsequently provides the intensive care physician with a patient that can be turned, moved and mobilized as required to improve the investigation and management of the central nervous and the pulmonary systems.

Complications following trauma

Precautions

Prophylaxis against deep venous thrombosis is recommended for all patients requiring bed-rest. The best prophylaxis is probably physiotherapy and early mobilization but claims for pharmacological techniques have been made. The use of antibiotics is controversial and the rationale is the reduced immune response in old age. As a guideline for any operation on the skeleton lasting for more than 1 h intravenous antibiotics (second or third generation cephalosporins) should be administered peroperatively. In cases with an increased risk such as diabetic patients,

antibiotics should be used for up to 5 days. The same applies to patients with open fractures (for classification see Gustilo and Anderson, 1976).

Local complications after trauma

All local complications described in younger patients can be encountered in old age too. With the skin becoming atrophic and the subcutaneous soft tissues being reduced, wound infection becomes more frequent. In patients with peripheral vascular disease this can be a major problem. Thrombophlebitis is also a well recognized complication.

The incision chosen has to respect the compromised blood supply of the skin and soft tissues. It should be more generous than in younger patients to avoid tearing of the edges and the handling of skin with forceps has to be gentle.

General complications after trauma

General complications are related to immobilization with pneumonia, urinary tract infection and pressure sores being the most common ones (Kolbow *et al.*, 1975; Haeske-Seeberg, 1988). Peroperative myocardial infarction has been reported (Haeske-Seeberg, 1988). In 94 elderly multiple trauma victims the most frequent complication was shock (37%) followed by renal failure (28%), pneumonia (19%) and cerebral oedema (16%). Sepsis accounted for 5% as did wound infection and osteomyelitis. The cause of death was head injury in 34%, shock in 32% and pulmonary complications in 24% (Haeske-Seeberg, 1988). The key to avoid these complications is expeditious treatment which facilitates early mobilization. It is very unlikely that a patient with multiple injuries will improve during a prolonged period of management by bed-rest alone. In general, the patient will deteriorate day by day with complications increasing in number and severity until operation is either impossible or aimless. An increased incidence of general complications leading to a longer stay on the intensive care unit and in hospital has been reported in younger patients with delayed stabilization of femoral fractures when compared with early management (Bone, Johnson and Weigelt, 1989). This experience can be easily extrapolated to elderly patients.

Fracture stabilization – technical considerations

Intramedullary techniques

The use of an interlocking nail is very attractive with the medullary canal mechanically supporting the device. Exposure of the actual fracture is not required and the intraoperative blood loss is minimal (Moran, Gibson and Cross, 1990). The locking technique relies on the intramedullary nail to align the fracture and the proximal and distal locking screws to prevent shortening and rotational deformities (Kempf, Grosse and Beck, 1985). The locking screws gain their purchase at a distance from the fracture site and part of the preoperative planning involves the placement of these screws. If poor purchase is to be expected or intraoperatively encountered in the distal femur, the Grosse–Kempf locking nail allows the use of the larger diameter proximal bolts in the distal holes. An alternative is the Vecsei expanding screw (Moran, Gibson and Cross, 1990) which is part of the same instrumentation. The placement of the distal locking should be precise and the use of a target device is recommended to avoid multiple attempts (Pennig, Brug and Kronholz, 1990). If further stability is required, the femoral canal may be filled with acrylic cement and the screws inserted rapidly after its instillation (Moran, Gibson and Cross, 1990). Proximal locking should be performed by placing the screw through the calcar rather than through the lesser trochanter and the nail end has to protrude about 10 mm above the tip of the greater trochanter for this. An augmentation with cement is an alternative.

Locked nailing can be used in the tibia and with the Seidel nail in the humerus (Brug and Pennig, 1988). In all cases it is advisable to select large diameter nails because of the increased width of the medullary canal in elderly persons.

A recent variation of the locking nail is the Gamma nail (Boriani and Bettelli, 1990) which allows placement of a large diameter screw through a short locking nail into the femoral neck and head. The reaming of the medullary canal should never be excessive to prevent thinning of the cortices. However, it is important to consider that the reaming products that are spread in the fracture site act as an intramedullary bone graft and the canal therefore should not be rinsed (Brug and Pennig, 1988). It is

advisable to lock all nails proximally and distally to prevent shortening due to collapse of the buttress. Should the locking screws cause local irritation they may be subsequently removed under local anaesthesia and the nail left in place but routine implant removal is neither required not recommended.

Another intramedullary technique uses Ender's nails, which are introduced via the medial supracondylar region of the femur and driven up into the femoral neck and head (Harper and Walsh, 1985). In osteoporotic bone nail migration is a common observation and bone cement can be used at the entry point to improve purchase. A minimum of four nails should be employed in a stable intertrochanteric fracture, whereas in unstable or reversed intertrochanteric fractures the Gamma locking nail seems to be superior.

With these nailing techniques at least partial weight bearing is possible immediately and full weight bearing is reached within 4–6 weeks with most fractures.

Plating techniques (Müller *et al.*, 1979; Schatzker and Tile, 1987)

The basic concept of plating involves exposure of the fracture site, anatomical reduction of the fracture and screw fixation. In osteoporotic bone it can be exceedingly difficult to obtain purchase with the screws. The correct drill size must be used and tapping should always be performed manually and in a very gentle way. In younger subjects, screw purchase in six cortices above and below the fracture seems to be sufficient whereas in osteoporosis eight or ten cortices may be required. Any cement used for augmentation purposes should be of medium viscosity and semi liquid and the implant used with it has to be trial fitted before the cement is applied. To improve the purchase of screws only the near cortex should be drilled with the exception of the most proximal and/or distal screw holding the implant in place. After that the cement should be instilled into the medullary canal through the screw holes. Drilling and tapping of the full screw length is performed afterwards and the screws are finally inserted. This technique produces better biomechanical results than insertion of the screws into still soft cement. Another advantage is that cement does not leak through already present drill holes in the far cortex.

An alternative method is the use of nuts on the side opposite the plate to secure the screws but in general weight bearing has to be delayed until union occurs. With the exception of the humerus, there is a recommendation to remove heavy plates electively to avoid fractures above or below the implant (Schatzker and Tile, 1987). However, whereas this may be essential in young, active individuals this is not necessarily the case in the elderly.

External fixation

It is important to realize that many elderly patients have difficulty in coming to terms with an external fixator and find the necessary pin care somewhat of a problem. Based on recent innovations (Bastiani, Aldegheri and Renzi-Brivio, 1984) there is an advantage in unilateral external fixation. The pins used should have a minimum diameter of 5 mm and the tapered design advocated seems to be beneficial. The use of cortical and cancellous screws is an advantage but it must be remembered that osteoporotic bone requires the use of a greater number of screws in comparison with younger patients. Again it is important to use the correct drill size and in severe osteoporosis a slightly smaller drill bit (e.g. 4.5 mm instead of 4.8 mm for cortical screws) can be employed. In the tibia, three screws per clamp are recommended (Figure 11.2) and in the femur up to four screws should be used. If a screw does not provide the required purchase it should be resited and subsequent pin care has to be meticulous to avoid pin site sepsis and loosening.

In cases where a fixator is applied in very ill patients as the most expeditious way to effectively stabilize a femoral, tibial or humeral fracture one has to consider at a later date changing the device to an intramedullary nail to facilitate rehabilitation. This should be performed no later than 2–4 weeks after which time pin tract sepsis innevitably occurs. The compliance required from the patient is much less after a statically locked nailing than with a fixator and while fracture healing takes place the nail supports the weight of the patient. However, mobilization can be undertaken with a suitable fixator with even partial weight bearing being possible (Bastiani, Aldegheri and Renzi-Brivio, 1984). In these cases the fixator should be dynamized after 2 weeks in stable fractures and full weight bearing should be achieved after a

further 4 weeks. In unstable fractures partial weight bearing in general is possible (20 kg) and dynamization should be delayed for 6–8 weeks depending on the callus formation (Bastiani, Aldegheri and Renzi-Brivio, 1984).

Cerclage and K-wires

The use of cerclage wires in the diaphysis of long bones is not advised because of its compromising effect on the periosteal blood supply which is of course necessary for fracture healing (Pennig, 1990). With the locked nailing technique described above it is certainly not necessary to use them since the fracture is adequately controlled by the implant alone (Brug and Pennig, 1988; Kempf, Grosse and Beck, 1985).

The method of tension banding has certain merits but the K-wires used should not be too small in diameter (1.5–2.0 mm) and neither should the tension band (1.2–1.4 mm). The K-wires do not obtain any purchase in the medullary canal or the metaphyseal bone and penetration of both cortices together with parallel placement are advisable. Correct tightening of the tension band should prevent migration of the K-wires, the ends of which should be bent through 180 degrees and the resulting hook should be driven cautiously into the cortex.

Cast and brace (Sarmiento and Latta, 1981)

In general below-knee casts are reasonably well tolerated by the elderly if weight bearing is permitted but the presence of peripheral vascular disease or venous ulcers must be noted. A long leg cast however leads to the immobilization of these patients with a heavy requirement for nursing. An alternative should therefore be sought. Naturally the use of lighter synthetic materials is beneficial whenever a cast is deemed necessary but with osteoporosis already present and the soft tissues altered by ageing, the problems of 'fracture disease' tend to be more pronounced. Functional bracing certainly has its merits but the mechanics of the method rely on an adequate soft tissue envelope. If as is frequently the case in the elderly there is marked atrophy, failures are likely to be encountered. The technique has the advantage that it leaves the adjacent joints free and provided the patient cooperates well and is adequately supervised it is a sensible conservative treatment option for

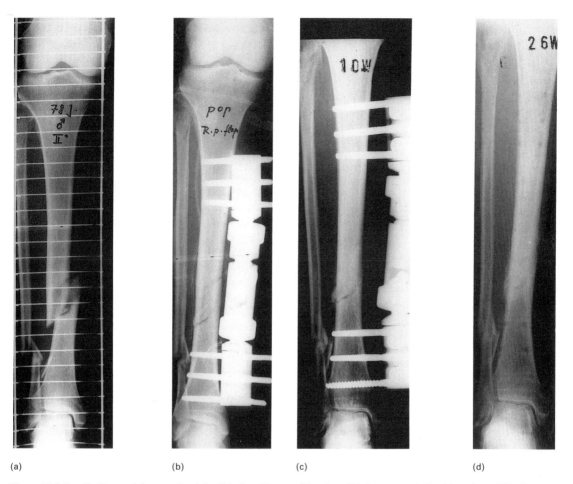

(a)   (b)   (c)   (d)

Figure 11.2 Gustilo II open injury to the right tibia in a 78-year-old male multiple trauma victim (a); early stabilization with a unilateral Orthofix external fixator using three pins instead of two per clamp and a random pattern flap to cover the exposed bone (b); periosteal callus formation after 10 weeks and full weight bearing (c); removal of the fixator after 4 months; (d) radiograph 6 months after the injury

fractures of the humerus and tibia. Frequent check-ups are however advisable.

A cast may also be used temporarily to protect the soft tissues after a surgical intervention.

Bone grafting and bone substitutes

The osteoporotic rarefication which affects the metaphyseal region of elderly patients also affects the typical bone donor sites (Heuck, 1979; Lane and Vigorita, 1983) and it is not uncommon that both iliac crests have to be used instead of one as is the case in younger subjects. When harvesting bone care must be taken not to apply too great a mechanical force on the pelvis in order to avoid fracture. The most suitable bone is found in the posterior part of the ileum and the use of this donor site should be considered for large defects and weighed against the possible complications. The cortex in this site in the elderly is thin and bone should be taken as corticocancellous chips to provide more matrix for integration of the graft. Compared with the volumes used in younger subjects the grafting should be more generous. When placing the graft one has to consider the blood supply required for the incorporation of the material and in the lower leg it is advantageous to pack the graft at the posterolateral surface of the tibia.

To fill a metaphyseal cavity or defect material from a bone bank or a bone subsitute (e.g. Interpore Coral Bone Substitute; Holmes, Bucholz and Mooney, 1986) can be used either alone or mixed with autologous bone. In general, however, this is not as successful as using the patient's own bone.

Acrylic cement (Bartucci *et al.*, 1985)

It is important to recognize that methylmethacrylate should not be placed at the fracture itself as it will prevent periosteal callus formation and subsequent union. Should its use be unavoidable at this site then an additional bone graft should also be placed at the fracture site to promote healing (Muhr, Tscherne and Thomas, 1979).

Bone cement can be used to improve the anchorage of an implant, e.g. in the femur to assist with distal locking (see above). In pathological fractures due to secondaries a more generous use of methylmethacrylate is possible since the aim is immediate stability for the remaining life span which is usually short.

The acrylic cement used should be of medium viscosity and it should be injected in a semi-liquid state (Bartucci *et al.*, 1985). Care must be taken to prevent the cement extruding through the fracture site or draining into a joint cavity.

Special features of fractures

Fractures of the upper extremity are dealt with in chapters 13 and 14.

Femur – proximal fractures

Most of the femoral fractures treated in old age are located proximally (Zimmermann, 1984) and those fractures of the neck are dealt with in chapter 12.

Pertrochanteric fractures are the second largest group of femoral fractures and when treating them a clear distinction must be made between stable and unstable injuries (Jensen, 1980). A more detailed analysis is also required with regard to the degree of the osteoporosis (Singh, Nagrath and Maini, 1970) which has a bearing on the anchorage of implants in the

femoral neck and head (Figure 11.3). In stable fractures associated with relatively little porosis Ender's nails (four or more), a dynamic hip screw or the Gamma nail can be used. Whichever method is employed, a traction table for anatomical reduction and an image intensifier should be available. The Ender technique is simple and associated with very little blood loss (Harper and Walsh, 1985) and may even be performed under local anaesthesia (though the author's preference is epidural or general anaesthesia). Immediate weight bearing is possible on the day after the operation. In stable fractures with more severe osteoporosis the addition of acrylic cement can be recommended together with the hip screw or the Gamma nail (Boriani and Bettelli, 1990). Since the anchorage of the nail portion of the latter device is provided by the medullary canal, the nail does not have to rely on screw purchase like the hip screw. The purchase in the femoral head and neck is however critical for both types of implants and this is reflected by a mechanical failure rate of 16% in a series of 230 intertrochanteric fractures (Davis *et al.*, 1990). The cut-out rate was also affected by the quality of fracture reduction and the misplacement of the implants (Mainds and Newman, 1989). In those cases with severe osteoporosis the anchorage of any implant in the head and neck will be problematical and the instillation of acrylic cement into the femoral neck will provide a better purchase (Bartucci *et al.*, 1985). The medium viscosity/ semi-liquid cement is injected into the neck ensuring that none extrudes through the fracture site or enters the hip joint which could happen if the guide wire is advanced beyond the cortex of the femoral head. Before the cement is used, the placement of the implant has to be trial-tested, subsequently removed and replaced rapidly after the cement is in place. When treating unstable fractures combined with the severe osteoporosis implant of choice is the Gamma nail because of its mechanical advantage regarding intramedullary anchorage (Figure 11.3). Acrylic cement can be added with the nail portion already in place and the neck/head screw is introduced after the cement instillation. The key to success for any implant in the proximal femur however seems to be an anatomical reduction of the fracture which is impossible without a traction table (Bartucci *et al.*, 1985; Davis *et al.*, 1990). The operation has to

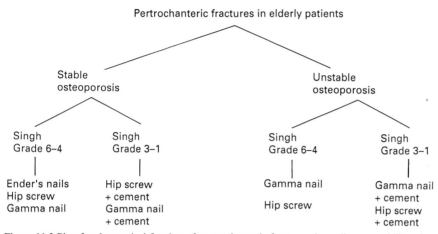

Figure 11.3 Plan for the surgical fixation of pertrochanteric fractures depending on stability of the injury and the degree of osteoporosis as assessed by the Singh index: Grades 1–3 = severe; grades 4–6 = mild

be performed as soon as possible after the injury since most patients will deteriorate with bed-rest.

If pain relief is the sole aim of surgery for bed-ridden patients, the mechanical considerations described above are irrelevant and Ender's nails are the quickest way of stabilization to facilitate nursing care.

Femur – shaft fractures

When dealing with isolated fractures of the shaft the most efficient form of stabilization is that of locked nailing (Kempf, Grosse and Beck, 1985; Bone, Johnson and Weigelt, 1989; Moran, Gibson and Cross, 1990) and the same is true when the injury is part of a multiple trauma. In those cases when the patient is haemodynamically unstable or otherwise considered unfit for nailing, unilateral external fixation (Bastiani, Aldegheri and Renzi-Brivio, 1984) applied on a standard orthopaedic table is an alternative method with which to quickly stabilize the femur. After subsequent improvement in the patient's condition there is the option of exchanging the fixator for a nail.

For standard nailing the patient is positioned supine on a traction table and unless the fracture is unusually distal a condylar Steinmann pin is used for skeletal traction. If hip pathology is present with a flexion contracture the patient may be positioned with advantage in lateral decubitus. The elasticity of the cortex in elderly people is reduced and the nailing technique has to allow for this. The point of entry should be precisely at the bottom of the piriform fossa and overreaming of 1.5 mm instead of 1 mm is advisable (Brug and Pennig, 1988). The purpose of this is to reduce the stress on the bone and protect the femur from iatrogenic fractures, e.g. Moran, Gibson and Cross (1990) described two femoral neck fractures in a series of 24 elderly patients. The proximal locking screw should cross the calcar rather than the soft bone of the lesser trochanter. The orientation of the nail in the frontal plane has to take account of the anteversion of the femoral neck and the implant should be turned so that the proximal screw is introduced 15 degrees anterior to the frontal plane. If purchase still seems to be poor cement augmentation can be performed with the nail *in situ*. The cement is inserted through the hole drilled for the proximal screw and deposited in the medullary canal on the medial and lateral side of the nail (Figure 11.4). The distal locking requires a precise targeting technique (Pennig, Brug and Kronholz, 1988) to avoid multiple attempts and when using the GK nail a 4.5 mm drill should be used for both cortices in elderly patients instead of the larger standard drill bit. Other possible solutions for sound distal locking in soft bone include use of the Vecsei expanding screw and cement augmentation (Moran, Gibson and Cross, 1990). The latter is used in the same way as described for the proximal screw (Moran, Gibson and Cross, 1990). The aim of nailing is to make full weight-bearing possible at a very early stage taking into account the limited compliance encountered in these patients. The

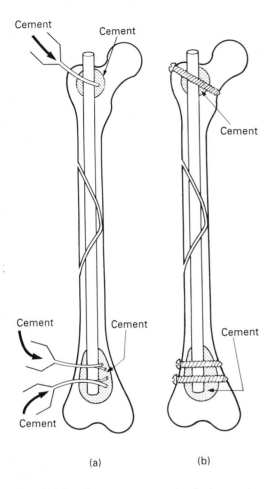

Figure 11.4 Acrylic cement augmentation for improved anchorage of the proximal and distal locking screws in severe osteoporosis (Singh grade 3–1). The nail is in place and the lateral but not the medial cortex is drilled prior to introduction of the cement to avoid cement leakage (a); *after* polymerization, the medial cortex is drilled and the locking screws are placed (b)

proximal limit for the use of a locking nail is an intact lesser trochanter in diaphyseal fractures (Brug *et al.*, 1988) and in these cases the point of entry has to be about 5 mm medial to the piriform fossa to avoid fractures of the medial cortex. Overreaming by 2 mm is advisable in these very proximal injuries. The distal limit is discussed below.

Following the satisfactory introduction of the locking nail, plating techniques are no longer seen as a rational alternative. However, in fractures below a hip prosthesis a plate is a sensible but not necessarily an easy solution. Screw fixation through eight cortices above and below the

fracture are biomechanically necessary to provide the required stability.

In those uncommon cases when the use of a traction table is not considered advisable, for example a combination of a femoral fracture and an unstable fracture of the thoracolumbar spine, a unilateral external fixator (Bastiani, Aldegheri and Renzi-Brivio, 1984) is a treatment option which can be applied on a standard table.

Fractures of the condylar region

Whenever possible, supracondylar fractures are best treated with the locking nail. The minimal distance from tip of the nail to the more proximal of the two distal holes in the GK nail is 45 mm and this is the portion of the nail that has to be distal to the fracture. Most supracondylar fractures are suitable for nailing and in extreme cases the nail tip can be sawn off to allow more distal placement of the nail. The difficult combination of a femoral shaft or supracondylar fracture together with an undisplaced percondylar or an undisplaced/displaced transcondylar fracture can also be nailed provided the necessary expertise of this technique is available (Baranowski and Pennig, 1988). The nailing is commenced after the reduction (if necessary) of the intra-articular fracture and cancellous lag screws are inserted. Placement of these screws must not obstruct the very distal path of the nail. Overreaming of the medullary canal by 2 mm is advisable to allow the nail to be pushed rather than hammered down.

If nailing is impossible, AO condylar plates or the AO DCS system can be used (Schatzker and Tile, 1987). If there is no medial buttress, bone grafting should be simultaneously performed. One may be tempted when treating these injuries to use acrylic cement but it is important to remember that union will not occur if cement spreads at the fracture site. With the soft supracondylar bone shortening of the fracture is not uncommon. It is certainly better to accept some longitudinal shortening rather than to attempt to fully restore length at the expense of creating a bone defect and possible non-union.

Fractures of the patella

Crack fractures without displacement of the articular surface are frequently seen in elderly patients and do not require surgery. If lifting the extended leg is too painful the limb should be immobilized with a lightweight cylinder leaving the ankle free. In transverse or Y-shaped fractures, most secure purchase is provided by two K-wires penetrating two cortices each and a loop type tension band. Screws rarely have sufficient purchase. If there is comminution the two main fragments can be fixed with the tension band and early joint movement commenced. When treating a severely comminuted fracture, a conservative approach with physiotherapy and continuous passive motion can be justified. If pain subsequently develops a patellectomy can be electively performed and interestingly, elderly patients rehabilitate faster following a delayed patellectomy when compared to a primary procedure.

Figure 11.5 Unstable proximal tibial fracture associated with severe osteoporosis. The fracture line extends into the tibial tuberosity (a); statically locked GK nail with the most distal locking screw being an expanding screw for better purchase in soft bone (b); nail removal after uneventful consolidation, irritation of the patellar tendon (c).

(a)

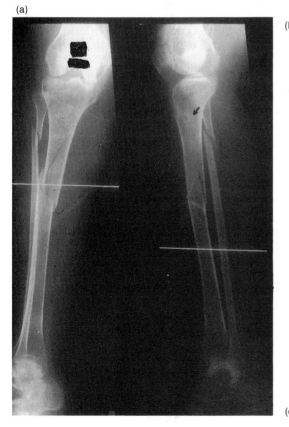

(b)

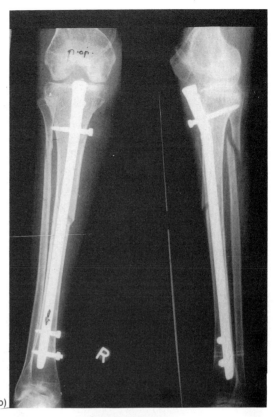

(c)

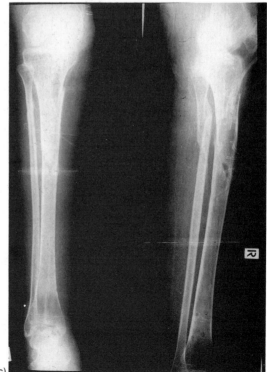

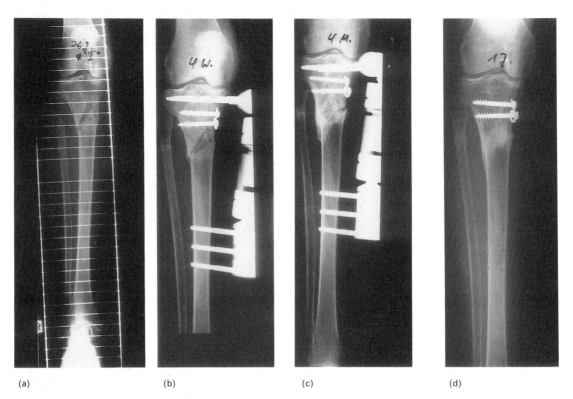

(a)   (b)   (c)   (d)

Figure 11.6 A 76-year-old female with a compound proximal intra-articular tibial fracture, Gustilo I(a). Step 1: the intra-articular fracture was temporarily secured with a percutaneously applied bone clamp prior to insertion of two 6.5 mm AO lag screws with washers through a stab incision. Step 2: application of the unilateral Orthofix external fixator to stabilize the main fracture (b); periosteal bone healing after 4 months (c); final result after 1 year (d)

Fractures of the tibia

Using the same rationale as described for the femur, tibia shaft fractures are best treated with a static locking nail (Figure 11.5). Exceptions would be the haemodynamically unstable patient following multiple trauma and those with severely compound and complicated fractures (Gustilo and Anderson, 1976) in which a unilateral external fixator is recommended (Bastiani, Aldegheri and Renzi-Brivio, 1984). Similarly proximal fractures with or without an intra-articular extension can be managed effectively with a combination of a unilateral fixator and limited internal fixation (Baranowski, Pennig and Borchardt, 1990) (Figure 11.6).

Fractures of the tibial plateau with depression of the joint elements benefit from open reduction and internal fixation (Schatzker and Tile, 1987). The aim is to realign the axis of the knee and to support the joint either by bone grafting or bone substitutes. A buttress plate should be used in these cases and if possible it should be placed on the lateral aspect of the tibia for improved soft tissue cover.

The very distal fracture without articular involvement should if at all possible be treated with a locked nail even if the tip of the nail has to be sawn off. With this closed technique the risk of a skin and wound breakdown is much reduced compared to open techniques. Shortening in the tibia should be accepted rather than vigorous attempts made to restore length resulting in a bone defect. Rapid union is the prime aim of treatment and a minor leg length discrepancy in old age is not difficult to deal with by footwear modification. In pilon fractures, plating is accompanied frequently by infection and wound breakdown and in this area a combination of external and internal fixation is recommended (Baranowski, Pennig and Borchardt, 1990). The fibula is fixed to restore length and limited internal fixation is carried out to reconstruct the tibial articulating surface. This is preferably performed after mounting the

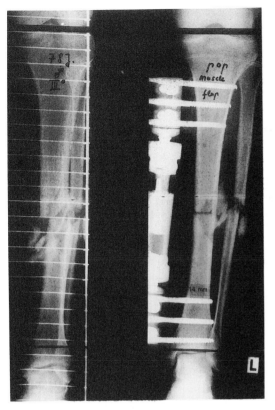

(a)   (b)

Figure 11.7 Transformation of an unstable Gustilo IIIB open tibial fracture (a) into a stable injury with good bony contact which will permit early weight bearing. This was achieved by a tibial shortening of 14 mm and removal of all avital bone pieces (b). A soleus flap was performed and bone healing without the need for grafting occurred after 22 weeks

fixator on the tibial shaft and the os calcis and applying axial distraction across the intact ligaments. Bone grafting may be necessary in these cases and should be performed as early as possible.

In severely compound injuries early stabilization is carried out using external fixation and the advice of a plastic surgeon should be sought regarding adequate soft tissue cover. If bone is exposed the likely outcome will be necrosis and infection. Shortening of up to 20 mm may be necessary to improve the soft tissue cover and to transform an unstable into a stable fracture with the benefit of early full weight bearing and rendering a bone grafting unnecessary (Figure 11.7).

Ankle fractures

In fit patients, the rationale for the treatment of ankle fractures is similar to that in younger subjects. An important difference however is the poorer bone quality and screw fixation alone or plate and screws together lack adequate purchase in the spongy bone of the medial or lateral malleolus. In both instances, a figure of eight tension band may be a better way, provided that both K-wires penetrate the opposite cortex. Migration of the K-wires is unlikely to occur if both branches of the cerclage wire are correctly tightened. The strongest bone on the medial side is just above the articular surface of the tibia and advantage should be taken of it. Screws ending in the medullary canal cannot be expected to gain any significant purchase.

For comminuted fractures of the lateral malleolus use of the tension band technique is not ideal. For a better hold, a plate should be applied to the posterior aspect of the fibula since with this placement two cortices can be held by each screw. With the usual technique of lateral plating, the distal screws cannot fully penetrate the medial cortex without entering and irritating the joint.

It is important to realize that an elderly patient has little or no time to adjust to a malunited ankle fracture. Accurate fixation performed correctly is the best line of action.

Fractures of the pelvis

Most pelvic fractures are stable and only require limited bed-rest, appropriate analgesics and early mobilization using a walking frame to prevent the general complications of prolonged immobilization. There would be no benefit from surgery (Tile, 1984). If however, there is involvement of the pelvic ring with marked disruption, the situation is totally different. In the absence of a vertical instability, a simple but rigid anterior fixator (Bastiani, Aldegheri and Renzi-Brivio, 1984; Pennig, Klein and Brug, 1989) may be used to allow the patient out of bed and to walk with a frame (Figure 11.8). The fixator pins (5/6 mm; 2 or 3 on either side) are best placed between the superior and inferior iliac spines (Pennig, Klein and Brug, 1989). The iliac crest is brittle and the ileum is very thin in osteoporosis of the elderly (Heuck, 1979; Lane and Vigorita, 1983) and pin anchorage is usually poor in these sites. In a disruption of the symphysis pubis, the

(a)

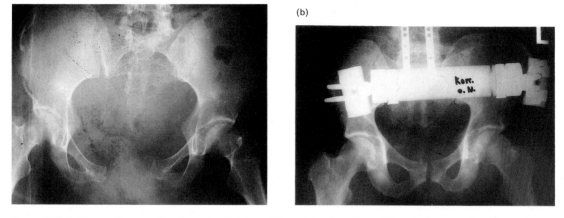

(b)

Figure 11.8 A 65-year-old man with a 'open book' injury of the pelvis, disruption of the anterior sacro-iliac ligaments on the right side; fracture dislocation of L4/5 (a); immediate closed reduction of the externally rotated right hemipelvis with a double T-clamp Orthofix external fixator; delayed posterior plating and grafting of the lumbar spine injury (b)

fixator should remain for 8 weeks but, if the pubic rami are fractured and displaced, 6 weeks should be sufficient. Fixation of the posterior ring as in fractures of the intra-articular portion of the ileum, displaced vertical sacral fractures and in disruption of the sacro-iliac joint is much more cumbersome. Adequate purchase for the screws is almost impossible to secure and a threaded sacral bar may be the only option (Tile, 1984). However, it must be stressed that the prime objective of treatment is the early mobilization of the patient and rigid anterior external fixation alone is likely to allow this in the majority of elderly cases even if a distortion of the pelvic ring persists. Since the posterior ring elements are hostile to surgical attempts, a successful compromise is better than damage done by an inevitable failure and the associated burden of a major surgical intervention.

Fractures of the spine

The vast majority of cervical spine fractures in the elderly may be best treated conservatively using braces, halo traction or cast (Kuhhit, Stoltze and Brinkmann, 1981). Whatever method is employed, the patient has to be able to be turned in the early days and later to be out of bed. Fractures of the thoracic spine are the most common variety in old age and they should be considered stable and require little treatment apart from analgesics. Injuries of the thoraco-lumbar spine are different and the fracture type has to be accurately analysed if necessary using computed tomography (Plane, 1981). Most fractures in this region are of the compression type in which it is more important to reassure the patient than to treat the condition. Often it is better to avoid speaking to the patient about the fracture because of the anxiety which it subsequently produces. The patient has to be warned about the pain and analgesics should administered. There is very little the attending physician can do to make the fracture worse and mobilization should commence after 3–4 days with support by the physiotherapists. A three-point brace may assist walking and keep the patient from involuntarily passing into a painful kyphosis. However, such orthoses are poorly tolerated by the elderly. The standard rule of bed-rest without pillows has to be eased to cater for the general condition of the patient and pillows may be allowed in some instances.

Unstable fractures of the spine such as fracture dislocations can benefit in experienced hands from surgery (Plane, 1981). The pedicular screws used in younger patients (Pennig and Brug, 1990) are not an attractive option in elderly subjects because of the poor purchase which they can achieve. A possible solution is sublaminar wiring with a Hartshill rectangle which makes use of the strongest part of the vertebra but this is only justified in patients who would otherwise be subjected to prolonged bed-rest. If surgery is considered prudent arrangements have to be made for it to be performed expeditiously before general complications have developed.

Indications for early amputation

Amputation of the upper extremity for trauma is an extremely unusual occurrence and reconstruction should be attempted for both functional and cosmetic reasons. All dead tissue has to be completely excised and it is worth remembering that even young patients can be lost due to complications of a crush syndrome in the forearm.

In the lower extremity the key issue is whether the patient will be able to achieve full weight bearing and the number and magnitude of surgical interventions required to achieve this. The biological response of the soft tissues will be less favourable than in younger patients because of the poorer vasculature. Whereas a single patent artery in the lower leg may be sufficient in a young person, a single vessel with atherosclerosis is a situation in which success is unlikely. If a substantial risk of failure is involved the decision to amputate has to be made early and a second opinion from an experienced colleague is worthwhile in these cases. With the satisfactory limb fitting facilities available in the western world an elderly patient can be expected to rehabilitate satisfactorily after a below-knee knee amputation (see chapter 9). In those cases in which amputation has been delayed the level of amputation when it is eventually performed will be higher, the stay in hospital longer and the emotional upset more pronounced (Bondurant *et al.*, 1988). As already mentioned good chances for rehabilitation exist for patients with below-knee and through-knee amputations but a 75-year-old patient with an above-knee amputation is a very difficult if not impossible rehabilitation task.

Conclusion

To the uninitiated the approach outlined in this chapter may seem to be unusually aggressive and very surgically oriented. However, the published results of this form of operative treatment in younger patients assists in the evaluation of its relative merits and possible drawbacks in elderly persons. For the reasons given, early mobilization must be the goal of treatment in order to prevent the sequelae of prolonged bedrest. If this can be achieved without surgery by using a lightweight cast or brace then it is obviously advantageous. However, if an operative procedure is the only way to reach this aim, then it should be carefully considered soon after the injury by an appropriate team. A femoral fracture represents an emergency with regard to the elderly patient as a whole. The input of an experienced anaesthetist as well as advice from a geriatrician may be sought as well as a second opinion from another experienced orthopaedic surgeon. The objectives in management are to allow early mobilization, to restore function and to avoid disability. The active patient possesses most of his available physiological resources on the day of admission, and these are likely to diminish day by day with bed-rest. A prompt decision about treatment will therefore be beneficial for both the patient and the attending surgeon. If delayed for too long, the option of surgical management may no longer exist. Common sense dictates that it is better to have a choice, and successful operative treatment clearly has advantages. Correctly balanced with the existing risks, an early and technically sound operation is likely to enhance the patient's recovery from his trauma.

References

Albrecht, F. (1985) Unfallchirurgie im Alter *Alterschir. Chirurg. Praxis*, **34**, 133–160

Baker, S.P., O'Neill, B., Haddon, W. Jr *et al.* (1974) Injury severity score: a method for describing patients with multiple injuries and evaluating emergency care. *J. Trauma*, **14**, 187–196

Baranowski, D., Pennig, D. and Borchardt, W. (1990) Komplementär–Osteosynthese und dynamisch-axiale Fixation an der distalen Tibia. *Unfallchirurg.*, **93**, 270–274

Baranowski, D. and Pennig, D. (1988) Grenzindikationen der Verriegelungsnagelung. *Osteosynthese International* (eds H.C. Nonnemann, V. Vecsei, R. Lindholm), Schnetztor-Verlag, Konstanz, pp. 402–405

Bartucci, E.J., Gonzalez, M., Cooperman, D.R., Freedberg, H.I., Barmada, R. and Laros, G.S. (1985) The effect of adjunctive methylmethacrylate on failures fixation in patients with intertrochanteric fractures and osteoporosis. *J. Bone Joint Surg.*, **76A**, 1094–1107

Bastiani, G., De, Aldegheri, R. and Renzi-Brivio, L. (1984) Treatment of fractures with a dynamic axial fixator. *J. Bone Joint Surg.*, **66B**, 538–545

Bondurant, F.J., Cotler, H.B., Buckle, R., Miller-Crotchett, P. and Browner, B.D. (1988) The medical and economic impact of severely injured lower extremities. *J. Trauma*, **28**, 1270–1273

Bone, L.B., Johnson, K.D., and Weigelt, J. (1989) Early versus delayed stabilization of femoral fractures. *J. Bone Joint Surg.*, **71A**, 336–340

Boriani, S., and Bettelli, G. (1990) The Gamma nail. *Chirurg. Org. Mov.*, **75**, 67–70

Brug, E., Pennig, D., Gähler, R. and Haeske-Seeberg, H. (1988) Polytrauma und Femurfraktur. *Akt. Traumatol.*, **18**, 125–128

Brug, E. and Pennig, D. (1988) Standortbestimmung der Verriegelungsnagelung. In *Jahrbuch der Chirurgie* (ed. H. Bünte), Regensberg & Biermann, Münster, pp. 145–160

Davis, T.R.C., Sher, J.L., Horsman, A., Simpson, M., Porter, B.B. and Checketts, R.G. (1990) Intertrochanteric femoral fractures *J. Bone Joint Surg.*, **72B**, 26–31

Devas, M. (1977) *Geriatric Orthopaedics*, Academic Press, Oxford

Friedebold, G. and Wolff, R. (1986) Unfallverletzte Patienten höheren Alters. *T. Orthop.*, **124**, 462–465

Friedel, B. (1985) Der alte, der behinderte und der kranke Mensch und seine Tüchtigkeit als Teilnehmer am Straßenverkehr. *Hefte Unfallheilk*, **174**, 135–169

Gustilo, R.B. and Anderson, J. T. (1976) Prevention of infection in the treatment of 1025 open fractures of long bones. *J. Bone Joint Surg.*, **58A**, 453–458

Haeske-Seeberg, H. (1988) Die Gesamtanalyse des Polytraumas Dissertation Medizinische Fakultät Westfälische Wilhelms-Universität Münster, Germany

Harper, M.C. and Walsh, T. (1985) Ender nailing for pertrochanteric fractures of the femur. *J. Bone Joint Surg.*, **67A**, 80–88

Heuck, F. (1979) Qualitative und quantitative radiologische Analyse des Knochens. In *Lehrbuch der Röntgendiagnostik*, (eds H.R. Schrinzetz, W.E. Baensch, W. Frommhold, R. Glauner, E. Uehlinger, J. Wellauer). Thieme Verlag, Stuttgart, Vol. II/1 pp. 145–212

Holmes, R.E., Bucholz, R.W. and Mooney, V. (1986) Porous hydroxyapatite as a bone graft substitute in metaphyseal defects. *J. Bone Joint Surg.*, **68A**, 904–911

Jensen, J.S. (1980) Classification of trochanteric fractures. *Acta Orthop. Scand.*, **51**, 803–810

Kempf, I., Grosse, A. and Beck G. (1985) Closed locked intramedullary nailing. *J. Bone Joint Surg.*, **67A**, 709–720

Kolbow, H., Schmit-Neuerburg, K.P., Suren, E.G. and Wilde, C.D. (1985) Komplikationen und Probleme bei mehrfachverletzten alten Menschen. *Hefte Unfallheilk*, **121**, 167–170

Knottenbelt, J.D., James, M.F. and Bloomfield, M. (1991) Intrapleural bupivacaine analgesia in chest trauma: a randomised, double-blind controlled trial. *Injury*, **22**, 114–116

Kuhhit, M.E., Stoltze, E. and Brinkmann, K. (1981) Die Behandlung der instabilen HWS-Frakturen beim alten Menschen mit der Halo-Extension. *Orthop. Praxis*, **5**, 409–412

Lane, J.M. and Vigorita, V.J. (1983) Osteoporosis. *J. Bone Joint Surg.*, **65A**, 274–278

Mainds, C.C. and Newman, R.J. (1989) Implant failures in patients with proximal fractures of the femur treated with a sliding screw device. In *injury*, **20**, 98–100

Moran, C.G., Gibson, M.J. and Cross, A.T. (1990) Intramedullary locking nails for femoral shaft fractures in elderly patients. *J. Bone Joint Surg.*, **72B**, 19–22

Muhr, G., Tscherne, H. and Thomas, R. (1979) Comminuted trochanteric fractures in geriatric patients. *Clin. Orthop.*, **138**, 41–44

Müller, M.E., Allgöwer, M., Schneider, K. and Willenegger, H. (1979) *Manual of Internal Fixation*, Springer, Berlin, Heidelberg, New York

Nankhonya, J.M., Turnbull, C.J. and Newton, J.T. (1991) Social and functional impact of minor fractures in elderly people. *Br. Med. J.*, **303**, 1514–1515

Oreskowich, M.R., Howard, J.D., Copass, M.A. and Carviro, C.J. (1984) Geriatric trauma: injury pattern and outcome. *J. Trauma*, **24**, 565–569

Pannike, A., Siebert, H., Kron H., and Weidner, R. (1981) Behandlungsgrundsätze und Prioritäten des Polytraumas in der Unfallchirurgie. *Unfallchirurgie*, **7**, 76–85

Pennig, D., Brug, E. and Kronholz, H.L. (1988) A new distal aiming device for locking nail fixation. *Orthopedics*, **11**, 1725–1727

Pennig, D. and Brug, E. (1990) A target device for implant placement in the thoracolumbar vertebral pedicles. *J. Bone Joint Surg.*, **72B**, 886–888

Pennig, D. and Brug, E. (1989) Femoral fractures in multiply injured patients. In *La Fissazione Esterna* (ed. F. Pipino), OIC Medical Press, Firenze, pp. 213–216

Pennig, D., Bünte, H., Klein, W., Haeske–Seeberg, H. and Brug, E. (1990) Die Bedeutung des Thoraxtraumas bei Polytraumatisierten: eine Analyse von 388 Patienten. *Hefte Unfallheilk* (in press)

Pennig, D., Klein, W. and Brug, E. (1989) Pelvic ring disruption. (eds R. Coombs, S. A. Green, A. Sarmiento) *In External Fixation and Functional Bracing*, Orthotext, London, pp. 191–195

Pennig, D. (1990) Zur Biologie des Knochens und der Knochenbruchheilung. *Unfallchirurg*, **93**, 488–491

Plane, R. (1981) Die Behandlung der Wirbelfrakturen beim alten Menschen. *Orthop. Praxis*, **5**, 401–408

Rehn, J. (1979) *Der alte Mensch in der Chirurgie*. Springer, Berlin, Heidelberg, New York

Sarmiento, A. and Latta, L. (1981) *Closed Functional Treatment of Fractures*. Springer, Berlin, Heidelberg, New York

Schatzker, J. and Tile, M. (1987) *The Rationale of Operative Fracture Care*. Springer, Berlin, Heidelberg, New York

Singh, M., Nagrath, A.R. and Maini, P.S. (1970) Changes in trabecular pattern of the upper end of the femur as an index of osteoporosis. *J. Bone Joint Surg.*, **52A**, 457–467

Tile, M. (1984) *Fractures of the Pelvis and Acetabulum*, Williams and Wilkins, Baltimore

Voigt, G.E. and Ottosson, A. (1985) Verkehrsunfälle älterer Menschen mit tödlichem Ausgang. *Hefte Unfallheilk*, **174**, 169–178

Waydhas, C., Nast-Kolb, D. and Betz, A. (1985) Der geriatrische Notfall in der Traumatologie. *Münch. med. Wschr.*, **127**, 794–796

Zimmermann, H.G. (1984) Operationstaktik in der Unfall-chirurgie im höheren Lebensalter: *Standardverfahren und Alternativen Chirurg*, **55**, 87–94

12

Fractures of the femoral neck

Jack Stevens

'We come into the world under the brim of the pelvis and go out through the neck of femur' reflects the defeatist attitude that has long been held by medical and lay personnel towards proximal femoral fractures (DeLee, 1984). The history and the development of treatment of femoral neck fractures parallel the historical development of orthopaedic surgery itself. Specific milestones have included the principle of reduction by dynamic traction, the importance of anatomical reduction and its maintenance by casts, the subsequent development of stable internal fixation devices and finally, the introduction of arthroplasty techniques. In spite of these advances in the management of femoral neck fractures we often still refer to this entity as 'the unsolved fracture' in certain situations (Speed, 1935).

Classification of femoral neck fractures

These are usually classified as intracapsular (subcapital or high) and extracapsular (intertrochanteric or low) fractures. There is also a borderline type of fracture occurring at the base of the neck which has some of the features of both of these injuries. However, since it tends to behave more like an intracapsular fracture it is usually considered with them.

The clinical features of these two fracture types are quite different and this is a reflection of their different biologies and biomechanics. Whereas the blood supply to the head is frequently prejudiced in intracapsular fractures, it hardly ever is in extracapsular fractures. The former, once they are reduced and held with a device, will only occasionally lose position,

whereas extracapsular fractures tend to collapse into varus. Furthermore, while non-union is common in intracapsular fractures, it is almost unknown in extracapsular injuries.

This chapter will concern itself solely with intra- and extracapsular fractures of the femoral neck and will not include the more distal subtrochanteric injury.

Intracapsular (high) fractures

Although there is probably no real difference in the behaviour of subcapital transcervical and mid-cervical fractures attempts have been made to differentiate them with regard to their likelihood of healing and the development of complications. Several classifications are available and these tend to be based either on the angle or the displacement of the fracture. For example the classification by Pauwels (1935) described the direction of the fracture line across the femoral neck with regard to the horizontal plane. However, the classification of Garden (1974) is based upon fracture displacement and is the one most widely accepted (Figure 12.1). It is as follows:

Stage I – incomplete or impacted fracture.
Stage II – complete fracture without displacement.
Stage III – complete fracture with some displacement.
Stage IV – complete fracture with total displacement.

It is possible to abbreviate this classification into two groups only – undisplaced and displaced – since stage II fractures are quite rare (Barnes *et al.*, 1976) and stage III and IV fractures tend to behave in much the same way.

138

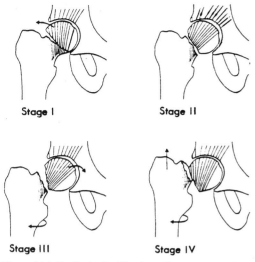

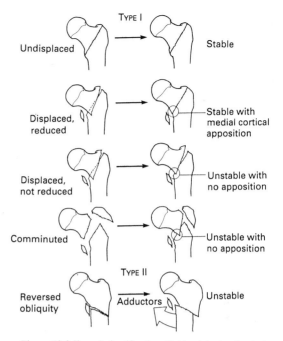

Figure 12.1 Garden's classification of intracapsular fractures of the neck of the femur. *Stage I*—incomplete or impacted fracture. The trabeculae of the inferior neck may remain intact. The femoral head is tilted in a posterolateral direction. *Stage II*—complete fracture without displacement. The weight-bearing trabeculae are interrupted by a fracture line across the entire neck of the femur but their alignment is generally undisturbed. *Stage III*—complete fracture with some displacement. The trabecular pattern of the femoral head does not align with the trabecular pattern of the acetabulum demonstrating incomplete displacement between the fracture fragments. *Stage IV*—complete fracture with total displacement. All continuity between the proximal and distal fragments is disrupted and therefore the trabecular pattern of the femoral head aligns with the trabecular pattern of the acetabulum. (*Source:* modified after Butt, 1990)

Figure 12.2 Evans' classification divides intertrochanteric fractures into two main types depending on the direction of the fracture. In type I the fracture line extends upwards and laterally from the lesser trochanter whereas in type II the fracture line demonstrates a reversed obliquity. Stability in type I fractures is obtained by anatomical medial cortical reduction. Type II fractures have a tendency towards medial displacement of the femoral shaft and hence retain their degree of instability. (*Source:* DeLee, 1984)

Intertrochanteric (low) fractures

There is some confusion as to the difference between intertrochanteric and pertrochanteric but if one believes that all low fractures are of a similar nature then this confusion is obviated. Several classifications have been proposed which relate the possibility of obtaining a primary stable and anatomical fracture reduction as well as allowing the surgeon to at least partly predict the risk of secondary loss of this position. The most well-known classifications have been discussed by DeLee (1984) and the most contemporary ones include those of Müller *et al.* (1990) and Gustilo (1991). The Evans' classification (1949) however is perhaps the easiest to understand and use in clinical practice since it divides fractures into 'stable' and 'unstable' groups. It further divides the unstable fractures into those in which stability can be restored by anatomical or near anatomical reduction and those in which anatomical reduction does not

create stability (Figure 12.2). From the standpoint of simplicity and accuracy the Evans' concept of classification based upon stability is the most satisfactory.

Incidence and epidemiology of proximal femoral fractures

There is evidence to suggest that the incidence and type of fracture may vary from country to country and indeed between different cities within the same country (Stevens, 1988). Similarly, there is some difference in the sex-specific and rate-specific hip fracture rates (Kellie and Brody, 1990). An alteration in the age-specific incidence in elderly patients between 1983/4 and 1973/4 has also been demonstrated but this did not affect the rural population (Larsson, Eliasson and Hansson, 1989). Zetterberg, Elmerson and Anderson (1984) were among the earlier reporters of a 'dramatic progressive increase in the incidence of cervical and trochanteric fractures' and based their figures on findings from 1940 to 1983. For example, from 1965 to 1983 the fracture rate increased by 109% but only 20% of this increase could be explained by the age factors of the population. They also indicated that the fracture incidence would double in 16 years for men and in 30 years for women.

One of the more important studies on this matter emanated from Sweden (Naessen *et al.*, 1989) where 29 277 hospital admissions for a first hip fracture were recorded in a population of 1.5 million. There was an increase in trochanteric fracture rates and a slight decrease in numbers of cervical fractures. However, this was in men only and the trochanteric fracture rate in women remained the same. The rate of cervical or trochanteric fracture increased in men compared with a decrease in women resulting in a decrease in the female:male ratio. It was reported that this finding of decreasing rates of hip fracture in women contrasted with the findings of most previous studies.

A similar article from Sweden (Jarnlo *et al.*, 1989) indicated a total incidence increase between 1966 and 1986 from 3.3 to 5.1 per 1000 over the age of 50 years. For persons over the age of 80 years the incidence almost doubled from 13.2 to 25.5. Again the urban population had a higher increase than the rural population. It was noted that the total incidence was higher in Sweden than in Denmark and Finland but lower than in Norway. Falch *et al.* (1985) found the highest reported age and sex incidence was in Oslo. Comparatively all other countries had a lower incidence. In Oslo the incidence was five times greater in 1982 than in 1950 and could not be explained by increased numbers of elderly persons. Similar findings were made by Finsen and Benum (1987) who suggested that the lower incidence in rural communities was related to the more physically active life style.

It has been estimated that there are 200 000 hip fractures each year in the USA and approximately 20% of these patients die. The cost of caring for these individuals exceeds $750 000 000 and it is believed that hip fracture is the fourth largest category in the list of causes of death in that country. Similarly, in 1980, Gallagher *et al.* indicated that the fracture rate doubled in each decade of life after the age of 50 years. It was greater in women than in men and by 90 years of age 32% of women and 17% of men had sustained such a fracture. Thus, approximately 113 000 women and 34 000 men over the age of 50 years will suffer a hip fracture each year. This represents a 'considerable cost' approaching $1 billion annually.

While noting that 20–40% of people who fractured their hips died within 6 months Rodrigues, Sattin and Waxweiler (1989) reinforced our belief that women were much more frequently involved than men especially at greater ages. Two reports from the Mayo Clinic (Melton *et al.*, 1982; Melton, O'Fallon and Riggs 1987) indicated that sex ratio changes could not account for the increased rate of hip fractures but in the second paper it was stated that no significant trends were noted for women within various age groups. It was noted that results for women seemed to conflict with other reports.

Boyce and Vessey (1985) indicated that in Oxford the incidence had doubled in both sexes and this increase was apparent at all ages. It was thought that some alteration in the aetiology of the fracture was responsible, at least in part, for this. Similarly, in 1983, Wallace found a disproportionate increase in fractures of the proximal femur in women over the age of 75 years. As a result of this he thought that 'work is urgently required to establish prophylactic treatment for this group of patients'.

In Denmark, Frandsen and Kruse (1983) indicated that between 1973 and 1979 there was a marked increase in hip fractures in females above what could be explained by demographic ageing processes alone. It was thought that this would lead to a threefold increase in the number of fractures over a 20-year period. Similar findings were reported by Caniggia and Morreale (1989). They, however, related the increase to climatic conditions. Lizaur-Utrilla *et al.* (1987) found that in Spain the incidence of the fracture was lower than in other countries but was increasing with time. They thought there was a relationship between osteopaenia and fracture type.

Trauma and biomechanics

Alfram (1964) reported that a fall from a sitting or a standing position (moderate trauma) was nine times as common as severe trauma in elderly female patients. This tendency for falling increases with age and estimates have been made that a previous history of fall was 35% more common in hip fracture patients than in controls

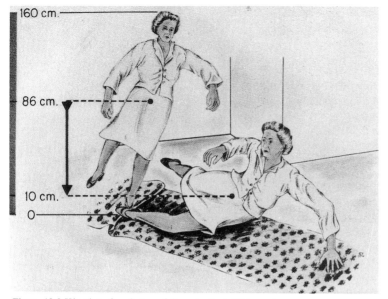

Figure 12.3 Kinetics of an indoor fall on to the left hip region

in the community (Prudham and Evans, 1981). Factors associated with this may include cerebrovascular or cardiac disease and the consumption of diuretics or tranquillizers.

Since 70% of elderly hip fracture patients have sustained their fall indoors, studies have been made (Hirsch and Frankel, 1960; Aitken, 1984) on the mechanics of such injuries. It appears that a combination of axial compression with a medially directed force on the hip is primarily responsible. When an individual falls from a standing position the potential energy available is the product of body mass and the distance that the centre of gravity of the body has moved (Figure 12.3). This value exceeds by many times the amount of force required to fracture a normal femur. The perplexing problem is why even more patients do not sustain femoral neck fractures after a fall. The answer comes at least in part from the dissipation of this potential energy by other means (particularly the energy absorbing movements of the upper limbs) and also elastic deformation in the soft tissues and other components of the skeleton (Frankel, 1974).

The fracture threshold is reduced by age-related osteoporosis which is more common and more severe as age increases. Locally the posterior rim of the acetabulum limits the range of external rotation of the femur and acts as an anvil causing comminution of the posterior cortex. Conversely the anterior cortex, which is

under tension, develops a single fracture line (Meyers, Harvey and Moore, 1973). This combination of fracture patterns is difficult to reproduce experimentally. It is now suggested that an increase in the bending component of the force producing the fracture is more likely to lead to a transcervical fracture (Frankel, 1960). Conversely, when the axial component is increased, a subcapital fracture is more likely.

Associated generalized conditions

Osteoporosis

This appears to be inversely correlated to bone strength and therefore it probably permits more fractures of the femoral neck to occur in elderly people. There are many studies concerning the correlation of osteoporosis with fractures including Stevens, Freeman and Nordin (1962) and Mazess and Barden (1988).

Techniques of assessing osteoporosis have become more sophisticated and currently the commonest method is dual-photon absorptiometry. Those systems based upon radiological measurements of metacarpals, femora and vertebrae are hardly used at all but the method of Singh, Nagrath and Maini (1970) based upon the trabecular pattern of the proximal femur has retained its popularity – probably because of its relative ease of use (Figure 12.4). Melton *et al.*

(1986) described a new approach to the assessment of fracture risk from bone mineral density measurement and indicated that osteoporosis was an important underlying cause of hip fracture. Conversely, Hogervorst *et al.* (1985) stated that the results of their transiliac biopsies were not consistent with a decreased bone mineralization in patients with hip fracture.

While there is undoubtedly a negative association between hip fracture and osteoarthrosis of the hip, there is no significant difference in the Singh index between patients resident in higher *versus* lower water aluminium areas (Wood, 1990).

The trouble with all of these methods of determining osteoporosis is that they have at least two major variables – one is the technique used in the particular unit reporting their results and the other is the variation from hospital to hospital of the patients admitted there. For example, Aitken (1984) found trochanteric fractures more commonly in severely osteoporotic women and cervical fractures in those who were not osteoporotic. He believed that the presence or absence of osteoporosis determined the type of fracture sustained. On the other hand Cummings (1985), after reviewing case-controlled studies, found that those with upper femoral fractures had less bone mass than those who did not sustain a fracture but these differences were small and overlapped. He assumed therefore that patients with hip fractures did not appear to be distinctly more osteoporotic than persons of similar age and that there may be other more important determinants of femoral neck fracture.

Quantitated computed tomography of the distal radius was used in women with spinal and hip fractures by Härmä *et al.* (1985) who subsequently described two forms of osteoporosis. One was characterized by excessive trabecular bone loss in the axial skeleton leading to spinal fractures and the second was due to combined axial and peripheral osteoporosis which was found in connection with hip fractures. Both groups of patients demonstrated reduced bone density compared with the controls.

Bohr and Schaadt (1983) concluded that the high incidence of femoral neck fracture with increasing age might be explained at least in part by a reduction in the bone mineral content of cortical bone. However, it was likely that other factors which reduced the strength of bone or increased the number of falls in elderly patients,

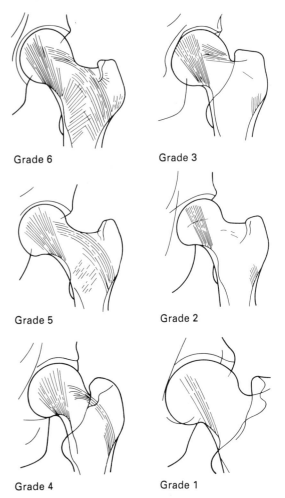

Grade 6   Grade 3

Grade 5   Grade 2

Grade 4   Grade 1

Figure 12.4 Singh's index of osteoporosis. *Grade 6*—all the normal trabecular groups are visible and the proximal femur seems to be completely occupied by cancellous bone. *Grade 5*—the structure of the principal tensile and compressive trabeculae is accentuated. Ward's triangle appears prominent. *Grade 4*—the principal tensile trabeculae are markedly reduced but can still be traced within the lateral cortex to the upper part of the femoral neck. *Grade 3*—there is a break in the continuity of the principal tensile trabeculae opposite the greater trochanter. This grade indicates definite osteoporosis. *Grade 2*—only the principal compressive trabeculae stand out prominently with the others more or less completely resolved. *Grade 1*—even the principal compressive trabeculae are markedly reduced in number and are no longer prominent

were also important. In a direct attack on the problem, Uitewaal, Lips and Netelenbos (1987) carried out a histomorphometric analysis and found that trochanteric fractures were associated with serious osteoporosis whereas cervical fracture patients constituted a more heterogeneous group. There was significant trabecular thinning in those with trochanteric fractures and there was a suggestion that decreased osteoblastic apposition was a prominent feature of patients with trochanteric fractures. However, using dual-photon absorptiometry on the proximal femur, Eriksson and Widhe (1988) found that bone mineral distribution in the proximal femur was essentially the same for the femoral neck fracture group as for the reference group of elderly women. Neither the Singh index nor measurements on the radius by single photon-absorptiometry provided a reliable estimate of the bone mineral density in the proximal femur. Following a study of considerable size Lester *et al.* (1990) concluded that single photon-absorptiometry appeared to be a useful tool for screening normal populations of asymptomatic women to predict the hip fracture risk.

These articles serve to indicate the uncertainty of the association of osteoporosis with hip fracture though there is a suspicion that patients with trochanteric fractures have less bone mass than 'normal'. Thus Cooper *et al.* (1987) indicated that above the age of 75 years the increasing risk of sustaining a fracture due to reduced bone mass was small and it was thought that the neuromuscular responses which protect the skeleton against this trauma may be more important than bone mass itself.

Physical activity is an important factor in reducing the risk of fracture of the femoral neck. Patients who undertake an average or greater than average amount of physical activity apparently have less chance of sustaining a fracture (Åström *et al.*, 1987; Boyce and Vessey, 1988).

The use of sodium fluoride may decrease osteoporosis and therefore the incidence of fracture but Riggs *et al.* (1987) reported that it made minimal difference. There is little doubt however that bone becomes more 'brittle' if fluoride is used in excess. Arnala *et al.* (1986) stated that fluoride content of bone samples correlated with drinking water fluoride concentrations. In a high fluoride area, osteofluorosis occurred in many patients but there was no association between this and hip fracture when patients from low fluoride areas, areas with fluoridated drinking water and high fluoride areas were studied. Conversely, Hedlund and Gallagher (1989) found that fluoride treatment increased the risk of hip fracture in osteoporotic women.

Whereas it had earlier been supposed that there was an increased incidence of osteomalacia in patients with hip fracture, it was later found that osteomalacia was not a contributory factor in the pathogenesis of this injury. On the other hand the consumption of thiazide diuretics appears to protect against hip fracture in the elderly.

Oestrogen lack has long been known to be associated with osteoporosis and it is recognized that hormone replacement therapy started around the time of the menopause, although inconvenient, will protect women against fracture (Keil *et al.*, 1987). Similarly, Weiss *et al.* (1980) found the risk of fracture was 50–60% lower in women who used oestrogen preparations for 6 years or more than in women who did not. Similarly, Johnson and Specht (1981) reported a reduction in the risk of hip fracture with post-menopausal oestrogen exposure.

The effects of vitamin D metabolites have also been investigated. For example, Al-Arabi, Elidrissy and Desrani (1984) studied the effects of the avoidance of sunlight on femoral neck fracture in elderly Saudi patients. They concluded that low levels of serum 25-(OH)D_3 may play a role in the pathogenesis of femoral neck fracture in elderly Saudis and this may be due to minimal exposure to ultraviolet irradiation. Similarly, Harju *et al.* (1985) found a low serum 25-(OH)D_3 in hip fracture patients and stated that osteoporosis was more common in these individuals. They also suggested that vitamin D supplementation should be an integral part of the treatment of the fracture. Lips *et al.* (1985) found that serum 25-(OH)D_3 was significantly lower in patients with hip fractures than in controls. However, they concluded that this preceded the occurrence of the fall whereas the lower serum 1,25(OH)$_2$ vitamin D was largely the result of the injury. Following an extensive study, Hordon and Peacock (1987) stated that the 1,25-(OH)$_2$ vitamin D response to oral 25-(OH) vitamin D was an unreliable guide to the presence of vitamin D deficient osteomalacia at the time of fracture. Active bone turnover was apparently still present 1 year later. Cooper *et al.* (1989) showed a small reduction in serum osteocalcin concentration in fracture patients and believed that this indicated that reduced osteoblast function may contribute to the osteoporosis which results in hip fracture.

Drugs

Stevens and Mulrow (1989) stated that the rise in hip fracture incidence paralleled the rate of prescription of drugs which affected overall stability and investigated this by a case control study. There was no significant difference between the two groups with regard to benzodiazepines, major tranquillizers, diuretics or other antihypertensives. The two groups did differ significantly in average body weight and the incidence of stroke.

The surgical treatment of proximal femoral fractures

The surgery of intra- and extracapsular fractures is radically different and will therefore be considered separately.

Intracapsular (high) fractures

Undisplaced fractures

These include Garden's stages I and II. Contemporary thought is that these fractures should be treated by internal fixation using the simplest possible technique to maintain stability. Garden screws, AO screws and Asnis screws (Figure 12.5) are used quite extensively in this situation. It is possible to treat this injury conservatively (Otremski *et al.*, 1990) but this is expensive with regard to hospital bed usage. Once treated by internal fixation the patients can be discharged home relatively early. Furthermore, surgical treatment is associated with a non-union rate of approximately 3% (Bentley, 1968) compared with approximately 9% with conservative therapy (Otremski *et al.*, 1990).

Displaced fractures

The ideal treatment for displaced femoral neck fractures is anatomical reduction and stable internal fixation since this results in better hip function than that noted in patients following prosthetic replacement (DeLee, 1984). Various techniques have been described for reduction of the displaced fracture but it is important to stress that the adequacy of the reduction is checked radiologically and the manipulative manoeuvre should be repeated if the radiograph shows an unsatisfactory position. The assessment is probably best performed using Garden's alignment index (1971) which is measured on both the anteroposterior and lateral radiographs. On the former radiograph the angle is

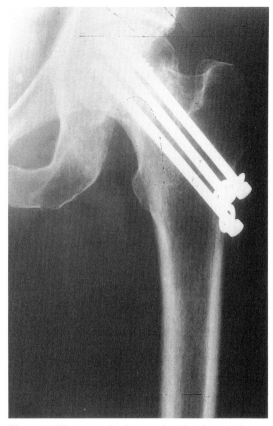

Figure 12.5 Intracapsular fracture held by three Asnis screws with washers

measured between the line of the medial trabecular stream in the femoral head and neck on the one hand and the medial cortex of the femoral shaft on the other. These normally form an angle of approximately 160 degrees and Garden suggested an acceptable value following manipulation to be between 155 and 180 degrees. On the lateral view the trabeculae proximal and distal to the fracture should theoretically be aligned perfectly but again Garden stated that the line of these trabeculae could be within 20 degrees of the theoretical straight line (Wood, 1990) (Figure 12.6).

Once a satisfactory reduction has been achieved the position can be held by several techniques including multiple screws (Figure 12.5) or a telescoping screw and plate device of either the Richards or AO variety (Figure 12.7). It must be emphasized that above all the surgeon must consider the age of the patient when planning treatment for a displaced subcapital fracture. In any patient with a significant life

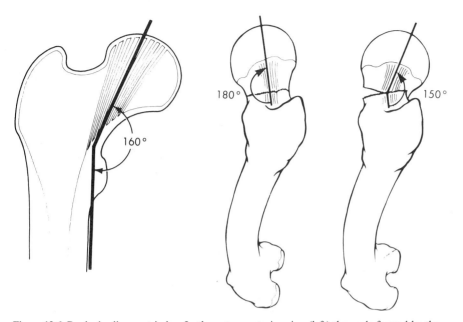

Figure 12.6 Garden's alignment index. In the anteroposterior view (left) the angle formed by the central axis of the medial trabecular system in the capital fragment and the medial cortex of the femoral shaft is measured. In the normal femoral head and neck this measures approximately 160 degrees. In the lateral view (centre) the central axis of the head and the central axis of the neck lie in a straight line at 180 degrees. According to Garden an acceptable reduction can be expressed as an alignment index when a figure of 160–180 degrees has been achieved on both the frontal and lateral planes. The figure on the right shows an unacceptable reduction in the lateral view. (*Source:* DeLee, 1984)

expectancy (more than 5 years) and a high level of activity consideration should be given to a procedure designed to salvage the femoral head, i.e. closed reduction and internal fixation. However, if a satisfactory reduction cannot be obtained or if the patient meets certain relative indications listed below a primary prosthetic hemiarthroplasty should be considered (Figure 12.8). The relative indications are as follows.

1. Displaced subcapital fractures in patients whose physiological age is advanced. Conventionally this refers to over 65–70 years but another way of looking at this is that the patient's life expectancy is less than 5 years.

2. Patients whose medical condition is so tenuous that a second salvage procedure for failure of the primary operation is not feasible.

3. Displaced fractures in patients who need to become fully ambulatory quickly because of other illnesses or debilities, e.g. blindness.

The operation of hemiarthroplasty may be performed through either a lateral or posterior approach and the Austin Moore and Thompson are the two most frequently used prostheses. The former may be fixed into the femoral canal using bone graft and acrylic bone cement is used with the latter. However, the role of cement in this situation is still debated. Sonne-Holm *et al.* (1987) performed a controlled trial of 112 patients divided between those treated with a cemented hemiarthroplasty and those who received a non-cemented prosthesis. The results at 6 months were significantly better in those patients treated with a cemented prosthesis particularly in relation to pain relief. This is perhaps not surprising considering the difficulty in achieving a secure cement-free fixation in the capacious proximal intramedullary canal of the elderly osteoporotic patient. Nonetheless, a significant number of these patients do require secondary revision surgery and the morbidity of this is significantly increased if acrylic cement has been used previously.

Hemiarthroplasty is contraindicated in the more active patient because of the painful, progressive cartilage erosion that occurs in the acetabulum. Thus, Hunter (1975) found that

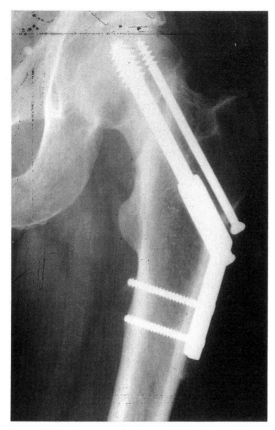

Figure 12.7 An intracapsular fracture held with an AO dynamic hip screw (DHS) with an anti-rotation screw placed proximal to it

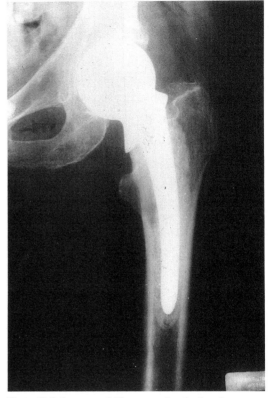

Figure 12.8 A cemented Thompson hemiarthroplasty

30% of patients experienced disabling pain 3 years following hemiarthroplasty and similar results have been reported in up to 50% of some other series (Coates, 1975). Barnes *et al.* (1976) however reported that almost 50% of their patients over the age of 84 years developed non-union and in these particularly elderly patients (and in this circumstance age depends more upon biology rather than chronology) a hemiarthroplasty is certainly justified. This must be accurately sized in order to fit the acetabulum which is not exactly hemispherical since the achievement of the maximum area of contact reduces the pressure and hence the concentration of stresses on the articular cartilage.

A modification of the Austin Moore or the Thompson prosthesis is the bipolar hemiarthroplasty which theoretically allows movement at two levels, i.e. between the metal cup and the cartilage of the acetabulum and between the much smaller metal head which is attached to the shaft of the femur and the polythene insert of the metal cup which fits the acetabulum. At the present time the Bateman prosthesis (Bateman, 1974) appears to be the most popular worldwide though in the UK the Hastings prosthesis is probably more widely used (Devas and Hinves, 1983; Franklin and Gallanaugh, 1983). However, doubt has been cast on the persistence of bipolar movement and 75% of 76 hip fractures treated with a bipolar device were found to be functioning as a unipolar device at 1 year.

There are few prospective trials which compare the outcome of elderly patients with displaced subcapital fractures that have been treated either by reduction and internal fixation or with hemiarthroplasty. Parker (1991) reported on 100 patients aged over 70 years who underwent reduction and fixation and 185 elderly patients with a similar fracture treated by hemiarthroplasty. When reviewed at 1 year from injury there was no significant difference between the two groups in the mortality, or for the survivors, in the degree of residual pain or change in mobility. However, for those patients treated by hemiarthroplasty the length of hospital stay was increased by an average of 10 days and their cost of treatment was approximately £300 more expensive than for those patients treated by internal fixation. However, only 9% of the arthroplasty group required further surgery compared with 23% of those patients treated by internal fixation. A more sophisticated economic analysis of the relative costs is therefore indicated in order that the cost-benefit ratio of the two surgical procedures can be evaluated. Clearly, however, the decision whether to salvage or sacrifice the femoral head carries with it significant financial consequences.

Total hip arthroplasty has been suggested for the primary treatment of elderly patients with displaced Garden III and IV femoral neck fractures. The rationale is to avoid the high incidence of complications following internal fixation of these displaced fractures such as avascular necrosis and the acetabular erosion and medial migration seen following a hemiarthroplasty. However, the results of total hip arthroplasty for osteoarthrosis and rheumatoid arthritis should not be confused with the much poorer results obtained when this operation is applied for the treatment of fracture. Sim and Stauffer (1980) showed that 81% of 85 patients with subcapital fractures were pain-free following primary total hip arthroplasty but the dislocation rate was 13% which is much higher than for routine hip replacement for osteoarthrosis. A similarly high dislocation rate was reported by Cartlidge (1981). Furthermore, though the mortality and postoperative infection rates were comparable to those following hemiarthroplasty, medical complications occurred in 21% and surgical complications in 22% when the total hip arthroplasty was used for femoral neck fracture (Sim and Stauffer, 1980).

It has been suggested (DeLee, 1984) that primary total hip arthroplasty be reserved for those patients with femoral neck fractures who have associated advanced hip joint disease and perhaps also those with contralateral hip disease. However, it needs to be shown in suitably controlled studies that such an aggressive surgical approach truly gives results which are significantly better than internal fixation or hemiarthroplasty in these patients.

Intertrochanteric (low) fractures

Early reports of the treatment of intertrochanteric fractures favoured closed treatment by means of skeletal traction with the aim not necessarily to gain an anatomical reduction but rather to allow the fracture to unite in a little varus (85–120 degrees) which subsequently required management with a shoe raise. Claims for increased mortality and morbidity associated with such conservative treatment led to recommendations for routine internal fixation of these fractures. It is difficult to compare accurately mortality figures for intertrochanteric fractures treated operatively with those treated conservatively since in most series those patients treated conservatively have tended to be older and with more associated medical problems. They were therefore higher risk surgical candidates. Recently, Hornby, Evans and Vardon (1989) performed a randomized trial in elderly patients in which surgical and conservative treatment was compared. They found the general complication rate to be similar in both groups with no difference with regard to mortality. It seems therefore that non-operative treatment may be suitable for the small proportion of patients who are unfit for operation but Hornby, Evans and Vardon (1989) showed that conservatively treated patients stayed in hospital for 26 days longer than those treated by surgery. This observation is relevant – particularly in the current financial climate. Other reports have claimed increased patient comfort, facilitation of nursing care and a better anatomical result demonstrated radiologically for patients treated surgically and the overwhelming majority of intertrochanteric fractures are now treated surgically.

Until recently the standard operation has been closed manipulation followed by internal fixation with a nail and plate device (Figure 12.9). However, the current trend is towards a telescoping screw system which accommodates the substantial collapse which may occur during the healing phase (Figure 12.7). Such screw devices give satisfactory results.

The vogue for treating this injury by multiple, flexible intramedullary nails (Ender, 1978) has waned. These are passed from a portal in the medial supracondylar region of the femur in a proximal direction to cross the fracture and enter the head (Figure 12.10). However, when this technique was compared with the dynamic hip screw, it was apparent that more of them required secondary operations (Sernbo *et al.*, 1988), the perioperative mortality was higher

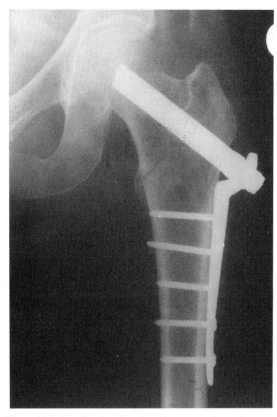

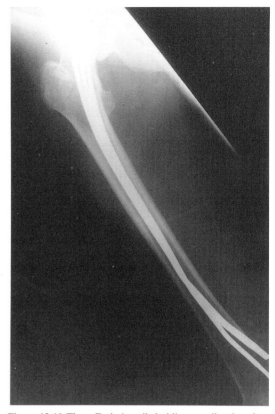

Figure 12.9 A well-reduced and stable intertrochanteric fracture internally fixed with a McLaughlin nail and plate

Figure 12.10 Three Ender's nails holding a well-reduced intertrochanteric fracture

and the maintenance of the anatomical reduction was poorer as was the final functional result (Juhn, Krimerhan and Mendes, 1988). Even when only patients with stable fractures were considered, there was still an unacceptably high level of complications (Cobelli and Sadler 1985). Conversely, Waddell, Czitrom and Simmons (1987) reported satisfactory results in terms of fracture healing, maintenance of reduction and functional activity after the use of condylocephalic nails with only six of their 144 surviving patients requiring revision of the fixation device. Wilson *et al.* (1980) audited the results in over 1000 patients who received the Jewitt nail plate after anatomical reduction and reported that more than 98% of the fractures united. They stated that the accuracy of the reduction and nail placement were critical factors with regard to fracture healing and the latter was emphasized by Mainds and Newman (1989). Esser, Kassab and Jones (1986) compared the Jewitt fixed angle nail plate with a dynamic hip screw and found no significant differences with regard

to pain, length of hospital stay, morbidity or mortality. However, by 6 months the use of the DHS had produced more mobile patients with significantly less loss of reduction.

Jensen, Sonne-Holm and Tondevold (1980) compared fixed angle nail plates, the sliding screw device and condylocephalic nailing (Ender, 1978). After the treatment of 1071 patients they stated that the sliding screw device was the most suitable technique for the treatment of unstable trochanteric fractures. More recently intermedullary devices such as the Gamma nail have been introduced. These have obvious theoretical advantages which remain to be proved in clinical practice.

The unstable intertrochanteric fracture is a serious and difficult problem and its inherent lack of stability often results in significant complications including failure of the fixation device, delayed or non-union and penetration of the device through the femoral head (see below). In an attempt to create some inherent bony

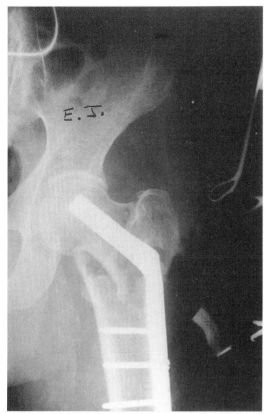

Figure 12.11 An intertrochanteric fracture held in the Dimon-Hughston position by a fixed angle nail plate

stability displacement osteotomies have been described in both varus and valgus directions (Dimon and Hughston, 1967, Figure 12.11). Such procedures are difficult and are associated with inherent complications and it has been shown that the use of a sliding compression screw alone gives superior results than a displacement osteotomy (Davis *et al.*, 1988). The use of acrylic cement to augment the osteotomy has been reported both in association with the Dimon–Hughston technique (Chow *et al.*, 1987) and with the Sarmiento procedure (Pun *et al.*, 1987) and it is possible that the former osteotomy performed slightly better. However Hornby *et al.* (1989) stated that 'unless the operating theatre environment can be shown to have an overall infection rate close to zero, for example less than 2%, it is difficult to justify, what is, effectively, elective surgery in these patients'.

Mortality rates

The reported mortality rate following hemiarthroplasty for displaced subcapital fractures varies from 10% to 40%. However, there is obvious difficulty in comparing such published statistics since some authors only report hospital mortality whereas others report their observations at 6, 9 or 12 months following the fracture. Similarly, when considering mortality figures one must be careful to ensure that the two groups of patients are truly comparable and the data must be compared against the expected mortality rate of an aged-matched group of patients in the area without fracture. Recent series have demonstrated little (DeLee, 1984) or no difference (Parker, 1991) in the mortality rates between patients with subcapital fractures treated by primary internal fixation with those undergoing prosthetic replacement. However, it has been emphasized that if specific indications are adhered to, then patients undergoing hemiarthroplasty should theoretically be older and more debilitated than those undergoing primary internal fixation. They therefore should have a slightly higher mortality rate.

Original reports stated that intertrochanteric fractures were associated with a higher mortality figure than subcapital fractures – possibly because the patients were older. If these age differences are corrected no difference in mortality exists between these two groups of patients.

Attempts have been made to predict which patients are likely to die with the aim of basing treatment options on this prediction. Ions and Stevens (1987) indicated that the presence of dementia and advanced age were good predictors of a poor outcome. The objective assessment of dementia can be difficult but they used a simple 10-question test which took only 2 min to assess cognitive function (Blessed, Tomlinson and Roth 1968) (Table 12.1). The maximum number of points obtained on this questionnaire was 13. Patients who scored more than 7 points were regarded as being normal or near normal and those with less than 3 points were generally assessed as unfit for operation and rehabilitation. They were therefore treated conservatively. In a study of 531 patients with a mean age of 77 years, by Wood (1990) 21% were considered unfit for surgery based upon their mental test score and were treated conservatively, 25% were cognitively impaired with scores between 3 and 10 and 53% were considered to

Table 12.1 The assessment of cognitive function by means of the 'mental test score'

Question	Points
1. Age to within 1 year	0,1
2. Time to the nearest hour	0,1
3. Address for recall (42, West Street)	0,1,2
4. Date	0,1,2,3
5. Day of the week	0,1
6. Name of the hospital	0,1
7. Date of birth	0,1
8. Year of the First World War	0,1
9. Name of the present monarch	0,1
10. Count backwards from 20	0,1

The maximum score possible is 13

be normal or near normal with scores between 10 and 13. Their conclusions were that the most discriminating variables for mortality at 6 months in order of significance were dementia, postoperative chest infection, neoplasia, age and wound infection. Thus, 74% of demented patients over the age of 85 years were dead within 6 months compared with 20% for similar patients over 75 years of age. However, for those under 75 years the mortality rate was only 7%.

Preoperative management of intracapsular and extracapsular hip fracture patients

It used to be thought that delaying surgery for more than a day or so had a deleterious effect on the outcome of patients with femoral neck fractures. This may not always be the case – at least for high fractures (Wood, 1990). It is possible, and certainly advantageous in some cases to spend a short time improving the general medical condition of these patients to make them as fit as possible before surgery. Their state of dehydration may be corrected and their cardio-respiratory status improved by physiotherapy, antibiotics and drug therapy before anaesthesia and surgery are performed. A preoperative blood transfusion may be necessary but a day or two must elapse before the transfused blood becomes capable of delivering a significant amount of oxygen. This is due to the relatively slow synthesis of adequate amounts of 2,3-diphosphate. In those patients in whom this 'medical' treatment is necessary the operation becomes one of 'semi-election' rather than a

'true emergency'. Nonetheless, the aim should be for the majority of patients to undergo surgery in the first day following their trauma and the medical management for the remaining patients should be performed as expeditiously as possible. For example, in a survey by Gilchrist *et al.* (1988) 78% of patients underwent surgery without problem in the first 24 h and even more impressive figures have been published by Sikorski, Davis and Senior (1985).

If prophylactic measures such as graduated compression stockings and low dose heparin are considered indicated for the prevention of deep venous thrombosis – and this is something still hotly debated in the UK – they should be initiated as soon as possible following the admission of the patient to the hospital. However, the prophylactic antibiotics which are routinely used for all patients undergoing hip fracture surgery should not be started until the induction of anaesthesia.

Postoperative management

Current practice is for the patient to be mobilized out of bed within a day or so of the operation. In this connection it must be remembered that these patients are somewhat weaker than normal and that walking with two crutches demands more energy than walking with a Zimmer frame. It also means manipulating two aids instead of one and for this reason it is the author's preference to keep these patients on a walking frame until such time as they can move easily on to two and preferably one walking stick. However long it takes them to change over to a single stick is of no consequence. What really matters is that the patients are up and mobile. If by any chance the reduction is not satisfactory and the internal fixation device has not been as rigidly successful as one would have hoped, then there may be theoretical advantage in keeping these patients non-weight bearing on the affected leg. Elderly patients however frequently find it impossible to adhere to such a regime and partial weight bearing is just as difficult even with a Zimmer frame. Let us therefore not deceive ourselves that in this population of patients there is much difference between weight bearing and non-weight bearing. Furthermore, the internal generation of forces by muscles across the hip is largely uninfluenced by weight bearing and the author has seen internal fixation devices bend after insertion into a patient who has not yet been out of bed!

Postoperative complications

Considering that the typical femoral neck fracture patient is elderly and often frail it is not surprising that many or all of them develop some generalized postoperative complications. These include bronchopneumonia, deep venous thrombosis, pulmonary embolism, constipation, urinary retention, urinary tract infection and confusion. Some of these complications are discussed in other chapters of this book and this section will only consider deep venous thrombosis and pressure sores in addition to the specific complications of intra- and extracapsular fractures.

Deep venous thrombosis

By far the commonest postoperative complication is deep venous thrombosis which has been demonstrated venographically to occur in 40–50% of patients. The thrombosis can occur in the calf veins, the thigh veins or both but it is the proximal thrombi which tend to lead to pulmonary embolism. This occurs in approximately 3% of patients with deep venous thrombosis and causes death in less than one-third of these.

It is for this reason that routine prophylactic anticoagulation of all patients with hip fractures is considered unreasonable by many but for those who wish to use it, there are many regimes available though convincing published evidence of their efficacy is often hard to find. Similarly, graduated compression stockings are in routine use in many centres though objective evidence of their true benefit is limited.

It is the author's preference not to use prophylactic anticoagulants since the complications that arise from the bleeding tendency tend to outdo the potential benefits of reducing the incidence of deep venous thrombosis and pulmonary embolism. However, once there is a clinical suggestion of these conditions they must be diagnosed objectively, i.e. venographically and/or by ventilation/perfusion scans. Once the diagnosis has been confirmed treatment with a regimen of heparin and subsequently warfarin is

indicated. However, a problem arises regarding the length of treatment. On the one hand there are those who believe it should be prescribed for 3 months only and on the other those who consider it should continue for life. It is the author's belief that a period of 3–6 months is appropriate. It does seem a little 'unreal' to keep elderly patients on systems where their clotting times are increased and to have them attend the hospital at regular intervals for haematological check-ups.

Should a massive, near fatal, pulmonary embolus occur, it should be treated non-operatively and there is no place for heroic procedures (e.g. Trendelenberg operation) in these patients.

Pressure sores

These are an expensive and totally preventable complication following fracture of the proximal femur. They are a manifestation of ischaemia of the local skin and subcutaneous tissue and the commonest sites are the sacrum, heels and buttocks. They can readily be prevented by turning the patient 2-hourly in appropriate cases, or getting them to turn themselves.

Patients with pressure sores stay in hospital much longer than those without and many appliances (more or less expensive) have been devised to 'spread the load' of the patient's weight (see chapter 18). Although pressure sores are relatively infrequent in a well-run surgical unit, they still occur and they obviously occur much more commonly where patients with this sort of fracture are given no special treatment. Versluysen (1985) showed that approximately one-third of patients admitted to a London teaching hospital for femoral neck fracture developed a pressure sore within the first 2 weeks and thought the cause of the sores was multifactorial. In the hip fracture unit in Newcastle, the incidence of pressure sores is only 2% and this low figure is the result of careful nursing, the use of appropriate low pressure surfaces and early and maintained mobilization.

Specific complications associated with intracapsular (high) fractures

The major complications specific to intracapsular fractures are avascular (or aseptic) necrosis and non-union in those patients in whom internal fixation is used and dislocation, loosening and pain in those in whom the head is sacrificed and a hemiarthroplasty inserted.

Avascular necrosis

This has long been studied but when discussing this subject it is important to differentiate it from late segmental collapse. The term avascular necrosis refers to the infarct that occurs early following a femoral neck fracture and is secondary to the fracture itself, the reduction manoeuvre or the size of the internal fixation device (Linde *et al.*, 1986). In contrast, segmental collapse identifies the change in shape in the femoral head that occurs late in the course of the avascular insult. The incidence of late segmental collapse is considerably less than that of avascular necrosis. For example, Barnes *et al.* (1976) showed that only 27% of united fractures underwent late segmental collapse whereas Catto (1965) found that 80% of all subcapital femoral fractures demonstrated evidence of at least partial avascular necrosis.

The radiological signs of avascular necrosis vary during the course of its natural history. In the early phase of hyperaemia plain radiographs show rarefaction of the surrounding bone with no change in the density of the avascular part. Later the dead bone apparently increases in density and this may be secondary to new bone being laid down on necrotic bony trabeculae or the calcification that may occur in the necrotic marrow (Figure 12.12). Segmental collapse appears as flattening and may be associated with fracture in the subchondral bone and articular cartilage overlying the infarct (Figure. 12.13). This produces joint incongruity and subsequent painful degenerative arthropathy requiring total hip arthroplasty in 16% (Kofoed and Alberts, 1980).

Manninger *et al.* (1989) reported a significant difference in the time and 'quality' of union and the incidence of collapse of the head of the femur between those treated within 6 h and those treated between 6 and 24 h. At the present time other than expeditious surgery there is little to combat the complications of avascular necrosis and segmental collapse with the exception of the wholesale removal of all femoral heads. This is obviously undersirable especially when one considers that fewer than 30% of patients who

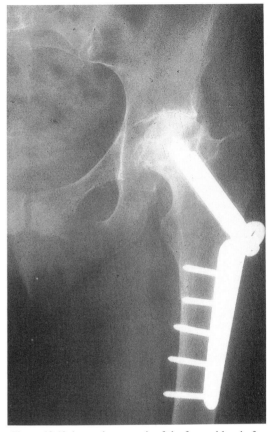

Figure 12.12 Avascular necrosis of the femoral head after fixation of an intracapsular fracture

develop late segmental collapse exhibit symptoms sufficient to warrant further surgery (Barnes *et al.*, 1976; Kofoed and Alberts, 1980). Attempts to determine the viability of the femoral head at the time of surgery have not been rewarding. These include the measurement of oxygen tension, venography, isotope clearances (Alberts, 1990) and intraosseous pressure measurement. All indicate a significant degree of disturbance of the vascular supply of the femoral head following the fracture but the correlation between the vascular findings and the clinical end result have never been more than approximately 80% accurate. Consequently, these techniques must still be considered research tools and of little practical value in the treatment of individual patients with femoral neck fractures.

Non-union

Non-union may occur in up to one-quarter of intracapsular fractures and this may or may not

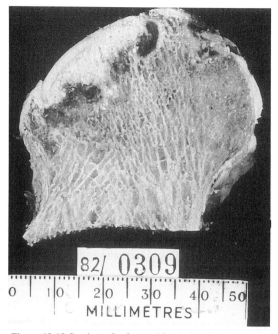

Figure 12.13 Section of a femoral head showing late segmental collapse due to avascular necrosis following healing of the fracture

be complicated by avascular necrosis of the femoral head. The groups of patients in which non-union particularly occurs are those with markedly displaced fractures and with poor reductions. For example, Kofoed and Alberts (1980) reported that 97% of Garden's stage I fractures united compared with 28% of stage IV injuries. Of those patients with painful non-union 75% required a further operation. Whereas in the younger, fitter adult bone grafting may be indicated, in the elderly patient the second operation must be definitive and with the least possible risk of complication. Hemiarthroplasty is possible but a total hip replacement is indicated if secondary changes have occurred in the acetabular side of the joint.

Dislocation

The incidence of dislocation following hemiarthroplasty varies in reported series between 1% and 10% (DeLee, 1984) and factors associated with it include excessive anteversion or retroversion of the prosthesis and excessive flexion or adduction of the operated limb postoperatively. It is also important to remember that infection is a frequent cause of dislocation and is said to be present in up to one-third of

dislocated femoral heads (DeLee, 1984). In the absence of a definite mechanical aetiology infection must therefore be excluded.

With prompt recognition and reduction, dislocation is unlikely to jeopardize the end result. Immediate reduction under anaesthesia is indicated followed by a period of immobilization in abduction and extension until soft tissue healing occurs. The use of an abduction hip brace may enable the patient's hip to be held in a safe position and still allow mobilization.

Pain

Pain is the principal long-term complication of hemiarthroplasty. Though good long-term results of this operation have been reported in over 85% of patients in some series (Hinchey and Day, 1964) other authors report the presence of pain reducing the chances of good long-term results to only 50% of patients (Coates, 1975).

Hip pain may be present without X-ray changes or may be associated with signs of prosthetic loosening or with distal or proximal prosthetic migration. Loosening on a radiograph is detected by the presence of a radiolucent zone around the prosthesis. Distal migration is best assessed by comparing recent with earlier radiographs when calcar resorption or a change in the distance from the collar of the prosthesis to the lesser trochanter may be seen. Proximal migration of the prosthesis is noted as protrusio acetabulae which is often associated with a concomitant loss of joint space.

If the clinical signs and symptoms are significant revision to a total hip arthroplasty may be indicated. However, it is important to recognize that some prostheses remain painful without radiological signs of sepsis, migration or loosening and in these patients it is possible that articular cartilage wear and the involvement of the underlying bone are the causes of pain.

Finally, it must be mentioned that fracture of the femoral shaft may occur just distal to the tip of the hemiarthroplasty stem.

Specific complications associated with inter-trochanteric (low) fractures

Complications are much less frequent in patients with intertrochanteric fractures when compared with equivalent individuals with sub-capital fractures. For example, avascular necrosis occurs in less than 1% (Sisk, 1987) as does non-union (DeLee, 1984). However, shortening and rotational deformities are well recognized problems especially in the unstable fractures. Varus displacement is associated with failure of implant fixation in the proximal fragment and failure to obtain a stable reduction. It is often accompanied by implant bending, breaking and cutting out of the femoral head or pulling away from the lateral aspect of the femoral shaft.

The shortening associated with varus displacement can usually be at least partially overcome by means of a shoe raise, and re-operation in this elderly group of frail patients is only indicated if the implant cuts out and is the source of severe pain.

Implant penetration into the hip joint following fixation of intertrochanteric fractures may account for up to one-third of treatment failures. It is usually due to using an excessively long screw or nail and not taking account of the fact that up to 15 mm of collapse can occur at the fracture site during the healing phase. The use of a sliding screw device should obviate this problem providing the screw slides appropriately within its barrel. Fortunately, implant penetration does not always prejudice the end result and the nail or screw should be left in position until union is certain. Only then should consideration be given to its removal but Wilson *et al.* (1980) noted that only 1.3% of cases of nail penetration required subsequent implant removal.

Unexplained discomfort may persist following healing of the fracture. It may be due to the presence of the implant, to residual deformity altering hip joint biomechanics or to low grade sepsis. Apart from the last condition further surgery is rarely indicated.

Pathological fractures of the hip

Pathological fractures occur after minimal force is applied across abnormal bone. Using this definition the majority of hip fractures must be considered pathological since in more than 90% of cases evidence of osteoporosis, osteomalacia or both can be detected. Conventionally, however, osteoporosis is excluded from the definition and will not be considered further.

Pathological fracture due to metabolic disease

This includes Paget's disease, parathyroid disorders and osteonecrosis due to previous irradiation. This used to be not uncommon following intracavity radiotherapy of cervical and endometrial carcinoma but is now virtually unknown.

Fractures associated with Paget's disease probably start as pseudo-fractures which then develop into a complete fracture. These pseudo-fractures occur on the convexity of the bone (tension side) and therefore appear on the lateral aspect of the femur or the superior aspect of the neck. The fractures themselves are usually perpendicular to the long axis of the femur. The commonest site around the hip for fracture in association with Paget's disease is the subtrochanteric region but subcapital fractures also occur. They present considerable difficulty in management and a review by Grundy (1970) showed that all such fractures failed to unite. Other authors have reported a non-union rate for subcapital femoral fractures of approximately 75% with refractures occurring after apparent healing in 10% (chapter 10).

At surgery Pagetic bone may be hard, soft or normal – with each type of bone presenting its own problems. Soft bone may not engage screws and sclerotic bone may be so hard that it is almost impossible to drill. Excessive haemorrhage from Pagetic bone may also occur especially if it is an 'active' phase.

Exactly which operation should be performed is a difficult decision but prosthetic replacement of the femoral head is recommended in subcapital fractures since the non-union rate is so high. It is the author's preference to perform a total hip replacement though he accepts that some patients will do as well with a cemented hemiarthroplasty. Internal fixation for trochanteric and subtrochanteric fractures can be performed but a screw system is preferable to a nail plate since the hammering associated with the latter technique may produce further iatrogenic fracture.

Generalized disorders causing predisposition to fracture of the femoral neck

The most common generalized disorder which causes a predilection to femoral neck fracture in the elderly is rheumatoid arthritis. This may be because of the associated osteoporosis or some other factor and indeed the frequency of bilateral hip fractures in this disorder is greater than in the normal population. Hadden, Abernethy and Haw (1982) treated 122 patients with hip fractures associated with rheumatoid disease (73 high and 49 low fractures) and compared the results with those obtained in 152 non-rheumatoid patients. Undisplaced fractures of the neck did much the same in both groups but when displaced fractures were considered (Garden stages III and IV) the rheumatoid patients achieved significantly less favourable results. Furthermore, only one acceptable result was achieved in the nine patients who had involvement of the hip joint itself by the rheumatoid process. In those patients with extracapsular fractures there was no real difference between the patient group and the control group.

A similar experience was reported by Strömqvist, Kelly and Lidgren (1988) who found that only one patient out of 20 with a displaced cervical fracture developed signs of union without evidence of ischaemic necrosis: 14 of the remainder required a secondary total hip arthroplasty and these figures were significantly poorer than those recorded in the control group. They therefore advocated primary hip arthroplasty in this group of patients. Stephen (1980) found similar results and confirmed that displaced fractures treated by reduction internal fixation did not unite in this group of patients with rheumatoid disease.

Benign tumorous conditions

These are quite a rare cause of hip fracture in the elderly but conditions such as simple bone cysts have been reported in the femoral neck. They should be treated by internal fixation with cement augmentation or hemiarthroplasty as appropriate.

Malignant bone tumours

Though pathological fractures through primary bone tumours have been reported in elderly patients these are excessively rare. Much more common is a fracture through a metastasis (Figure 12.14). Behr, Dobozi and Badrinath (1985) showed that the commonest primary tumour which gave rise to metastases around the hip was of the female breast and this accounted for 45% of pathological fractures; 20% were due to myeloma and 11% to bronchial tumours.

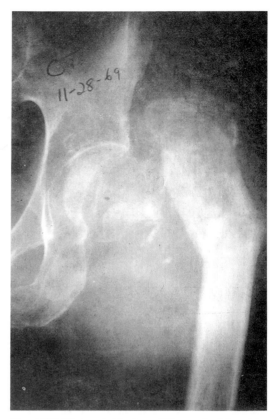

Figure 12.14 Segmental fracture of the proximal femur due to advanced metastatic disease

Similar figures have been published by Haberman *et al.* (1982).

Levy, Sherry and Siffert (1982) stated that the aims of treatment of such patients were to relieve pain and restore function by the use of a device or technique with an anticipated life which should exceed the patient's life expectancy. They considered prosthetic replacement to be a successful method for fractures of the head and neck but advised intramedullary techniques of internal fixation for trochanteric and subtrochanteric fractures. Suitable implants would be the Zickel or gamma nails. They emphasized the beneficial effect of the concomitant use of methylmethacrylate bone cement and this was also the opinion of Haberman *et al.* (1982) who analysed the results of treatment of 283 pathological fractures of the hip; 196 were treated by internal fixation or prosthetic replacement with methylmethacrylate and 110 were treated by similar measures but without the use of acrylic cement. They reported that pain relief, the ability to walk and the survival rates were all enhanced by the use of the cement. They found that bronchial metastases were associated with the worst prognosis but overall 59% of their patients survived 6 months and 48% survived 12 months.

Technical considerations regarding surgery for pathological fractures around the hip are described in chapter 15 together with the management of patients with fractures and terminal illness. The role of prophylactic fixation is also considered.

References

Aitken, J.M. (1984) Relevance of osteoporosis in women with fractures of the femoral neck. *Br. Med. J.,* **288** 597–601

Al-Arabi, K.M., Elidrissy, A.W. and Desrani, S.H. (1984) Is avoidance of sunlight a cause of fractures of the femoral neck in elderly Saudis? *Trop. Geogr. Med.,* **36**, 273

Alberts, K.A. (1990) Prognostic accuracy of preoperative and postoperative scintimetry after femoral neck fracture. *Clin. Orthop.,* **250**, 221–225

Alfram, P.-A. (1964) An epidemiological study of cervical and trochanteric fractures of the femur in an urban population. *Acta Orthop. Scand.,* **65** (Suppl), 1–109

Arnala, I., Alhava, E.M., Kivivouri R. and Kauranen, O. (1986) Hip fracture incidence not affected by fluoridation. Osteofluorosis studied in Finland. *Acta Orthop. Scand.,* **57**, 344–348

Åström, J., Ahnqvist, S., Beertema E., J. and Johnson, B. (1987) Physical activity in women sustaining fracture of the neck of the femur. *J. Bone Joint Surg.,* **69B**, 381–383

Barnes, R., Brown, J.T., Garden, R.S. and Nicoll E.A. (1976) Subcapital fractures of the femur. A prospective review. *J. Bone Joint Surg.,* **58B**, 2–24

Bateman, J.E. (1974) Single-assembly total hip prosthesis – preliminary report. *Orthop. Dig.,* **2**, 15

Behr, J.T., Dobozi, W.R. and Badrinath, K. (1985) The treatment of pathological and impending pathological fractures of the proximal femur in the elderly. *Clin. Orthop.,* **198**, 173–178

Bentley, G. (1968) Impacted fractures of the neck of the femur. *J. Bone Joint Surg.,* **50B**, 551–561

Blessed, G., Tomlinson, B.E. and Roth, M. (1968) The association between quantitative measures of dementia and of senile change in the cerebral grey matter of elderly subjects. *Br. J. Psychiat.,* **114**, 797

Bohr, H. and Schaadt, O. (1983) Bone mineral content of femoral bone and the lumbar spine measured in women with fracture of the femoral neck by dual-photon absorptionmetry. *Clin. Orthop.,* **174**, 240

Boyce, W.J. and Vessey, M.P. (1985) Rising incidence of fracture of the proximal femur. *Lancet,* **i**, 150–151

Boyce, W.J. and Vessey, M.P. (1988) Habitual physical inertia and other factors in relation to risk of fractures of the proximal femur. *Age Ageing,* **17**, 319–327

Butt, W.P. (1990) Fractured neck of femur. (ii) Radiological evaluation. *Curr. Orthop.,* **4**, 156–164

Caniggia, M. and Morreale, P. (1989) Epidemiology of hip fractures in Siena, Italy, 1975–1985. *Clin. Orthop.,* **238**, 131–138

Cartlidge, I.J. (1981) Primary total hip replacement for displaced subcapital femoral fractures. *Injury,* **13**, 249–253

Catto, M. (1965) The histological appearances of late segmental collapse of the femoral head after transcervical fracture. *J. Bone Joint Surg.,* **47B**, 777–791

Chow, S.P., Tang, S.C., Pun, W.K., Lee, P.C., Lau, H.K., Lim, J. and Leong, J.C. (1987) Treatment of unstable trochanteric fractures with Dimon-Hughston osteotomy displacement fixation and acrylic cement. *Injury,* **18**, 123–127

Coates, R.L. (1975) A retrospective survey of eighty-one patients with hemi-arthroplasty for subcapital fracture of the femoral neck. *J. Bone Joint Surg.,* **57B**, 256

Cobelli, N.J. and Sadler, A.H. (1985) Ender rod versus compression screw fixation of hip fractures. *Clin. Orthop.,* **201**, 123–129

Cooper, C., Barker, D.J., Morris, J. and Briggs, R.S. (1987) Osteoporosis, falls and age in fracture of the proximal femur. *Br. Med. J.,* **295**, 13–15

Cooper, C., McLaren, M., Wood, P.J., Coulton, L. and Kanis, J.A. (1989) Indices of calcium metabolism in women with hip fractures. *J. Bone Min. Res.,* **5**, 193–200

Cummings, S.R. (1985) Are patients with hip fractures more osteoporotic? *Am. J. Med.,* **78**, 487–494

Davis, T.R.C., Sher, J.L., Checketts, R.G. and Porter, R.B. (1988) Intertrochanteric fractures of the femur: a prospective study comparing the use of the Kuntscher Y-nail and a sliding hip screw. *Injury,* **19**, 421–426

DeLee, J.C. (1984) Fractures and dislocations of the hip. In *Fractures in Adults* (eds C.A. Rockwood and D.P. Green), Lippincott, London, Vol. 2 pp. 1211–1356

Devas, M. and Hinves, B. (1983) Prevention of acetabular erosion after hemi-arthoplasty for fractured neck of femur. *J. Bone Joint Surg.,* **65B**, 548–551

Dimon, J.H. and Hughston, J.C. (1967) Unstable intertrochanteric fractures of the hip. *J. Bone Joint Surg.,* **49A**, 440–450

Ender, H.G. (1978) The treatment of pertrochanteric and subtrochanteric fractures of the femur with Ender nailing. *Proc. Hip Soc.,* Mosby, St Louis, p. 187

Eriksson, S.A and Widhe, T.L. (1988) Bone mass in women with hip fracture. *Acta. Orthop. Scand.,* **59**, 19–23

Esser, M.P., Kassab, J.Y. and Jones, D.H.A. (1986) Trochanteric fractures of the femur. A randomised prospective trial comparing the Jewitt nail-plate with the dynamic hip screw. *J. Bone Joint Surg.,* **68B**, 557–550

Evans, E.M. (1949). The treatment of trochanteric, fractures of the femur *J. Bone Joint Surg.,* **31B**, 90–203

Falch, J.A., Ilebeck, A. and Slungaard, U. (1985) Epidemiology of hip fractures in Norway. *Acta Orthop. Scand.,* **56**, 12–16

Finsen, V. and Benum, P. (1987) Changing incidence of hip fractures in rural and urban areas of central Norway. *Clin. Orthop.,* **218**, 104–110

Frandsen, R.A. and Kruse, T. (1983) Hip fractures in the county of Funen, Denmark. Implications of demographic aging and changes in incidence rates. *Acta. Orthop. Scand.*, **54**, 681–686

Frankel, V.H. (1960) In *The Femoral Neck Function, Fracture Mechanisms and Internal Fixation*, Charles C. Thomas, Springfield, IL

Frankel, V.H. (1974). In *Surgery of the Hip Joint* (ed. R.G. Tronzo), Lea & Febiger, Philadelphia

Franklin, A. and Gallanaugh, S.C. (1983) The biarticular hip prosthesis for fractures of the femoral neck: a preliminary report. *Injury*, **15**, 159–162

Gallagher, J.C., Melton, L.J., Riggs, B.L. and Bergstrath E. (1980) Epidemiology of fractures of the proximal femur in Rochester, Minnesota. *Clin. Orthop.*, **150**, 163–171

Garden, R.S. (1971) Malreduction and avascular necrosis in subcapital fractures of the femur. *J. Bone Joint Surg.*, **53B**, 183–197

Garden, R.S. (1974) Reduction and fixation of subcapital fractures of the femur. *Orthop. Clin. N. Am.*, **5**, 683–712

Gilchrist, W.J., Newman, R.J., Hamblen, D.L. and Williams, B.O. (1988) Prospective randomised study of an orthopaedic geriatric in-patient service. *Br. Med. J.*, **297**, 1116–1118

Grundy, M. (1970) Fractures of the femur in Paget's disease of bone. *J. Bone Joint Surg.*, **52B**, 252–263

Gustilo, R.B. (1991) *The Fracture Classification Manual*, Mosby Year Book Inc., St Louis

Haberman, E.J., Sachs, R., Stern, R.E., Hirsh, D.M. and Anderson, W.J. (1982) The pathology and treatment of metastatic disease of the femur. *Clin. Orthop.*, **169**, 70–82

Hadden, W.A., Abernethy, P.J. and Haw C. (1982) Hip fractures of rheumatoid arthritis. *Clin. Orthop.*, **170**, 252–259

Harju, E., Sotaniemi, E., Puranen, J. and Lahti, R. (1985) High incidence of low serum vitamin D concentration in patients with hip fracture. *Arch. Orthop. Trauma Surg.*, **103**, 408–416

Härmä, M., Karjalainen, D., Hoikka, V. and Alhava, E. (1985) Bone density in women with spinal and hip fractures. *Acta Orthop. Scand.*, **56**, 380–385

Hedlund, L.R. and Gallagher, J.C. (1989) Increased incidence of hip fractures in osteoporotic women treated with sodium fluoride. *J. Bone Min. Res.*, **4**, 223

Hinchey, J.J. and Day, P.L. (1964) Primary prosthetic replacement in fresh femoral neck fractures. *J. Bone Joint Surg.*, **46A**, 223–240

Hirsch, C. and Frankel, V.H. (1960) Analysis of forces producing fractures of the proximal end of the femur. *J. Bone Joint Surg.*, **42A**, 633–640

Hogervorst, E.J., Lips, P., De Blieck-Hogervorst, J.M., Van Der Vijgh, W.J. and Netrenbos, J.C. (1985) Bone mineral contents of transilial biopsies in patients with hip fractures. *Bone*, **6**, 297–299

Hordon, L.D. and Peacock, M. (1987) Vitamin D metabolism in women with femoral neck fracture. *J. Bone Min. Res.*, **2**, 413–426

Hornby, R., Evans, J.G. and Vardon, V. (1986) Trochanteric fractures in the elderly. *J. Bone Joint Surg.*, **68B**, 157

Hornby, R., Evans, J.G. and Vardon, V. (1989) Operative or conservative treatment of trochanteric fractures of the femur. A randomised epidemiological trial in elderly patients. *J. Bone Joint Surg.*, **71B**, 619–623

Hunter, G.A. (1975) The results of operative treatment of trochanteric fractures of the femur. *Injury*, **6**, 202–205

Ions, G.K. and Stevens, J. (1987) Prediction of survival in patients with femoral neck fractures. *J. Bone Joint Surg.*, **69B**, 384–387

Jarnlo, G.B., Jakobsson, B., Ceder, L. and Throngren, K.-G. (1989) Hip fracture incidence in Lund, Sweden, 1966–1986. *Acta. Orthop. Scand.*, **60**, 278–282

Jensen, J.S., Sonne-Holm, S. and Tondevold, E. (1980) Unstable trochanteric fractures: a comparative analysis of four methods of internal fixation. *Acta Orthop. Scand.*, **51**, 949–962

Johnson, R.E. and Specht (1981) The risk of hip fracture in postmenopausal females with or without estrogen drug exposure. *Am. J. Publ. Hlth*, **71**, 138

Juhn, A., Krimerhan, J. and Mendes, D.G. (1988) Intertrochanteric fracture of the hip. Comparison of nail-plate fixation and Ender's nailing. *Arch. Orthop. Traum. Surg.*, **107**, 136

Keil, D.P., Felson, D.T., Anderson, J.J., Wilson, P.W. and Moskowitz, M.A. (1987) Hip fracture and the use of estrogens in postmenopausal women. The Framingham study. *N. Engl. J. Med.*, **317**, 1169–1174

Kellie, S.E. and Brody, J.A. (1990) Sex specific and race specific hip fracture rates. *Am. J. Publ. Hlth*, **80**, 326

Kofoed, H. and Alberts, A. (1980) Femoral neck fractures. 165 cases treated by multiple percutaneous pinning. *Acta Orthop. Scand.*, **51**, 127–136

Larsson, S., Eliasson, P. and Hansson, L.-I. (1989) Hip fractures in northern Sweden, 1973–1984. A comparison of rural and urban populations. *Acta Orthop. Scand.*, **60**, 567–571

Lester, G.E., Anderson, J.J., Tylavsky, F.A., Sutton, W.R., Stinnett, S.S., Demas, R.A. and Talmage, R.V. (1990) Update on the use of distal radial bone density measurements in prediction of hip and Colles' fracture risk. *J. Orthop. Res.*, **8**, 220

Levy, R.N., Sherry, H.S. and Siffert, R.S. (1982) Surgical management of metastatic disease of bone at the hip. *Clin. Orthop.*, **169**, 62–69

Linde, F., Andersen, E., Hvass, I., Madsen, F. and Pallesen, R. (1986) Avascular femoral head necrosis following fracture fixation. *Injury*, **17**, 159–163

Lips, P., Bouillon, R., Jongen, M.J., Van Ginkel, F.R., Van Der Vijgh, W.J. and Netelenbos, J.C. (1985) The effect of trauma on serum concentrations of vitamin D metabolites in patients with hip fracture. *Bone*, **6**, 63

Lizaur-Utrilla, A., Puchades Orts A., Sanchez Del Campo, F., Anta Barrio, J. and Gutierrez Carbonel, P. (1987) Epidemiology of trochanteric fractures of the femur in Alicante, Spain. *Clin. Orthop.*, **218**, 24–31

Mainds, C.C. and Newman, R.J. (1989) Implant failures in patients with proximal femoral fractures treated by a sliding screw device. *Injury*, **20**, 98–100

Manninger, J., Kazar, G., Fekete, G., Fekete, K., Frenyo, S., Gyarfas, F., Salacz, T. and Varga, A. (1989) Significance of urgent (within 6 h) internal fixation in the management of fractures of the neck of the femur. *Injury*, **20**, 101–105

Mazess, R.B. and Barden, H.S. (1988) Measurement of bone by dual-photon absorptionmetry (DDA) and dual-energy X-ray absorptionmetry (DEXA). *Ann. Chir. Gynaecol.*, **77**, 197–203

Melton, J.L., Ilstrup, D.M., Riggs, B.L. and Beckenbaugh, R.D. (1982) Fifty-year trend in hip fracture incidence. *Clin. Orthop.*, **162**, 144–149

Melton, J.L., Wahmer, H.W., Richelson, L.S., O'Fallon, W.M. and Riggs, B.C. (1986) Osteoporosis and the risk of hip fracture. *Am. J. Epidemiol.*, **124**, 254–261

Melton, J.L., O'Fallon, W.M. and Riggs, B.L. (1987) Secular trends in the incidence of hip fractures. *Calcif. Tissue Int.*, **41**, 57–64

Meyers, M.H., Harvey, J.P. and Moore, T.M. (1973) Treatment of displaced subcapital and transcervical fractures of the femoral neck by muscle pedicle bone graft and internal fixation. *J. Bone Joint Surg.*, **55A**, 247–254

Müller, M.E., Nazarian, S., Koch, P. and Schatzker, J. (1990) *The Comprehensive Classification of Fractures of Long Bones*, Springer–Verlag, London

Naessen, T., Parker, R., Persson, I., Zack, M. and Adami, H.O. (1989) Time trends in incidence rates of first hip fracture in the Uppsala health care region, Sweden. 1963–1983. *Am. J. Epidemiol.*, **130**, 289–299

Otremski, I., Katz, A., Dekel, S., Salama, R. and Newman, R.J. (1990) Natural history of impacted subcapital femoral fractures and its relevance to treatment options. *Injury*, **21**, 379–381

Parker, M.J. (1991) Choice of treatment of the elderly patient with a displaced sub-capital fracture. Reduction or replacement. Br. Orthop. Ass., Brighton

Pauwels, F. (1935) *Der Schenkenholsbruck, Em Mechanisches Problem*, Beilagehft Zur Zeitschrift Fur Orthopaedische Chirurgie, Ferdinand Enke, Stuttgart

Prudham, D. and Evans, J.G. (1981) Factors associated with falls in the elderly. A community study. *Age Ageing*, **10**, 141–146

Pun, W.K., Chow, S.P., Chan, K. C., Ip, F.K., Tang, S.C., Ling, J. and Leong, J.C. (1987) Treatment of unstable intertrochanteric fractures with Sarmiento valgus osteotomy and acrylic cement augmentation. *Injury*, **18**, 384–389

Riggs, B.L., Baylink, D.J., Kleetlekoper, M., Lane, J.M., Melton, J.L. and Meunier P.J. (1987) Incidence of hip fractures in osteoporotic women treated with sodium fluoride. *J. Bone Min. Res.*, **2**, 123–126

Rodrigues, J.G., Sattin, R.W. and Waxweiler, R.J. (1989) Incidence of hip fractures, United States, 1970–1983. *Am. J. Prev. Med.*, **5**, 175–181

Sernbo, I., Johnell, O., Gentz, C.F. and Nilsson, J.A. (1988) Unstable intertrochanteric fractures of the hip. Treatment with Ender pins compared with a compression hip-screw. *J. Bone Joint Surg.*, **70A**, 1297

Sikorski, J.M., Davis, N.J. and Senior, J. (1985) The rapid transit system for patients with fractures of the proximal femur. *Br. Med. J.*, **290**, 439–443

Sim, E.H. and Stauffer, R.N. (1980) Management of hip fractures by total hip arthroplasty. *Clin. Orthop.*, **152**, 191–197

Singh, M., Nagrath, A.R. and Maini, P.S. (1970) Changes in the trabecular patterns of the upper end of the femur as an index of osteoporosis. *J. Bone Joint Surg.*, **52A**, 457–467

Sisk, T.D. (1987) In *Campbell's Operative Orthopaedics* (ed. A.H. Crenshaw), C.V. Mosby, St Louis, Vol. 3, Ch. 44

Sonne-Holm, S., Nordkild, P., Dyrbye, M. and Jensen, J.S. (1987) The predictive value of bone scintigraphy after internal fixation of femoral neck fractures. *Injury*, **18**, 33–35

Speed, K. (1935) The unsolved fracture. *Surg. Gynecol. Obstet.*, **60**, 341–351

Stephen, I.G. (1980) Subcapital fractures of the femur in rheumatoid arthritis. *Injury*, **11**, 233–241

Stevens, A. and Mulrow, C. (1989) Drugs affecting postural stability and other risk factors in the hip fracture epidemic – case control study. *Commun. Med.*, **11**, 27

Stevens, J. (1988) Unpublished observations

Stevens, J., Freeman, P.A. and Nordin, B.E.C. (1962) The incidence of osteoporosis in patients with femoral neck fractures. *J. Bone Joint Surg.*, **44B**, 520–527

Strömqvist, B., Kelly, I. and Lidgren L. (1988) Treatment of hip fractures in rheumatoid arthritis. *Clin. Orthop.*, **228**, 75–78

Uitewaal, P.J., Lips, P. and Netelenbos, J.C. (1987) An analysis of bone structure in patients with hip fracture. *J. Bone Min. Res.*, **3**, 63–73

Versluysen, M. (1985) Pressure sores in elderly patients. The epidemiology related to hip operations. *J. Bone Joint Surg.*, **67B**, 10–13

Waddell, J.P., Czitrom, A. and Simmons, E.H. (1987) Ender nailing in fractures of the proximal femur. *J. Trauma*, **27**, 911

Wallace, W.A. (1983) The increasing incidence of fractures of the proximal femur: an orthopaedic epidemic. *Lancet*, **i**, 1413–1414

Weiss, N.S., Ure, C.L., Ballard, J.H., Williams, A.R. and Daung, J.R. (1980) Decreased risk of fracture of the hip and lower forearm with postmenopausal use of estrogen. *N. Engl. J. Med.*, **303**, 1195–1198

Wilson, H.J., Rubin, B.D., Helbig, F.E., Fielding, J.W. and Munis, G.L. (1980) Treatment of intertrochanteric fractures with the Jewett nail: experience with 1015 cases. *Clin. Orthop.*, **148**, 186–191

Wood, D. (1990) MS Thesis. University of London

Zetterberg, C., Elmerson, S. and Anderson, G.B. (1984) Epidemiology of hip fractures in Goteborg, Sweden, 1940–1983. *Clin. Orthop.*, **191**, 43–52

13

Shoulder injuries in the elderly

Paul G. Stableforth

A shoulder that functions normally allows the hand to be placed comfortably and strongly in the best position for the activities of daily living. This includes domestic and leisure pursuits as diverse as writing, housework, driving and gardening as well as the more 'physical' of sporting activities. In addition the elderly person with spinal or lower limb disorders needs stable, strong and painless shoulders to help him rise from a lying or sitting position, to transfer from one position to another and to walk. A significant shoulder injury may therefore lead to temporary or permanent loss of self-care and independence.

Fractures and dislocations around the shoulder form some 5–10% of all bone and joint injuries but for the elderly patient they may cause major functional impairments and hence have an importance out of all proportion to their relative infrequency.

Dislocation of the shoulder (usually anterior or subcoracoid) may follow a fall onto the outstretched hand and a fracture of the proximal humerus may follow a sideways fall onto the shoulder. Injuries of the clavicle, the scapula and the acromioclavicular joint are rare in the older patient unlike tears of the rotator cuff which are not infrequently seen.

This chapter will first discuss the clinical features and treatment of those bony injuries of the shoulder girdle which are commonly sustained by elderly members of the population. Pathological fractures will also be described as will some painful and disabling conditions of the soft tissues around the shoulder.

Fractures and dislocations of the shoulder girdle

Causes of disability

Everyday non-sporting activities can be performed without difficulty with a total shoulder range of movement of 95 degrees of flexion, 50 degrees of extension and 45 degrees of internal and external rotation. However, scapulothoracic movement alone can provide up to 45 degrees of flexion and 20–30 degrees of total rotation. Therefore, though true glenohumeral movement is often restricted after shoulder injury, stiffness of this joint is not often a cause of significant disability. The latter is usually due to pain or instability particularly after the more severe proximal humeral fractures.

Pain may arise from impingement of displaced bone fragments against the coraco-acromial arch, glenoid or acromioclavicular joint, from damage to the articular surfaces, from fibrous glenohumeral ankylosis, from fracture non-union or from post-injury algodystrophy (Sudek's atrophy).

Instability may follow articular, capsular or ligamentous damage, may be a sequel to nerve damage or may more commonly occur as a result of the transient muscle atony that follows bone or joint injury.

Examination of the shoulder

The normal bony landmarks should be seen and palpated in turn. Flattening of the shoulder contour, undue prominence of the humeral head anteriorly and any other localized or diffuse

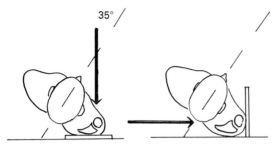

Figure 13.1 Positioning for anteroposterior and axial radiographs of the shoulder. These two radiographic projections can be taken with the patient lying down or standing and are the minimum needed for management of a fractured proximal humerus. The heavy arrow indicates the direction of the X-ray beam (Modified after Neer, 1970a)

swellings that alter or obscure these landmarks are noted. The deltoid muscle should be felt to contract as the patient is asked to push the elbow away from the side as this is resisted by the examiner's hand. The scapula is then steadied as the patient tries to move the arm in each direction. Restriction of active movements and any associated pain are noted.

The elbow, forearm and hand are then examined for motor, sensory, reflex or vascular abnormality.

An A-P view of the shoulder together with an axial view of the scapula (Neer and Rockwood, 1984) and an axillary view are the essential radiographic projections needed after injury (Figure 13.1). Many other projections are available and are sometimes of benefit.

Aims of treatment

The basic principles underlying the treatment of fractures and dislocations around the shoulder include the necessity of joint surfaces to be made congruous, displaced fracture fragments to be aligned without soft tissue interposition or impingement and the joint capsule and ligaments to be protected or repaired. Rehabilitation following a significant shoulder injury may be prolonged and it is desirable that the patient starts his programme of exercises as soon as pain permits.

The first 4 or 5 days and nights will be much more comfortable if the patient rests or sleeps propped up in a chair or in bed with the elbow well supported by pillows. An early start on shoulder exercises aids absorption rather than organization of post-traumatic haematoma and oedema. Our studies have shown that a delay of

up to two weeks will delay the return to self-care for a similar period but does not affect the final range of motion. An elbow-supporting broad-fold (broad arm) sling is therefore applied, the patient is encouraged to use the arm and hand for self-care and the shoulder is safely rested until the acute pain of injury has eased.

By the end of the first week the arm should be taken out of the sling regularly, used at meal-times and the elbow, forearm, wrist and hand put through a full range of movements. The patient sits or stands leaning forwards and starts 'pendulum' exercises with the arm hanging freely at the shoulder and is encouraged to use the whole arm as normally as pain and stiffness allow. The emphasis is on the functionally important movements of flexion, extension and internal and external rotation with the elbow and hand at waist height.

By the end of the second week active assisted flexion, extension and rotation exercises are begun with the patient initially lying supine.

Exercises against gravity and graded resistance are started at about 4 weeks and continue with increasing vigour for 6–12 weeks or longer.

Clavicular and acromioclavicular joint injuries

These injuries usually follow a tumbling fall or a fall from a height onto the 'point' of the shoulder and are relatively uncommon in the elderly.

There is bruising that is localized initially to the acromioclavicular joint or clavicle but later spreads down the arm and the chest wall. Soft tissue swelling occurs locally but usually there is little other deformity. The thin, elderly skin sometimes splits over the site of injury and may need to be held with Steristrips.

The diagnosis is confirmed by A-P radiographs of the shoulder and clavicle.

Treatment is by shoulder support and rest in a broadfold sling and suitable analgesics are prescribed until the pain eases over the first 4–5 days. Functional range of movement exercises are then encouraged and recovery takes 12–16 weeks.

Late pain or deformity are rare.

Glenohumeral dislocation

A sideways fall onto a braced, outstretched arm may force the humeral head forwards and tear the anterior shoulder joint capsule and ligaments to result in subcoracoid (or anterior) dislocation of the humeral head.

In the thin patient the flattening of the normal deltoid curve together with the fullness caused by the displaced humeral head lying below the lateral third of the clavicle and the slightly abducted and internally rotated arm makes the diagnosis easy. In the more obese patient the deformities may be concealed by the subcutaneous fat and the diagnosis can only be made by biplanar radiography.

In the elderly the supraspinatus part of the rotator cuff may be stretched or torn at its insertion. It heals poorly and may be a cause of continuing shoulder stiffness or discomfort even after early reduction of the dislocation (Johnson and Bayley, 1981; Astley, 1986). The greater tuberosity, the tendon's attachment to the upper humerus, may be avulsed but this bone fragment usually realigns itself during reduction of the dislocation. Occasionally it does not and open reduction and screw fixation of the tuberosity is indicated if rotator cuff function is to be restored. Tuberosity displacement may be immediate or may occur several days after reduction of the dislocation and therefore it is prudent to take further radiographs 7–10 days later.

The axillary nerve is damaged in 25–35% of anterior dislocations and this is associated with weakness or paralysis of the deltoid and inconsistent numbness over its insertion (Brown, 1952; Blom and Dahlbäck, 1970). Spontaneous recovery is usual but the 2–3 month delay before muscle power returns may be a cause of persistent shoulder stiffness.

The dislocated humeral head should be reduced into the glenoid as soon as possible; the greater the delay the more difficult will be the reduction and the greater the likelihood of persistent shoulder stiffness or pain. While a short general anaesthetic may be needed, most dislocations can be reduced by gentle manipulation under analgesic sedation. Ideally the weight of the arm hanging over the side of a trolley or bed is allowed to draw the humeral head into joint (Stimson, 1900). However, in my experience the 15–20 min of prone lying needed for this is poorly tolerated by the elderly. The Hippocratic or the Kocher's manoeuvre are therefore usually required (Neer and Rockwood, 1984).

In the former the operator's foot or a towel is placed against the axillary fold and slow and gentle traction is applied to the arm; very gentle rocking of the arm into internal and external rotation may ease reduction. In the Kocher's method the flexed elbow is steadied by the patient's side, the arm is gently, slowly but firmly externally rotated, then adducted to bring the elbow in front of the chest. The arm is then internally rotated and a soft thud is felt as the dislocation is reduced. Rapid or forced external rotation of the arm, or an attempt to reduce a dislocation that is more than a week old may cause a spiral fracture of the humeral shaft.

When clinical reduction has occurred biplanar radiographs should be taken to confirm congrous and concentric reduction of the humeral head.

Recurrent anterior dislocation, so commonly a problem in the young, is rare in the older patient, and although the arm and elbow should be supported in a broadfold sling shoulder movements may be safely encouraged as soon as comfort permits.

Independence for self-care is usual by 4–6 weeks and the final range of movements by 4–6 months. Full recovery of motion is rare but although persistent shoulder stiffness or weakness may make hand use at or above shoulder height impossible, disabling stiffness is uncommon.

Aching discomfort in inclement weather, with arm use under load or away from the body may last 12–18 months.

Recurrent subcoracoid dislocation

This is an uncommon injury in the elderly (Rowe and Sakellarides, 1961). It is possible that in this age group the weak anterior capsule tears during the acute dislocation and the resulting fibrous scar provides a barrier to recurrent dislocation (Reeves, 1968). The clinical presentation is the same as in younger patients with an initial acute traumatic dislocation and later episodes of painful instability that occur with little force or from incautious or inadvertent elevation or external rotation of the arm, often during sleep or self-care.

Apprehension of dislocation when the arm is moved passively into elevation and external rotation may be the only positive finding on clinical examination.

If the condition proves disabling anterior stabilization of the shoulder by plication of the anterior capsule and the subscapularis muscle will usually prevent further episodes of dislocation. Rarely an anterior glenoid deficiency or a large posterior humeral head defect may make a bone block procedure or humeral rotation osteotomy more appropriate.

Chronic, unreduced subcoracoid dislocation

Persistent dislocation after an unremembered fall may be the cause of shoulder stiffness and pain. Deformity may not be apparent but all glenohumeral movement is painfully restricted. It is therefore wise to take biplanar shoulder radiographs of any elderly patient who presents with a 'frozen shoulder' before physiotherapy is started.

If the pain is intrusive open reduction of the dislocation should be considered. The procedure is often taxing as the tissue planes are distorted and adherent, the glenoid needs to be cleared of soft tissue and a large indent fracture on the posterior aspect of the humeral head may compromise stability and make it necessary to transfix the humeral head and glenoid with stout guide wires for 6 weeks to maintain reduction.

Although rest and motion pain are usually eased the final range of movement is often disappointing as a result of rotator cuff rupture, subdeltoid and infraglenoid adhesions and the necessary prolonged postoperative immobilization.

Sometimes the presentation is atypical with little pain at rest or on movement. With this 'painless stiffness' it is probably prudent to leave the dislocation unreduced, though on occasion a humeral rotation osteotomy may improve function.

Fracture of the proximal humerus

This injury is common following a sideways fall onto the shoulder. Its incidence progressively rises from the fifth to eighth decades (Figure 13.2) both as a result of the inability of a tripping elderly person to check a fall and of the ease with which the increasingly brittle bone of age-related osteoporosis breaks (Figure 13.3).

Following fracture of the proximal humerus pain in the shoulder and subdeltoid regions is immediate and swelling occurs within hours. Bruising may be delayed and is usually seen in the lower arm around the elbow and in the upper chest wall and breast as blood tracks from

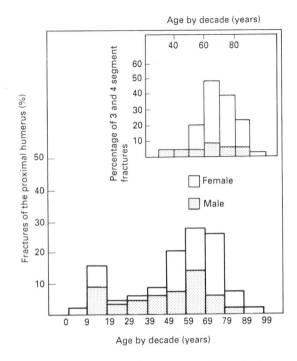

Figure 13.2 Age distribution of patients with proximal humeral fractures; incidence by age and sex. The lower graph refers to patients with all fractures of the proximal humerus and the upper graph refers to those patients with three and four segment fractures only (author's personal experience in Bristol)

under the deltoid muscle. All shoulder movements are pain-inhibited and crepitus may be evident.

Most fractures are little displaced and damage to the circumflex humeral or to the axillary vessels is rare. However, early surgical exploration may occasionally be needed to decompress a tensely swollen axilla or repair a major arterial tear resulting in hand or forearm ischaemia. The severest fractures can be associated with dislocation of the humeral head which may compress the median nerve or more rarely branches of the brachial plexus. This produces a major sensorimotor disturbance in the hand and forearm from which neurological recovery is very slow despite intensive treatment (Stableforth, 1984).

The fracture type and displacement are established by biplanar radiography and classification by the four-segment system popularized by Neer (1970a) aids decisions on management (Figure 13.4). In this classification a 'segment' is

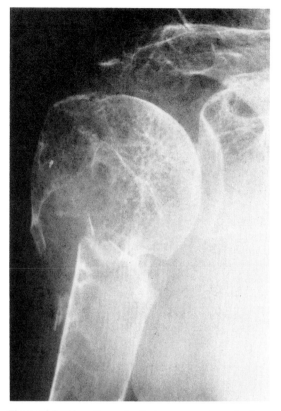

Figure 13.3 This radiograph of a two-segment proximal humeral fracture in a 90-year-old shows the extreme osteoporosis often seen at this age

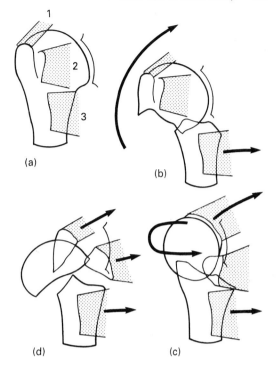

Figure 13.4 Proximal humeral fractures. The four-segment classification. (a) This shows the normal anatomy with the insertion of the supraspinatous tendon (1) into the greater tuberosity, the subscapularis (2) into the lesser tuberosity and the pectoralis major (3) into the proximal part of the humeral shaft. The pull of these muscle groups determines the direction of displacement of the bony fragments following (b) a two-segment fracture, (c) a three-segment fracture, and (d) a four-segment fracture

defined as either a tuberosity, an articular element or the humeral shaft and a 'part' is a bit or fragment of bone of which there can be any number.

In 85% of fractures the bone fragments are little displaced and do not require manipulation or surgery (Figure 13.5). The patient is assured that the severe pain and sleep disturbance rarely last more than 4 to 5 days, warned that 4–6 weeks will pass before he (or more frequently she) will achieve the activities of daily living and told that shoulder mobility and strength will improve gradually over a period of 4–6 months and sometimes longer. Conversely, in 15% of proximal humeral fractures the bone segments are grossly displaced or malrotated. Since the outcome of functional (conservative) treatment may be poor for these injuries closed manipulation or open reduction with internal fixation should be considered (Figure 13.6).

If, with two-segment fracture, the proximal segment is not in contact with the humeral shaft soft tissue interposition and consequent non-

union is likely. Manipulation under anaesthesia will usually restore the anatomy but the use of an external fixator to capture the proximal segment and secure a reduction which will not redisplace may be necessary.

Conservative treatment of the displaced three-segment fracture in which the articular segment is often grossly malrotated and the isolated tuberosity avulsed commonly results in painful shoulder dysfunction. The fracture is difficult to reduce by manipulation alone and the treatment of choice is an external fixator as described above. Open reduction and internal fixation may sometimes be indicated but the surgery is technically demanding and the postoperative regimen prolonged.

In the uncommon four-segment fracture the articular segment is stripped of its soft tissue attachments and both tuberosities widely displaced from their beds. Shoulder stiffness is usual and pain common following conservative

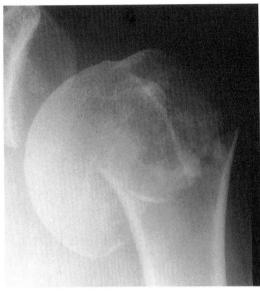

Figure 13.5 This three-segment fracture does not require manipulation since there is no soft tissue interposition. The fracture will unite without articular damage, malrotation or impingement and the subluxation will correct (*cf.* Figure 13.6)

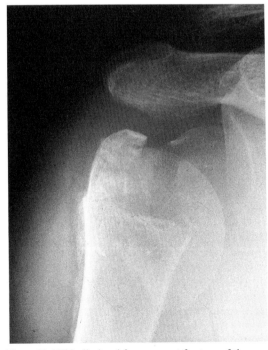

Figure 13.6 This displaced four-segment fracture of the proximal humerus has been managed non-operatively. The subluxation will correct but the greater tuberosity will probably impinge against the undersurface of the acromion in abduction. The lesser tuberosity has been avulsed by the subscapularis

therapy (Stableforth, 1984). The results of treatment of this otherwise devastating injury have been markedly improved by the advent of prosthetic reconstruction. The combination of appropriate surgery, intensive and prolonged aftercare and a cooperative patient will result in a comfortable and functional shoulder (Neer, 1963 and 1970b).

Pathological fracture of the proximal humerus

Metastases, most commonly from a primary breast or bronchial carcinoma, and less frequently from a thyroid, renal or other tumour, may erode and destroy the humeral head, neck or proximal shaft to cause painful shoulder dysfunction. The proximal humerus may also undergo necrosis following radiotherapy of the breast or axilla for malignant disease. This complication may present some 15–20 years after this form of treatment.

The onset may be insidious with constant, dull aching pain in the upper arm, present at rest, disturbing sleep and sometimes exacerbated by use of the upper limb. Conversely, the onset may be sudden with severe pain that prevents use of the arm. This usually indicates a pathological fracture through the weakened bone.

The patient may be known to have a primary tumour but on occasion the metastasis may be the first sign of malignancy.

Examination may reveal a little, diffuse soft tissue swelling, local tenderness and shoulder movements slowed by discomfort. Obvious swelling, bruising and painful loss of function may accompany a pathological fracture. Radiographs will show bony destruction with cortical erosion and occasionally subperiosteal callus.

Clinical examination of the patient for a primary tumour, urine analysis for blood, chest radiography and a radionuclide bone scan to identify other skeletal metastases should be performed expeditiously. If the diagnosis is in doubt and, certainly, if no primary tumour is found, the edge of the lesion should be biopsied and material sent for histological and bacteriological examinations. X-ray-guided needle biopsy techniques are now readily available in many centres so obviating the need for open biopsy under general anaesthesia.

If more than one-third of the humeral cortex has been destroyed but fracture has not yet occurred prophylactic bone splintage of some sort is advisable. This is because it is likely that fracture will occur prior to radiotherapy or chemotherapy causing tumour regression and bony reconstitution. Once fracture occurs it is associated with pain and loss of independence. This represents a severe blow to the patient's morale which may already be low. Surgical stabilization is essential and worthwhile and the technical considerations concerning both prophylactic and therapeutic fixation are discussed in chapter 15. At all times the aim of management of pathological fractures around the shoulder in the elderly is to preserve independence, self-care and mobility for as long as possible. The surgical procedure chosen must therefore allow or restore use of the arm for these activities as quickly as possible.

Painful soft tissue conditions around the shoulder

Tears of the rotator cuff

This condition may arise either insidiously or acutely following trauma. In the former case it is secondary to a chronic degeneration of the supraspinatus tendon which is common in older male manual workers. It may also occur in patients with rheumatoid arthritis or without obvious cause in patients of either sex with increasing age. The tendon thins close to its insertion into the greater tuberosity and develops small attrition tears within its substance or on its surface. These lesions may gradually extend until the tendon totally wears away. This leads from the insidious onset of nagging discomfort in the shoulder and upper arm, to a gradual reduction of strength and mobility or to a combination of the two. Sleep disturbance and difficulty with self-care are common.

The shoulder joint may be a little swollen and tender with active movements restricted and more painful the further the arm is moved away from the body. Conversely, passive movements are much more comfortable.

The acute type of cuff tear may follow unguarded shoulder use or a fall with the arm outstretched and is a common complication of subcoracoid dislocation without greater tuberosity fracture in the older patient. Examination reveals marked local swelling and tenderness with all shoulder movements grossly restricted by pain. Radiographs however show no evidence of acute bony or joint injury.

A satisfactory though incomplete functional recovery from cuff tears is usual and pain relief with a return to self-care and domestic routine follow non-operative treatment. The arm is initially rested in a broadfold sling and effective analgesics are prescribed. As the pain eases active shoulder rotation with the hand at waist height is encouraged and passive and active assisted flexion exercises are started. Gentle exercises against resistance are introduced after 4–6 weeks.

In some cases the pain remains severe and independence for self-care is not restored in the expected time. In these cases a course of subacromial injections of steroid and local anaesthetic (sometimes combined with manipulation of the shoulder under general anaesthesia), may speed recovery.

Sleep disturbance, difficulty with self-care, and pain when the arm is used away from the body or above shoulder height may persist if cuff thinning allows upward migration of the proximal humerus causing the greater tuberosity to impinge against the undersurface of the acromion. This mechanical problem is not helped by repeated steroid injections and is best treated surgically by an anterior acromioplasty, in which the underside of the acromion and the coracoacromial ligament are excised (Neer, 1972). This overcomes the painful impingement and predictably eases pain and increases mobility. Self-care is restored within 3 or 4 weeks though up to 6 months may elapse before the full benefits conferred by this procedure are achieved.

Adhesive capsulitis

Adhesive capsulitis, often associated with some adhesive subacromial bursitis, is a common end result of many different shoulder disorders. It is frequently secondary to rotator cuff degeneration with small tears and sometimes follows an inflammatory bursitis. Occasionally, it is the end result of a constrictive capsulitis.

It frequently presents in older patients with intrusive pain around the shoulder, sleep disturbance and restriction of shoulder mobility resulting in problems with self-care. A thorough history may allow one to differentiate the underlying aetiology. For example, a history of preceding unusual physical activity followed by local tenderness and restriction of shoulder movements may suggest a cuff degeneration whereas concomitant inflammatory changes in other joints may indicate that the shoulder condition is secondary to a subacromial bursitis. Pain and tenderness in the shoulder preceding the stiffness by many weeks is suggestive of constrictive capsulitis.

Physical examination reveals limitation of both passive and active shoulder movements in all directions by at least 50% but the radiological examination is normal.

The initial treatment is rest and anti-inflammatory medications followed as comfort increases by progressive mobilization exercises. Administration of an intra-articular injection of steroid and local anaesthetic often speeds the return of comfort and self-care and both manipulation under anaesthesia and distension injections of the glenohumeral joint have been suggested.

References

Astley, T. (1986) Dislocation of the shoulder in the elderly. *J. Bone Joint Surg.*, **68B**, 676.

Blom, S., Dahlbäck, L.O. (1970). Nerve injuries in dislocation of the shoulder joint and fractures of the neck of the humerus. A clinical and electromyographical study. *Acta. Chir. Scand.*, **136**, 461–466

Brown, J.T. (1952) Nerve injuries complicating dislocation of the shoulder. *J. Bone Joint. Surg.*, **34B**, 526

Johnson, J.R. and Bayley, J.I.L. (1981) Loss of shoulder function following acute anterior shoulder dislocation. *J. Bone Joint Surg.*, **63B**, 633

Neer, C.S. (1963) Prosthetic replacement of the humeral head; indications and operative technique. *Surg. Clin. N. Am.*, **43**, 1581–1597

Neer, C.S. (1970a) Displaced proximal humeral fractures. Part I. Classification and evaluation. *J. Bone Joint Surg.*, **52A**, 1077–1089

Neer, C.S. II, (1970b) Displaced proximal humeral fractures. Part II. Treatment of four part and three part displacement. *J. Bone Joint Surg.*, **52(A)**, 1090–1103

Neer, C.S. (1972) Anterior acromioplasty for the chronic impingement syndrome in the shoulder. A preliminary report. *J. Bone Joint Surg.*, **54(A)**, 41–50

Neer, C.S. II and Rockwood, C.A. (1984) Fractures and dislocations of the shoulder. In *Fractures in Adults* (eds C.A. Rockwood and D.P. Green), 2nd edn, J.B. Lippincott, Philadelphia; Toronto, pp. 675–985

Reeves, B. (1968) Experiments on the tensile strength of the anterior capsular structures of the shoulder in man. *J. Bone Joint Surg.*, **50B**, 858–865

Rowe, C.R. and Sakellarides, H.T. (1961) Factors related to the recurrence of anterior dislocation of the shoulder. *Clin. Orthop.*, **20**, 40–48

Stableforth, P.G. (1984) Four part fractures of the neck of the humerus. *J. Bone Joint Surg.*, **66B**, 104–108

Stimson, L.A. (1900). An easy method of reducing dislocations of the shoulder and hip. *Med. Rec.*, **57**, 356–357

14

Wrist fractures

Joseph J. Dias

The outstretched hand protects the falling body from sustaining major injury since a proportion of the impact is borne by the hand and wrist. It is therefore not surprising that wrist fractures, in particular the Colles' fracture, constitute a significant problem in the management of the elderly patient.

Incidence

In men the incidence of wrist fractures does not change with age and varies between 5 and 20 per 10 000 population per year (Alffram and Bauer 1962; Miller and Grimley Evans, 1985). In women however there is a sharp increase in the incidence rate between the ages of 45 and 60 years which peaks to 95 per 10 000 population per year. At approximately the age of 65 years and then thereafter, the rate of wrist fractures show a series of fluctuations but no general upward trend (Figure 14.1). In addition there appears to be an increase in the risk of falling among women over the age of 45 years (Winner, Morgan and Grimley Evans, 1989).

The pattern in old age of an increasing risk of proximal femoral fracture but a constant rate of wrist fracture may suggest that with increasing age a falling patient is less likely to throw her arm out in time to break the fall and is consequently more likely to fracture a hip. The interaction between the fall, the bone strength and the protective response of throwing out the arms during the fall (Grimley Evans, 1990) may help to interpret the changes in the incidence of wrist fractures in middle-aged women.

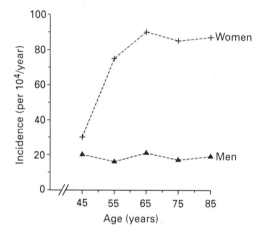

Figure 14.1 Incidence of distal radial fracture in British population samples (compare with Figure 17.1, which shows cumulative figures for Rochester, USA) (*Source:* Cooper, 1989, reproduced by permission of the author)

Osteoporosis and wrist fractures

There is considerable circumstantial evidence that wrist fractures occur more frequently in patients with osteoporosis. A female preponderance of 6:1 (Alffram and Bauer, 1962; Owen *et al.*, 1982), a peak incidence just after the menopause (Owen *et al.*, 1982a; Riggs and Melton, 1983), a significantly higher incidence of subsequent femoral neck fractures in patients sustaining a wrist fracture (Gay, 1974; Owen *et al.*, 1982b) and the fact that a Colles' fracture can result from a fall from standing height or less (Alffram and Bauer, 1962; Cummings *et al.*, 1985) have all been put forward as evidence of impaired bone quality.

It has been demonstrated (Dias *et al.*, 1987b) that 75% of patients with a Colles' fracture were

167

osteoporotic as assessed by measuring the width of the second metacarpal cortex. It is probable that the structural weakness of bone not only predisposes to such a fracture but also determines the amount of cancellous collapse at the time of injury, greater collapse occurring in osteoporotic bone. In the healing phase the bony deformity produced by the wrist fracture occurs to a greater extent in patients with osteoporosis than in those with good quality bone. This probably reflects an impairment, due to osteoporosis, in the ability to resist deforming forces in the healing phase. Thus, osteoporosis renders the bone more vulnerable to a fracture, determines the degree of cancellous compaction at the time of the injury, and adversely influences the progression of the bony deformity in the healing phase.

Clinical presentation

The patient usually presents having fallen onto the outstretched hand. She complains of pain and swelling around the wrist and inability to use the hand without considerable discomfort. If the injury is a few days old extensive bruising is common.

In the wrist is deformed the diagnosis is obvious (Colles, 1814; Smith, 1847). However, if there is no deformity, gentle palpation of the distal radius should be performed to establish the site of maximum tenderness (DaCruz and Dias, 1990). If this is in the region of the distal radius it is very probable that a fracture has occurred. The wrist and hand must be splinted and investigated.

In addition to the wrist, the impact of the fall can also injure the elbow, shoulder and neck. This injury can range from a slight wrench of the ligaments or muscles around these regions to an associated fracture. It is therefore important to enquire about additional sites of discomfort and to examine these regions.

Radiographic assessment

The clinical diagnosis is confirmed by radiographs of the distal radius, wrist and hand. A posteroanterior radiograph establishes whether the fracture extends into the joint, its displacement and whether there is an associated fracture of the ulna. A lateral radiograph distinguishes

between the very common Colles' fracture and the less common Smith's and Barton's fractures. The Colles' fracture (Figure 14.2) occurs within approximately 4 cm of the distal articular surface of the radius and tends to displace backwards creating the typical 'dinner fork' deformity. In the Smith's fracture, the distal fragment tends to displace forwards. The Barton's fracture is an intra-articular wrist fracture in which the anterior part of the distal articular surface of the radius displaces forwards and carries the carpus forwards with it (Figure 14.1).

Factors which determine treatment

The four key factors which determine treatment are the displacement and comminution of the fracture, the alignment of the carpal bones with the distal radius, the quality of bone, and the patient's functional requirement.

Fracture displacement

The fracture is considered to be undisplaced if the fracture line is undisplaced or minimally displaced without clinical wrist deformity. Displacement may occur at the metaphyseal fracture line, the articular fracture line or both.

Metaphyseal displacement

The distal articular surface of the radius is normally inclined forward towards the palm by 11 degrees. In a Colles' fracture the articular surface tends to lose this volar tilt and may even tilt backwards. The distal articular surface is also tilted towards the ulna. In a Colles' or Smith's fracture there is flattening of this tilt (Gartland and Werley 1951: Lindstrom, 1959; Van der Linden and Ericson, 1981) and, in addition, the distal fragment may be displaced backwards, forwards or radially. There may also be an overlap or impaction of the fracture with loss of length.

Articular displacement

The articular surface of the distal radius is triangular in shape with two main facets; the lateral articulates with the scaphoid and the medial articulates with the lunate. An intra-articular fracture usually separates these two

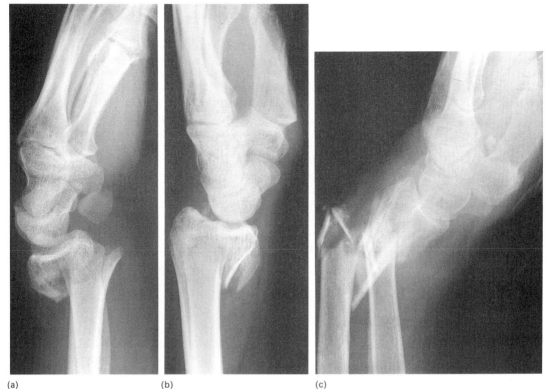

(a)   (b)   (c)

Figure 14.2 The lateral radiographs of (a) a Colles' fracture, (b) a Barton's fracture, and (c) a Smith's fracture. The thumb metacarpal establishes the orientation of the radiograph as it lies volar to the other metacarpals.

facets. In addition, the medial lunate facet is often split into anterior and posterior fragments determined by the strong ligamentous attachments at the anteromedial and posteromedial corners of the distal articular surface (Melone, 1984). Such a fracture results from axial impaction of the distal articular surface. If the displacement is considerable any reduction may be unstable.

Metaphyseal comminution

Gross comminution at this site is uncommon. When present it renders any reduction unstable especially if it occurs on the convex side of the deformity.

Carpal alignment

This aspect is of particular importance in a Barton's fracture subluxation of the wrist (Figure 14.2b). If the subluxation cannot be adequately reduced by closed methods (Mills, 1957; Thomas, 1957), surgical reduction and buttress plating must be considered (Ellis, 1957). Carpal malalignment may also occur as a consequence of the bony deformity in Colles' fractures (Dias and McMohan, 1988).

Bone quality

In addition to the influence of osteoporosis on the deformity during the healing phase, the quality of bone must be considered if any form of surgery is contemplated as any fixation is less likely to be satisfactory.

The patient's functional requirement

The patient's ability to use the hand may be impaired occasionally either by disease such as a stroke or by an alteration in their mental state and consequent dependence on others for their daily activities. In such patients the objectives for management may be few and the threshold for intervention high.

Management

The traditional management is closed reduction of the fracture and immobilization in a plaster-of-Paris below-elbow cast with the wrist in slight palmar flexion and ulnar deviation until the fracture has healed (Charnley, 1974).

Undisplaced fractures

These are stable and unlikely to displace significantly. They can be treated without immobilization (Dias *et al.*, 1987c) with rapid recovery of function (76% of wrist movement in 5 weeks) and without any greater pain and discomfort. The patient may be provided with a removable wrist splint but must be encouraged to remove the splint and use the hands within limits of comfort from the very outset.

Displaced fractures

These require reduction, especially if there is a clinical deformity, but the patient should not experience unneccessary pain during the manipulation. Several authors have recommended a haematoma block using 15–20 ml of 1–2% lignocaine but the analgesia obtained by this method is usually imperfect (Houghton and Bowes, 1989). The safest form of local anaesthesia for wrist fractures is the regional intravenous block using 30–40 ml of 0.5% prilocaine. Complications are uncommon provided that a safe and adequate tourniquet is used and kept inflated for at least 20 min to allow tissue fixation of the anaesthetic agent (Lee and Wildsmith, 1990). A general anaesthetic while equally effective requires a longer period of observation in hospital.

Reduction

After adequate analgesia has been obtained reduction is performed by applying longitudinal traction to disimpact the fracture and to regain length. Any coronal or sagittal displacement is reduced by moulding of the distal radius. A difficult reduction suggests that a large part of the periosteal sleeve is intact. Sustained traction in this case hinders appropriate reduction (Charnley, 1974) which can be better achieved by exaggerating the initial deformity until the cortices on the concave side of the deformity are aligned and then moulding the distal fragment

to correct any displacement. The fracture is then immobilized.

The reduction of the displacement is confirmed clinically and radiologically. The reduced position is maintained in a well moulded below-elbow plaster of Paris cast for 4–6 weeks.

If considerable swelling is present a dorsal plaster slab can be applied for the first few days. Following resolution this can be changed for a definitive cast.

Cast bracing for displaced Colles' fractures

While the value and safety of early mobilization for undisplaced Colles' fractures has been established (Dias *et al.*, 1987c) that for displaced fractures is less clear. Sarmiento *et al.* (1975) suggested that early mobilization of the wrist in a cast brace resulted in excellent functional recovery without deterioration of the bony position. Stewart *et al.* (1984) were unable to show any significant benefit 6 months following cast brace treatment. It has been demonstrated (Dias *et al.*, 1987c) that a plaster of Paris cast brace allowing early movement from the outset promoted both resolution of swelling and a rapid recovery of wrist and finger movement (54% of wrist movement at 5 weeks) in comparison with conventional treatment (28% wrist movement at 5 weeks). The position of the fracture deteriorated in the cast regardless of the method of cast immobilization (Gartland and Werley, 1951; Van der Linden and Ericson, 1981) and early mobilization did not adversely influence this deterioration (Dias *et al.*, 1987a). The cast brace, however, demands expertise and attention to detail in its application and requires close monitoring to ensure its proper use. Both these factors influence whether this method is commonly used.

The use of external fixators

Fractures of the distal radius caused by axial impaction with either displaced articular fragments or considerable metaphyseal comminution can be unstable (Riis and Fruensgaard, 1989) and are best immobilized in distraction (Figure 14.3) using an external fixator (Anderson and O'Neil, 1944; Cooney *et al.*, 1979; Johnson, 1983; Vaughan *et al.*, 1985; Riis and Fruensgaard, 1989). It must be stressed however that very few such fractures occur in the elderly

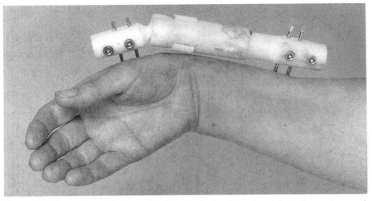

Figure 14.3 An external fixator with threaded pins introduced into the metacarpal shaft distally and the shaft of the radius proximally. The unstable wrist fracture is reduced using continuous traction and the fixator assembled. (The device shown is the 'Sheffield fixator'; courtesy of Mr J. Martindale)

and in addition the quality of bone in such patients often precludes the secure purchase of the fixator pins (Schuind *et al.*, 1989).

The need for remanipulation

While a redisplacement of the fracture in the first 2 weeks necessitates remanipulation, this is uncommon and accounts for only 5% of all manipulated Colles' fractures (Jenkins, 1989). The recurrence of deformity is more commonly insidious and occurs over the entire healing period (Dias *et al.*, 1987a). Remanipulation may not achieve the theoretical goal of anatomical bony position in the elderly (McQueen *et al.*, 1986). The four key factors which influence treatment and which have been discussed earlier must be considered before deciding to re-manipulate. A backwards tilt of the distal articular surface of the radius by 15 degrees is compatible with a very satisfactory functional outcome.

The care of the injured limb during the healing phase

The three principles of care in this period are the control of swelling, promotion of functional recovery and prevention of wrist deformity.

High elevation in a broad-arm sling and a carefully applied plaster cast, which may be split if considerable swelling is anticipated, are of paramount importance in preventing swelling of the hand and fingers. The injured limb must not be allowed to lie idle in a dependent position.

The patient must be encouraged to use the injured limb as much as possible, exercising the fingers, shoulder and elbow from the outset. When the cast is removed the patient must be reassured that the stiffness of the wrist, the weakness of the hand, and the ulnar styloid discomfort on forearm rotation are not uncommon and usually improve with time. If finger movement is compromised or if non-compliance is anticipated the patient will benefit from immediate supervised physiotherapy.

Displacement of the fracture tends to recur regardless of the method of conservative treatment (Gartland and Werley, 1951; Bacorn and Kurtze, 1953; Pool, 1973; Dias *et al.*, 1987c). This is gradual and continues even after the cast has been removed. Only those elderly patients with a backward tilt of greater than 15 degrees benefit from manipulation of their fracture (Dias *et al.*, 1987a). In the rest the fracture heals in a position similar to that before manipulation was undertaken. These patients are usually left with a hand that is slightly radially deviated and in whom the ulnar styloid is prominent.

Complications

While deformity, stiffness, weakness and ulnar styloid pain are common associations of wrist fractures in the elderly (Cooney *et al.*, 1980), once they have occurred they cannot be directly influenced by the treating doctor. There are however three complications which benefit from immediate recognition, the first one being carpal tunnel syndrome.

In this condition the median nerve is compressed at the wrist usually as a consequence of the fall or the resulting swelling (Lynch and Lipscomb, 1963; Sponsel and Palm, 1965). The patient complains of tingling or numbness in the thumb, index and middle fingers which often wakes her up at night. Approximately 17% of patients with a Colles' fracture display some clinical evidence of compression of the median nerve at the wrist at 3 months and 12% will have symptoms at 6 months. These patients are usually in their mid-60s. If the symptoms deteriorate or persist beyond 6 months the diagnosis may be confirmed on nerve conduction studies and the carpal tunnel must be released. This can be performed under general, regional or local anaesthesia and is required in approximately 3% of all cases (Stewart *et al.*, 1985).

Rupture of the extensor pollicis longus tendon tends to occur between 5–12 weeks following what is often a minimally displaced Colles' fracture (Trevor, 1950; Simpson, 1977). The patient is unable to extend the interphalangeal joint of the thumb. If this is considered functionally disabling tendon transfer to restore thumb extension must be considered.

The third complication which merits early recognition is reflex sympathetic dystrophy (algodystrophy, Sudek's atrophy). Progressive stiffness and swelling of the fingers and hand with pain in excess of what one would expect with a healing fracture must alert the treating doctor to the possibility of this condition. If neglected the resulting hand becomes stiff and functionless. It is an under-diagnosed disorder accounting for the published incidence figures from 0% (Stewart *et al.*, 1985) to 25% (Atkins *et al.*, 1989). Early aggressive treatment with repeated regional blocks and physiotherapy will often lead to a satisfactory result.

One particular late complication which deserves consideration relates to the ulnar head. Very occasionally after the fracture has united it may become a persistent source of pain and discomfort, especially on forearm rotation. In such patients excision of the head of the ulna (Darrach, 1927) may be considered.

Long-term disability after Colles' fractures in the elderly

There is little published information regarding the long-term disability after Colles' fractures in the elderly. Smaill (1965) reviewed 41 of 97 patients with such fractures over 5 years after injury and demonstrated that although more than half displayed a cosmetic deformity, most patients had very good wrist movement and were satisfied. In a recent prospective 6-year review of elderly patients with Colles' fractures 19% of the patients had moderate or severe pain and 17% had wrist stiffness. However, only 10% said they were bothered by the pain and 2% were bothered by the stiffness. Five per cent were concerned about the appearance of the hand although 23% had moderate radial deviation. The range of movement in all cases was better than 75% of that of the opposite side with a mean of 96%. The deformity did not correlate with the range of movement (personal unpublished study).

The disability was however considerable with one-third experiencing difficulty opening jars and a quarter not able to wring a cloth as a consequence of their wrist fracture. Many also had difficulty lifting a full kettle (16%) or a full saucepan (20%).

It appears therefore that although patients with a Colles' fracture recover their range of wrist and forearm movement almost completely, one in four patients with a Colles' fracture will have persisting disability which interferes in their ability to perform their daily tasks.

Conclusion

Wrist fractures are very common especially in elderly osteoporotic women. Malunion is common but providing adequate emphasis is given to functional recovery the outcome need not be poor. Undisplaced fractures do not require immobilization. This results in rapid recovery of function without the complications of a plaster cast. Long-term results indicate that one in four patients with Colles' fractures will have some wrist deformity and will have some disability in their daily activities although most will recover wrist and forearm movement.

References

Alffram, P. and Bauer, G.C.H. (1962) Epidemiology of fractures of the forearm. A biomechanical investigation of bone strength. *J. Bone Joint Surg.*, **44-A**, 105–114

Anderson, R. and O'Neil, G. (1944) Comminuted fractures of the distal end of the radius. *Surg. Gynecol. Obstet.*, **78**, 434–439

Atkins, R.M., Duckworth, T. and Kanis, J.A. (1989) Algodystrophy following Colles' fracture. *J. Hand Surg.*, **14B**, 161–164

Bacorn, R.W. and Kurtze, J.F. (1953) Colles' fracture. A study of two thousand cases from the New York State Workmen's Compensation Board. *J. Bone Joint Surg.*, **35A**, 643–658

Barton, J.R. (1838) Views and treatment of an important injury of the wrist. *Med. Exam..* **1**, 365

Charnley, J. (1974) *The Closed Treatment of Common Fractures*, Churchill Livingstone, Edinburgh, pp. 128–142

Colles, A. (1814) On fracture of the carpal extremity of the radius. *Edinburgh Med. J.*, **10**, 182–186

Cooney, W.P.III, Dobyns, J.H. and Linscheid, R.L. (1980) Complications of Colles' fractures. *J. Bone Joint Surg.*, **62-A**, 613–619

Cooney, W.P., Linscheid, R.L. and Dobyns, J.H. (1979) External pin fixation for unstable Colles' fractures. *J. Bone Joint Surg.*, **61A**, 840–845

Cooper, C. (1989) Osteoporosis – an epidemiological perspective: a review. *J. Roy. Soc. Med.*, **82**, 753–757

Cummings, S.R., Kelsey, J.L., Nevitt, M.C. and O'Dowd, K.J. (1985) Epidemiology of osteoporosis and osteoporotic fractures. *Epidemiol. Rev.*, **7**, 178–201

DaCruz, D. and Dias, J. (1990) Traumatic wrist pain. *Hosp. Update*, **16(8)**, 665–675

Darrach, W. (1927) Fractures of the lower extremity of the radius: diagnosis and treatment. *J. Am. Med. Ass.*, **89**, 1683–1685

Dias, J.J. and McMohan, A. (1988) Effect of Colles' fracture malunion on carpal alignment. *J. Roy. Coll. Surg. Edinb.*, 234–236

Dias, J.J., Wray, C.C. and Jones, J.M. (1987a) The radiological deformity of Colles' fractures. *Injury*, **18**, 304–308

Dias, J.J., Wray, C.C. and Jones, J.M. (1987b) Osteoporosis and Colles' fractures in the elderly. *J. Hand Surg.*, **12B**, 57–59

Dias, J.J., Wray, C.C., Jones, J.M. and Gregg, P.J. (1987c) The value of early mobilisation in the treatment of Colles' fractures. *J. Bone Joint Surg.*, **69B**, 463–467

Ellis, J. (1957) Smith's and Barton's fractures. A method of treatment. *J. Bone Joint Surg.*, **47B**, 724–727

Gartland, J.J.Jr and Werley, C.W. (1951) Evaluation of healed Colles' fractures. *J. Bone Joint Surg.*, **33-A**, 895–907

Gay, J.D.L. (1974) Radial fracture as an indicator of osteoporosis: a 10-year follow-up study. *Can. Med. Ass. J.*, **111**, 156–157

Grimley Evans, J. (1990) The significance of osteoporosis. In *Osteoporosis* (ed. R. Smith), Royal College of Physicians of London, London, pp. 1–8

Houghton, K. and Bowes, J.B. (1989) Surface and infiltration anaesthesia. In *Anaesthesia* (eds W.S. Nimmo and G. Smith), Blackwell Scientific, Oxford, p. 1113

Jenkins, N.H. (1989) The unstable Colles' fracture. *J. Hand Surg.*, **14B**, 149–154

Johnson, U. (1983) External fixation for redislocated Colles' fracture. *Acta Orthop. Scand.*, **54**, 878–883

Lee, A. and Wildsmith, J.A.W. (1990) Local anaesthetic techniques. In *Textbook of Anaesthesia* (eds A.R. Aitkenhead and G. Smith), Churchill Livingstone, Edinburgh, pp. 464–465

Lindstrom, A. (1959) Fractures of the distal end of the radius. A clinical and statistical study of end results. *Acta Orthop. Scand.*, Suppl. 41

Lynch, A.C. and Lipscomb, P.R. (1963) The carpal tunnel syndrome and Colles' fractures. *J. Am. Med. Ass.*, **185**, 363–366

McQueen, M.M., Maclaren, A. and Chalmers, J. (1986) The value of remanipulating Colles' fractures. *J. Bone Joint Surg.*, **68B**, 232–233

Melone, C.P. (1984) Articular fractures of the distal radius. *Orthop. Clin. N. Am.*, **15**, 217–236

Mills, T.J. (1957) Smith's fracture and anterior marginal fracture of radius. *Br. Med. J.*, **ii**, 603–605

Miller, S.W.M. and Grimley Evans, J. (1985) Fractures of the distal forearm in Newcastle: an epidemiological survey. *Age Ageing*, **14**, 155–158

Owen, R.A., Melton, L.J., Ilstrup, D.M., Johnson, K.A. and Riggs, B.L. (1982a) Colles' fracture and subsequent hip fracture risk. *Clin. Orthop.*, **171**, 37–43

Owen, R.A., Melton, L.J., Ilstrup, D.M., Johnson, K.A. and Riggs, B.L. (1982b) Incidence of Colles' fracture in a North American Community. *Am. J. Publ. Hlth*, **72**, 605–607

Pool, C. (1973) Colles' fracture: a prospective study of treatment. *J. Bone Joint Surg.*, **55B**, 540–544

Riggs, B.L. and Melton, L.J. (1983) Evidence for two distinct syndromes of involutional osteoporosis. *Am. J. Med.*, **75(6)**, 899–901

Riis, J. and Fruensgaard, S. (1989) Treatment of unstable Colles' fractures by external fixation. *J. Hand Surg.*, **14B**, 145–148

Sarmiento, A., Pratt, G.W., Berry, N.C. and Sinclair, W.F. (1975) Colles' fractures: Functional bracing in supination. *J. Bone Joint Surg.*, **57-A**, 311–317

Schuind, F., Donkerwolcke, M., Rasquin, C. and Burny, F. (1989) External fixation of fractures of the distal radius: A study of 225 cases. *J. Hand Surg.*, **14A**, 404–407

Simpson, R.G. (1977) Delayed rupture of extensor pollicis longus tendon following closed injury. *Hand*, **9**, 160–161

Smaill, G.B. (1965) Long-term follow-up of Colles' fracture. *J. Bone Joint Surg.*, **47B**, 80–85

Smith, R.W. (1847) *A treatise on fractures in the vicinity of joints and on certain accidental and congenital dislocation*, Hodges and Smith, Dublin, 162 pp.

Sponsel, K.H. and Palm, E.T. (1965) Carpal tunnel syndrome following Colles' fracture. *Surg. Gynec. Obstet.*, **121**, 1252–1256

Stewart, H.D., Innes, A.R. and Burke, F.D. (1984) Functional cast-bracing for Colles' fractures: a comparison between cast-bracing and conventional plaster casts. *J. Bone Joint Surg.*, **66B**, 749–753

Stewart, H.D., Innes, A.R. and Burke, F.D. (1985) The hand complications of Colles' fractures. *J. Hand Surg.*, **10B**, 103–106

Thomas, F.B. (1957) Reduction of Smith's fracture. *J. Bone Joint Surg.*, **39B**, 463–470

Trevor, D. (1950) Rupture of the extensor pollicis longus tendon after Colles' fracture. *J. Bone Joint Surg.*, **32-B**, 370–375

Van der Linden, W. and Ericson, R. (1981) Colles' fracture. How should its displacement be measured and how should it be immobilized? *J. Bone Joint Surg.*, **63A**, 1285–1288

Vaughan, P.A., Lui, S.M., Harrington, I.J. and Maistrelli, G.L. (1985) Treatment of unstable fractures of the distal radius by external fixation. *J. Bone Joint Surg.*, **67B**, 385–389

Winner, S.J., Morgan, C.A. and Grimley Evans, J. (1989) Perimenopausal risk of falling and incidence of distal forearm fracture. *Br. Med. J.*, **298**, 1486–1488

15

Management of bony metastases

Dietmar Pennig

In the course of the natural history of a malignant disease process the occurrence of skeletal metastases and in particular of pathological fracture is considered to be a serious development and a harbinger of impending demise (Galasko, 1986). The medical and surgical treatment have to be considered together with the limited life expectancy and the objectives of treatment must be clearly determined for each case by the attending surgeon. The primary malignancies which most commonly give rise to bony metastases originate in the breast (54.2%), kidney (12.2%) and bronchus (5.3%) and other sites include thyroid and prostate (Kunze *et al.*, 1984; Heinz, Stoik and Vecsei, 1989). Most fractures occur in patients aged 60 to 80 years and the female to male ratio is 2.5:1 (Heinz, Stoik and Vecsei, 1989). Spontaneous fractures or fractures with minimal trauma are the rule (76.5%;) (Heinz, Stoik and Vecsei, 1989) and they show little tendency for displacement (Parrish and Murray, 1970). Most pathological fractures are localized in the femur and humerus with the other bones accounting for only a minority (Figure 15.1). This chapter will describe the principles of the management of pathological fractures in the elderly due to bony metastases. It will also discuss the place of prophylactic fixation as well as the technical considerations regarding surgery of metastatic disease of the femur, tibia and humerus. Details regarding treatment of pathological fractures of the spine and femoral neck are described in chapters 8 and 12.

Patient selection for operation

There are three types of patients with fractures due to metastatic bone disease: those with diag-nosed malignancy but capable of walking; those with diagnosed malignancy but bed-ridden and those with undiagnosed malignancy.

In recent years progress has been made in oncology with an increased life expectancy achieved in some younger patients with certain malignancies. Skeletal metastases however predominantly occur in older patients and are considered in general as an almost final complication of the disease process (Rehn, 1979). When selecting patients for surgery information has to be obtained on the state of the primary tumour and its treatment, prognosis regarding life expectancy, the general medical condition including further secondaries and the anaesthetist's view on the proposed surgical intervention.

The local factors to be considered include the affected bone itself, the quality of the bone proximal and distal to the pathological fracture and the presence and type of other skeletal metastases. A technetium-99m scan is the most reliable way of detecting metastases in cancellous bone. On plain radiographs, more than 40% of the cortical bone has to be destroyed before metastases become visible (Cloyer, 1986). When a pathological fracture is present, the likelihood of further metastases is at least 60% (Heinz, Stoik and Vecsei, 1989). Multiple metastases appear to be the rule and this should be taken into account when radical skeletal surgery is being planned.

The aim of treatment can be either to mobilize a patient and render him capable of walking again or simply to facilitate the general management of a bed-ridden individual. The surgical approach will therefore be different in these two cases. With regard to timing of the operation similar principles have to be followed in this

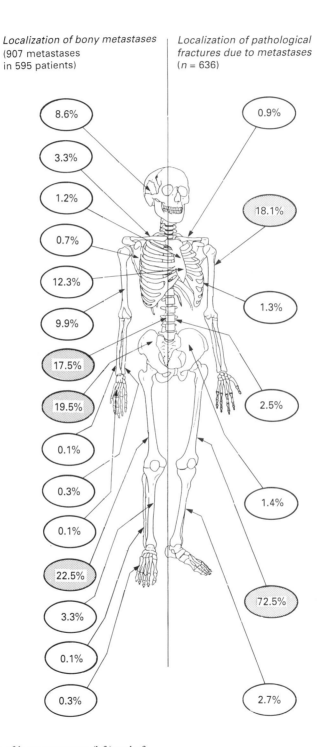

Figure 15.1 Localization of bony metastases (left) and of
pathological fractures due to metastases (right) (*Source:*
Heinz *et al.,* 1989)

group of patients as are conventionally applied to the treatment of traumatic fractures sustained by elderly patients. The earlier the operation is performed, the better the patient's general condition is likely to be. However, when dealing with pathological fractures due to an unknown primary tumour, an effort has to be made to reach a diagnosis before the fracture is dealt with. In a series of 595 pathological fractures, 76 (13%) presented with an unknown primary tumour (Heinz, Stoik and Vecsei, 1989). In only six of them was a diagnosis made by bone biopsy and this indicates that an attempt to find the primary tumour before dealing with the fracture is both justified and necessary.

Significant haemorrhage during the procedure must be expected, especially in those patients with a low platelet count as is frequently encountered in metastases due to renal or thyroid malignancies (Parrish and Murray, 1970).

The most important question however is the expected survival time for the patient to be treated. In bronchial malignancies, 83% die within 3 months of their fracture. In breast cancer the equivalent rate is 37% and after 1 year 76% have died (Heinz, Stoik and Vecsei, 1989). A consultation with an oncologist is very important when planning a procedure in these patients and a radiotherapist should also be involved to evaluate the use of local radiotherapy following stabilization of the fracture.

Technical considerations

An implant used alone or in combination with acrylic cement has to be capable of supporting the patient's expected activities. Generally, bone healing cannot be expected to assist the osteosynthesis and it is therefore important to assess both the remaining life span and the possible failure mode of the implant (Heinz, Stoik and Vecsei, 1989). When treating the bed-ridden patient the primary objective is to stabilize the individual in order to facilitate nursing and achieve significant pain relief. The mechanical requirements are a secondary consideration since most of these patients will not tolerate a major operation.

When treating a patient capable of walking the prime aim of treatment is to restore function as soon as possible.

An intramedullary technique such as a locking nail is theoretically the method of choice since it has the advantage of being supported throughout its length within the medullary canal (for further details refer to chapter 11). Always the critical surgical issue is the quality of the proximal and distal locking which must be anchored into strong, unaffected bone. Cement augmentation can be used to assist the purchase of the locking screws. A nail of the largest possible diameter (e.g. 15–17 mm in the femur) must be used to confer maximum stability (Kempf, Grosse and Beck, 1985; Brug and Pennig, 1988). An unslotted nail is more rigid than a slotted nail and will allow early weight bearing but static locking is mandatory. For reasons that are not clear the reaming does not apparently lead to a dissemination of viable malignant cells and initial worries on this account do not seem to have been substantiated (Parrish and Murray, 1970; Heinz, Stoik and Vecsei, 1989). Plating techniques will in most cases be combined with acrylic cement to provide better immediate stability (Ganz, Isler and Mast, 1984).

If reconstruction of the defect is not possible, a prosthesis has to be considered which allows replacement of a bone or joint (Kotz, 1983; Kotz and Engel, 1983; Schmit-Neuerburg and Klaes, 1990). However, this major type of surgery should obviously only be considered in fit patients with a reasonable life expectancy.

In practice plating is most commonly performed for pathological fractures followed by intramedullary techniques and prosthetic replacement (Figure 15.2). This is a direct function of the anatomical localization of metastases which is illustrated in Figure 15.1.

Special features of some pathological fractures

Femur

In more than 70% of cases the femur is affected (Figure 15.1) and in these individuals it is the proximal third which is the most common site (Heinz, Stoik and Vecsei, 1989). At least half of the medial cortex has to be destroyed for a spontaneous fracture to occur. The lesion has a minimum diameter of 30 mm in most cases and in more than 10% of patients there is a second metastasis in the affected bone. This obviously has an impact on the planned procedure and a full length radiograph is therefore mandatory.

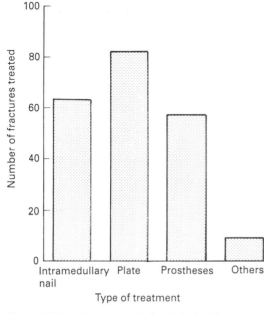

Figure 15.2 Surgical treatment of pathological fractures due to metastases (*n* = 211)

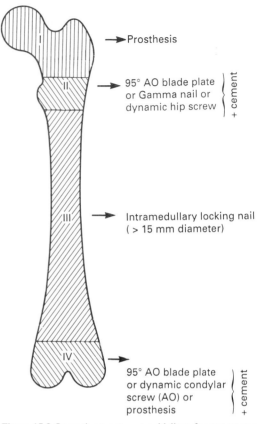

Figure 15.3 Operative treatment guidelines for metastases in the femur (incidence 72% of pathological fractures)

The treatment guidelines are illustrated in Figure 15.3. When the extent of the metastasis involves two areas, the one closer to a joint determines the technique to be used. To illustrate this, if areas II and III are affected, the treatment options for area II (blade plate, Gamma nail or hip screw) have to be used and the implants must be checked for adequate length to reach suitable bone distal to the fracture. In some of these cases a modular replacement system (Kotz and Engel, 1983; Kotz, 1983) may be the only suitable option for stabilization. If the fracture is localized in the head and/or neck (area I), a prosthetic replacement seems to be the treatment of choice.

The combination of a 95-degree blade plate with bone cement has been shown to achieve sufficient initial stability in the proximal femur (Figure 15.4). It is also biomechanically superior to the combination of a 130-degree blade plate or hip screw with cement. Stability in this site can also be improved by using a medial buttress plate (Mischkowski *et al.*, 1984; Schmit-Neuerburg and Klaes, 1990). The recently introduced Gamma nail is regarded as a good alternative which confers the benefits of intramedullary anchorage (Boriani and Bettelli, 1990). Cement augmentation should be used with this implant (for details of technique refer to chapter 11). The area between the innominate tubercle and the

lower border of the lesser trochanter (area II) is suitable for the 95-degree angled blade plate, the Gamma nail or the hip screw (again in combination with acrylic cement). With an intact and unaffected lesser trochanter, fractures of the diaphysis (area III) are a prime indication for a statically locked nail provided the proximal and distal locking can be achieved in unaffected bone (Figure 15.5). The proximal locking screw should penetrate the calcar rather than the lesser trochanter for better stability of the locking screw site and cement augmentation should be practised if severe osteoporosis is present. To combine nailing with cement augmentation in the diaphysis is technically difficult and increased mechanical stability has not been proved (Schmit-Neuerburg and Klaes, 1990). In very distal fractures or fractures of the condyles (area IV), the angled blade plate, the AO dynamic condylar screw system or a prosthesis may be employed (Ganz, Isler and Mast, 1984).

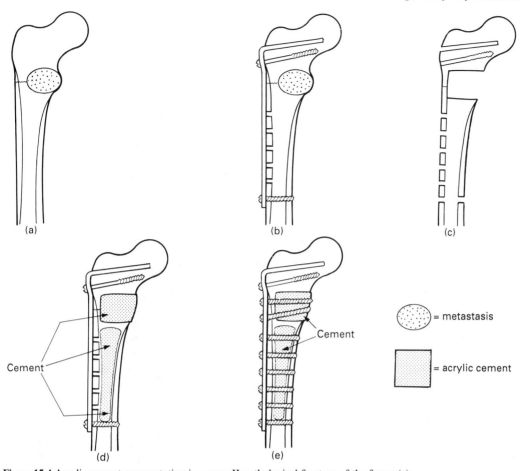

Figure 15.4 Acrylic cement augmentation in a zone II pathological fracture of the femur (a); reduction of the fracture and placement of a 95-degree angled blade plate with insertion of the most proximal and distal screw while for the other screws only the near cortex is drilled (b); removal of the implant and resection of the focus (c); reapplication of the plate and buttressing of the defect with acrylic cement. After polymerization of the cement block further cement is injected for improved anchorage of the plate screws (d); drilling and tapping of cement and far cortices followed by insertion of the screws (e)

In all cases the cement used should be of medium viscosity and semi-liquid and the implant has to be trial fitted before the cement is injected. The purpose of the cement is to replace the bone loss and to assist the purchase of the fixation device. Application of a plate is easier if it is temporarily applied before the bone ends are squared off and all implants should be in place before the cement is inserted. To improve the purchase of screws above and below the fracture only the near cortex should be drilled with the exception of the most proximal and/or distal screw for easier implant positioning. The cement should then be instilled in the medullary canal through the screw holes of either the plate or the locking nail. Drilling and tapping of the entire screw length is performed after polymerization and the screws are finally inserted. This produces better biomechanical results than insertion of the screws into the semi-liquid cement (Mischkowski *et al.*, 1984; Schmit-Neuerburg and Klaes, 1990). Another advantage of this technique is that the cement does not leak through drill holes present in the far cortex. The cement acts as an intramedullary peg in these cases.

In a bed-ridden patient, the simplest suitable method should be used to achieve the stability required for easier and painfree nursing. Ender's nails have a certain advantage and they are suitable for fractures in areas II and III. In fractures of areas I and IV, the life span and the

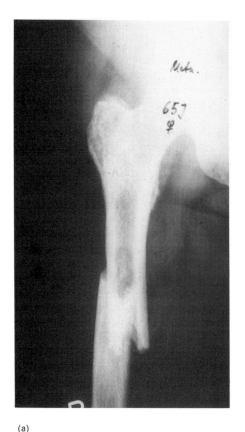

(a)

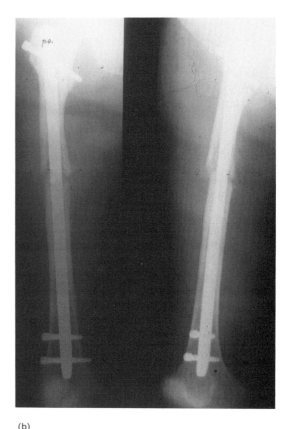

(b)

Figure 15.5 Pathological fracture of the femur in a 65-year-old female patient with breast cancer (a); closed GK nail statically locked; note the large nail diameter for immediate weight bearing (b)

chances of surviving a major operation have to be considered. A light-weight long leg cast may be applied in area IV cases to reduce pain.

Humerus

The indication to stabilize the humerus (incidence 18%; Figure 15.1) is pain relief and improvement of the quality of remaining life especially if the dominant arm is affected.

Fractures in area I (Figure 15.6) are best treated with a (Neer) prosthesis or by resection of the humeral head but for unfit patients a sling may be sufficient. In area II the use of plate(s) and cement is recommended. For lesions of the humeral shaft (area III) tensioned Rush pins have been used in the past primarily because of their ease of insertion. However, a modern intramedullary locking nail is to be preferred and can be inserted by a percutaneous technique with the radial nerve not being exposed and in danger (Seidel) (Figure 15.7). The medullary canal ends

about 50 mm above the joint line and the nail should have 30–40 mm of intact canal at its end. If anchorage is doubtful and in area IV, the combination of plate(s) and cement is a more secure method. Injury to the radial nerve must be avoided since it leaves the patient with a useless extremity even if function returns after 6–12 weeks. With a limited life expectancy this may ridicule the purpose of the intervention.

Casts and braces have a restricted application since fracture healing cannot be expected. In a bed-ridden patient however, a lightweight brace may be used for pain relief. In these patients surgery is indicated only if it can be performed expeditiously and with minimum exposure. A percutaneous intramedullary technique is really the only viable option in these cases.

Tibia

The incidence of pathological fracture in the tibia is much lower than in the femur and

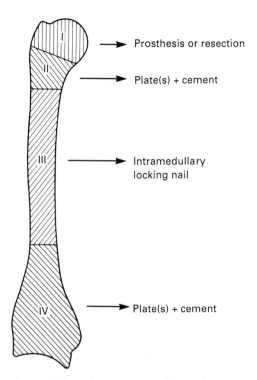

Figure 15.6 Operative treatment guidelines for metastases in the humerus (incidence 18% of pathological fractures)

humerus (3%). If areas I and II are affected, plate(s) and cement is the treatment of choice but in suitable cases a prosthesis may by a better solution (Figure 15.8). If the fracture is below the tibial tuberosity (area III), a large diameter (13–14 mm) locking nail provides the best biomechanical fixation which will permit early weight bearing. Cement augmentation may be required – especially for the proximal locking screws. For fractures in the distal 4 cm (area IV) plate(s) and cement may be used provided there is adequate purchase in the distal fragment. If not, a light weight below-knee cast should be applied to allow pain free walking.

Complications

Deep venous thrombosis may occur in patients with pathological fractures requiring even a short period of bed-rest. Some form of prophylaxis is essential and the best form is probably physiotherapy and early mobilization. The use of antibiotics to prevent infection around the implant is controversial and the rationale for its use is based upon the reduced immune response

seen in some patients with advanced malignancy. As a guideline when any operation on the skeleton lasts more than 1 h intravenous antibiotics (second or third generation cephalosporins) should be administered peroperatively. In those cases associated with a particular risk factor, e.g. diabetes mellitus, antibiotics should be exhibited for up to 5 days.

Any local complication of surgery encountered in young trauma patients can also be found in older patients with pathological fractures. In these individuals the skin thins and the subcutaneous soft tissue become atrophic, with wound slough and infection more frequent. In cases complicated with peripheral vascular disease this can be a major problem. Thrombophlebitis is also a well-recognized complication. Because of these considerations the incision has to respect the poorer blood supply of the skin and soft tissues. It should be more generous than in younger patients in order to avoid tearing of the wound edges and the handling of skin with forceps has also to be gentle. Systemic complications tend to be related to immobilization of the patients and include pneumonia, urinary tract infection and pressure sores. The key to avoid such complications is expeditious surgery aiming at early mobilization. In general, the patient will deteriorate steadily following the fracture with complications increasing in number and severity until finally an operation is either impossible or pointless.

The most serious complication is further spread of the metastic disease within the operated bone. This may cause a fracture above or below the implant or may allow the device to cut out. The incidence of this is 15% and accounts for the vast majority of all local complications (Heinz, Stoik and Vecsei, 1989). The implant failure rate when intramedullary techniques are used is significantly lower (Heinz, Stoik and Vecsei, 1989). The management of this complication requires detailed individual assessment, careful consideration of the magnitude of the proposed intervention and a consideration of its possible benefits. A major operation is usually required in these cases.

Prophylactic treatment of bone metastasis

Only for metastases in the lower extremity and perhaps the spine can a rationale be found for

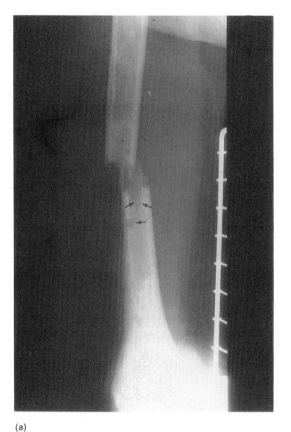

(a)

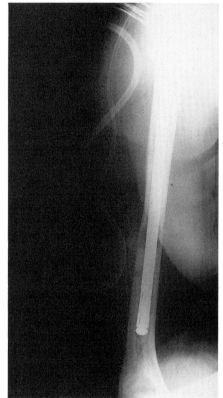

(b)

Figure 15.7 Pathological fracture of the humerus in a 64-year-old patient with breast cancer: note the second metastasis below the fracture involving the lateral cortex (a); stabilization with a Seidel locking nail. It is important that the nail gains 40–50 mm purchase in the distal fragment (b)

prophylactic stabilization. This policy is based on the fact that whereas only 22% of skeletal metastases occur in the femur, 72% of fractures due to metastases occur in this bone. The guidelines for patient selection are similar to those followed for patients with non-pathological fractures. In the femur, a metastasis of 30 mm diameter involving the medial cortex should be considered for surgery since the occurrence of a subsequent pathological fracture often precipitates the patient into a deep depression and the prognosis becomes more grim (Figure 15.9). The aetiology of the primary tumour must be known and consultation with an oncologist is mandatory. Generally, a bed-ridden patient should not be subjected to a prophylactic operation.

Conclusion

Longevity in a patient with a pathological fracture is short and time is precious. It is therefore rewarding to improve the quality of remaining life in these patients with a sensible, well-planned operation, no matter whether the aim is walking ability or pain relief. In a series of 190 patients subjected to operative treatment of their fractures, 24% were able to walk without support, 50% required some kind of aid and only 26% remained unable to walk (Heinz, Stoik and Vecsei, 1989). Since about three-quarters of the patients returned to some form of walking a surgically oriented attitude appears to be beneficial. The choice of implant depends on the affected area and cement augmentation is often performed to improve the mechanical stability.

The majority of patients show evidence of further skeletal metastases at the time of a pathological fracture and this is relevant with regard to the extent of the proposed surgery. Several techniques are available but the lower incidence of implant-related failures with use of

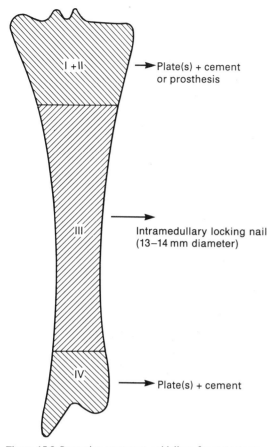

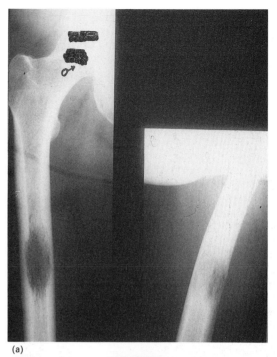

(a)

Figure 15.8 Operative treatment guidelines for metastases in the tibia (*Source:* Heinz *et al.*, 1989)

the locked intramedullary nail makes application of the latter method preferable whenever possible.

A multi-disciplinary team should be involved in deciding on the perioperative management of all patients with pathological fractures. Long-term results can hardly be expected with this group of elderly individuals but improvement in the quality of remaining life is a worthwhile aim.

References

Boriani, S. and Bettelli, G. (1990) The Gamma nail. *Chir. Org. Mov.*, **75**, 67–70

Brug, E. and Pennig, D. (1988) Standortbestimmung der Verriegelungsnagelung. In *Jahrbuch der Chirurgie* (ed. H. Bünte), Regensberg and Biermann, Münster, pp. 145–160

Cloyer, R.A. (1986) Surgical stabilization of pathological neoplastic fractures. *Curr. Prob. Cancer*, 117

Galasko, C.S.B. (1986) *Skeletal Metastases*, Butterworths, London

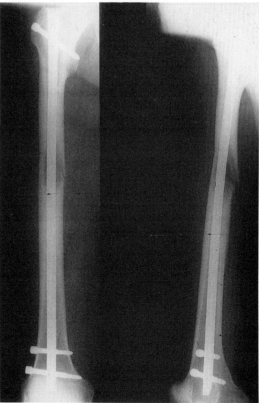

Figure 15.9 Prophylactic stabilization of a large metastasis in the femur with thinning of the medial cortex (a); closed GK nailing with static locking (b)

Ganz, R., Isler, B. and Mast, J. (1984) Internal fixation techniques in pathological fractures of the extremities. *Arch. Orthop. Trauma. Surg.*, **103**, 73–80

Heinz, Th., Stoik, W. and Vecsei, V. (1989) Behandlung und Ergebnisse von pathologischen Frakturen. *Unfallchirurg*, **92**, 477–485

Kempf, I., Grosse, A. and Beck, G. (1985) Closed locked intramedullary nailing. Its application to comminuted fractures of the femur. *J. Bone Joint Surg.*, **67A**, 709–720

Kotz, R. and Engel, A. (1983) Cement-free design of a tumour prosthesis for osteosarcoma of the distal femur and proximal tibia with a new fixation for the ligamentum patellae. In *Tumour Prosthesis for Bone and Joint Reconstruction*, Thieme and Stratton, New York

Kotz, R. (1983) *Modular femur and tibia reconstruction system* Product Information, Howmedica, Kiel, Germany

Kunze, KG., Rehm, K.E., Hofmann, D. and Jander, R. (1984) Die Behandlung pathologischer Frakturen and ihre Ergebnisse. *Aktuel. Traumatol.*, **14**, 48–53

Mischkowski, T., Schult, W., Friedl, W. and Gerber, B. (1984) Stabilitätsverhalten subtrochantärer Doppelplattenverbundosteosynthesen nach Kontinuitätsresektion. *Langenbecks Arch. Chir. Suppl.*, 201–205

Parrish, F.F. and Murray, J.A. (1970) Surgical treatment for secondary neoplastic fractures. *J. Bone Joint Surg.*, **52A**, 665–686

Rehn, J. (1979) *Der alte Mensch in der Chirurgie*, Springer, Berlin, Heidelberg, New York

Schmit-Neuerburg, K.P. and Klaes, W. (1990) Chirurgische Therapie bei pathologischen Frakturen. In *Jahrbuch der Chirurgie* (eds H. Bünte and Th. Junginger), Biermann, Münster, 151–169

Seidel, H. (1989) Humeral locking nail: a preliminary report. *Orthopaedics*, **12**, 219–226

16

Principles of modern inpatient and community rehabilitation

Richard Sainsbury

It is a sad fact that many elderly patients receive less than optimum rehabilitation after musculoskeletal trauma. In many cases those who complain loudest about elderly trauma patients (principally those with hip fractures) inappropriately occupying acute hospital beds are the very ones who create most of the problem by the poor medical care that they deliver. There is much to gain from a sound rehabilitation programme following both trauma and elective orthopaedic surgery not only in terms of reduced bed occupancy but also in terms of improved functional recovery which subsequently allows greater numbers of patients to return successfully to the community.

Early management

It is recognized that preoperative delay adversely affects the outcome of patients with hip fractures (Villar, Allen and Barnes, 1986). It is therefore regretful that a recent report of 100 consecutive unselected elderly patients with hip fractures admitted to a London hospital revealed that many patients lay on hard trolleys in the accident and emergency or radiology departments for up to $12\frac{1}{2}$ h (70% between 2 and 6 h). This observation may account for the fact that 66% of this group of patients subsequently developed pressure sores (Versluysen, 1987). Similarly, this study also found lengthy delays before operation with 48% of the patients waiting 2 or 3 days between admission and surgery. Only one-third reached theatre within 2 h of preoperative preparation with some patients starved and sedated for up to 14 h! This contrasts markedly with a study by Gilchrist et al.

(1988) in which 78% of hip surgery was performed within the first 24 h. This seems impressive until the so-called 'rapid transit system' is considered. Utilizing its principles 38% of patients underwent their hip fracture surgery and were returned to their homes having spent only one night or less in hospital (Sikorski, Davis and Senior, 1985).

Early involvement by a physician with a special interest in the elderly can be of assistance when dealing with medical problems in the perioperative period, such as confusion, which can cause much disruption in the orthopaedic and rehabilitation wards (Sainsbury and Benton, 1981). The physician also has a role in determining the cause of the patient's fall and this is discussed further in chapter 3.

What happens in the early days following trauma has a crucial influence on ultimate functional outcome. While it may be useful to divide the patient's stay into stages to identify where inappropriate delays may be occurring (Robbins and Donaldson, 1984) in practice this should be avoided as it is artificial and rehabilitation must be built into the patient's management programme from the outset (Irvine, 1985).

Rehabilitation versus convalescence

The aim of rehabilitation is to restore an individual to his (or her) fullest physical, mental and social capability (Mair, 1972) and theoretically the goal of restoring the person's former functional and environmental status should be achieved. If this is not possible then the aim must be to assist the person to live as full a life as possible. These aims should underlie all treatment in the elderly as geriatric medicine has been described as 'medicine with built-in rehabilitation' (Irvine, 1985). Rehabilitation has been described as an approach or a philosophy as much as it is a set of techniques. It is an active process involving a team approach with set goals and objectives. In this way it differs substantially from traditional convalescence defined as 'recovery from illness' which is a passive process. Passive convalescence for elderly patients is fraught with dangers. Old people are at high risk from postoperative complications and the hazards of bed-rest often result in chronic disability unless there is a positive programme for enabling functional recovery. Convalescence without a planned recovery programme may deprive the elderly person of the motivation to improve.

The need for an active programme underlies the principles of orthopaedic–geriatric rehabilitation enunciated by Devas and Irvine (Devas, 1977; Irvine 1982) which consider the patient's age, the surgery, the urgency and emphasize the patient and not the part.

Age

No patient is too old to be denied the relief of pain and improvement in mobility that may be expected to follow surgery. Only those who are likely to die within a day or two should be regarded as too ill for operation. The patient must have an operation at the soonest available opportunity.

Surgery

The second principle is that the operation must obviate the fracture so that it can be disregarded in the subsequent programme of rehabilitation. The patient must be able to bear weight and use the limb immediately postoperatively. Methods which do not allow immediate function and weight bearing but require the patient to remain immobilized in bed, in traction or in a cast should not be used primarily as they greatly increase postoperative complications and slow the processes of rehabilitation.

Urgency

There must be a sense of urgency not only with the surgery, but also in rehabilitation which must commence as soon as the fracture has been treated surgically. Prevention of pressure sores should start as soon as the patient is admitted and not when the sore is threatening. Delay in mobilization is deleterious both for the patient and for the family who may become convinced the patient may never walk again and make arrangements for institutional care. Devas frequently observed that 'bed-rest is rehabilitation for the grave'.

The patient and not the part

This means that the fracture should not be treated in isolation from other medical and social problems. It implies the need for a full medical, functional and social assessment – an approach which is the hallmark of good geriatric medicine. This is best achieved utilizing the skills of a multi-disciplinary team.

The team approach

Elderly patients following trauma or elective orthopaedic surgery may be rehabilitated in a variety of surroundings. These include the acute orthopaedic wards for the full duration of their hospital stay, in departments of medicine for the elderly alongside people with other conditions such as stroke, in specialized orthopaedic–geriatric rehabilitation units and early community rehabilitation. Where it occurs depends on both the availability of local resources and relationships between disciplines, particularly orthopaedic surgeons and physicians for the elderly. More important than the site of rehabilitation is the need to ensure that the principles enumerated above are followed and there is a team approach to the task.

The patient should be made to feel welcome on arrival and receive a careful explanation of the rehabilitation plan. The need for early ambulation must be understood and communication by staff should be in positive and encouraging terms. Patients need to understand that they will be up and dressed and relatives should be asked to bring in street clothes and walking shoes. They should also be encouraged to be part of the team. As rehabilitation of the elderly is sadly often performed in old buildings that are not purpose built there is an added responsibility on staff to provide a positive attitude even in adversity and when there may be severely

anol:l noit bl
ey

disabled or very confused patients also housed in the same ward.

Teamwork is of the essence. Apart from ward-round days there should be a multidisciplinary case conference to plan patient management. This is the key event of the week but is only effective if all disciplines are present, communicate freely, respect the role of others and have sufficient understanding to avoid conflict. All staff must be conversant with each patient's diagnosis, management and capabilities. This applies particularly to the nurses who at weekends and 'after hours' can consolidate gains made by the therapists. It is also useful for at least one ward round to be held at a time when relatives are present to give an opportunity to meet the team and pose questions. This is also a chance to encourage the patient to walk and demonstrate his/her abilities. This is far more preferable to spending visiting time with the patient in bed apparently still disabled. A family meeting may be necessary in the case of particularly frail patients to assist with discharge planning and to allay fears. The need for such a meeting may be reduced if staff have been readily available and approachable to the family throughout the admission.

Nursing

Good preventive care for pressure sores, awareness of pain and discomfort and skill in management of confused patients are the chief attributes required in orthopaedic rehabilitation nursing for the elderly. Equally important is an understanding of how to promote continence. The nurse has to be particularly alert to the problem of an increase in pain which may indicate an orthopaedic complication needing prompt attention and be conversant with the principles of wound care. The nurse has also to understand the need to extend the patient's rehabilitation by consolidating the work of the occupational therapist and physiotherapist. This includes assistance with dressing and feeding as well as and supervision of walking wherever possible (using appropriate aids if necessary) but without performing tasks that the patient can and should do for himself. The change from the nurse doing things for the patient to encouraging self-reliance is one that nurses, patients and relatives may all find difficult. This concept may be foreign to nurses

whose previous experience has been with acute or postoperative patients but it must be learned and practised in the interests of good teamwork.

Physiotherapy

The principal aims of physiotherapy are to maintain motivation, interest and cooperation and to help the patient regain confidence in order to maximize his or her functional independence and ability to return successfully to the community. The physiotherapist has a vital role in assessing the patient with regard to his or her social, domestic and working circumstances following which realistic goals may be set for each individual and reviewed regularly with the members of a multidisciplinary rehabilitation team.

The physiotherapist has to supervise a suitable programme of gait re-education and improvement in the patient's general mobility and endurance. Elderly patients quickly lose muscle bulk following trauma and/or surgery and this may make getting in and out of bed difficult. Thigh and calf strengthening exercises are required and the patient must be instructed on how to lift his operated limb off the bed unassisted and safely. This is particularly important following hemi- and total hip arthroplasty.

Those patients with post-operative balance or early weight-bearing problems may be assisted by the use of a tilting table. Walking between parallel bars is not now considered to be an effective form of gait rehabilitation in the elderly as it confers a false sense of security in an unrealistic situation. More appropriate is the use of a walking frame (Zimmer) with close supervision. The correct provision of walking aids of appropriate height is an essential function of the physiotherapist as is the timing of the transition from a frame to elbow crutches or a stick.

As well as improving the patient's general mobility and endurance the physiotherapist also plays an important role in other aspects of care such as treatment of possible pressure sores and respiratory complications. Home visits are undertaken in conjunction with the occupational therapist and any relevant members of the multidisciplinary care team. Close liaison with relatives is, of course, essential throughout the patient's rehabilitation.

Further improvement in mobility often occurs a considerable time after injury (Barnes and

Donovan, 1987; Kauffman, Albright and Wagner, 1987). Thus, it is necessary for the physiotherapist to advise on which patients would benefit from continuing rehabilitation in the day hospital, outpatient department or in their own home.

Occupational therapy

The role of the occupational therapist is to assist the patient to overcome the effects of any temporary or permanent disability due to his orthopaedic condition and to help him adjust to the varied demands of everyday living.

The therapist will undertake a comprehensive assessment which will include the level of independence prior to admission, the current functional, psychological and cognitive states as well as a consideration of the social situation and home environment. This information will be used to formulate an individual rehabilitation programme with particular attention to the activities of daily living. This includes:

Transfers: toilet management, in/out of bed, up/down from chair.

Personal: personal hygiene, dressing, eating and drinking.

Household: preparing hot drink/meal, shopping and housework.

Occupational therapy provides the patient with the opportunity to practise self-care skills. This is initially performed within the environment of the hospital, thus improving his self confidence and ability to manage at home following discharge. Equipment such as dressing aids and raises for bed, chair and toilet are provided where appropriate to ensure safety and independence with these specific tasks.

A home visit prior to discharge is necessary for many patients. This affords the opportunity to gain a much clearer picture of the circumstances in which he or she will have to cope. Possible hazards and problems may be identified and rectified. The therapist can assess the need for any adaptations to the home which may be required and liaise with the social services. Many families are understandably anxious about relatives being discharged home and therefore the opportunity may be taken during the domiciliary visit to reassure the family of the patient's level of independence.

If the visit is unsuccessful the multidisciplinary team can then discuss the rehabilitation and placement alternatives still available.

Social work

The social worker must be involved as part of the multidisciplinary team from the outset and not just called in as an afterthought because problems arise regarding discharge or resettlement. The person's prefracture level of function should be determined as well as the amount of help likely to be available from family and friends so that the rehabilitation team can set realistic goals.

The social worker further complements the skills of the multidisciplinary team by providing advice and assistance to both patients and medical colleagues regarding legal matters and welfare benefits as well as facilitating and organizing a wide range of social services. The social worker also has a valuable role in protecting the vulnerable patient by statutory intervention where appropriate.

If a community-based social worker or home-care worker is already involved with the patient he or she can be identified and invited to attend discharge planning meetings. If family carers (especially elderly spouses) are stressed, emotional support and counselling can be offered as well as a range of community support services. Advice and help with applications for appropriate statutory financial benefits or rehousing can be organized and will be appreciated by both patients and their family. If there is a need for long-term residential or nursing-home care then discussions with the patient and relatives can be coordinated at an early stage by the social worker to help prepare for this major change in lifestyle.

Illness and trauma often cause far-reaching changes in elderly patients – not only physically but also emotionally, socially and economically. Serious strains can be placed upon otherwise caring relationships and this is particularly so when there are increased and severe disability problems. At the same time as the patient's physical condition is treated the social situation also needs to be fully considered to ensure that it does not impede the patient's recovery and rehabilitation.

Ward environment

Rehabilitation is often carried out in acute wards or rehabilitation wards that are not purpose designed. The environment must therefore be organized so that it favours the patient's ability to mobilize and attend to his own self-care. Adjustable height beds are mandatory as are individual bedside wardrobes for storage of clothes and suitable footwear. Chairs must be of a height to allow the patient to raise from them easily and to sit in them without the chair tipping. A variety of heights should be available and the higher ones reserved for those patients who have recently undergone hip arthroplasty. Armchairs are particularly helpful for those with multi-joint arthritic involvement of the lower limbs. Tilt-back chairs and those with footplates are not only unsuitable but may be dangerous. Adequate stools must be available for the elevation of affected legs. Toilets must be accessible, within easy walking distance, clearly signposted and well designed. A night commode should be theoretically available for every bed. Walking aids are discussed in a separate chapter but these should also be readily available and appropriate to the patient's needs. Unfortunately, badly prescribed 'aids' are often a hindrance and may be frankly dangerous.

Rehabilitation is more than just getting people up and dressed. There must be a purpose for their being up and this means providing a day programme aimed at retraining home skills and an attractive lounge and day facilities.

Domiciliary services

Appropriate domiciliary services must commence immediately the patient is discharged. Delays may be costly in terms of loss of the patient's confidence and in the ward staff losing the trust of the family. It is particularly wasteful if a patient's discharge is delayed because of inadequate planning of domiciliary services. This can be prevented by good communication. In our unit a district nurse liaison officer attends the weekly case conference and arranges the services required (Sainsbury *et al.*, 1986). A follow-up service is provided by either a social worker or a district nurse to ensure the patient is coping satisfactorily and to identify those who may benefit from further domiciliary physiotherapy or day hospital treatment.

Orthopaedic–geriatric units

Some centres have developed combined orthopaedic–geriatric units in an attempt to improve the quality and speed of rehabilitation and to try and reduce acute orthopaedic bed occupancy by elderly patients following injury but especially those with femoral neck fractures. Advocates of these collaborative units in which geriatric physicians and orthopaedic surgeons work side by side with the same rehabilitative goal in mind are usually enthusiastic on the basis of reduced length of stay and reduced numbers needing continuing care (Irvine, 1982; Boyd *et al.*, 1983; Sainsbury *et al.*, 1986; Makai, 1990) but the results of the few controlled trials available are conflicting (Fordham *et al.*, 1986; Gilchrist *et al.*, 1988; Kennie *et al.*, 1988; Hempsall *et al.*, 1990). A detailed analysis of the methodology and results of such an approach to rehabilitation is presented in chapter 17 together with a discussion of other special collaborative rehabilitation schemes available to facilitate early discharge and rehabilitation in the patient's own home.

Day hospitals

Day hospitals form part of most geriatric departments and their function includes rehabilitation after trauma and acute illness as well as post-discharge, medical, nursing and social care (Brocklehurst and Tucker, 1980). While day hospital treatment is thought to reduce inpatient stay and prevent hospital admissions for elderly people requiring medical treatment or rehabilitation there is a paucity of publications to support this. A New Zealand study (Tucker, Davison and Ogle, 1984) compared day hospital patients with a group treated as they would have been before the day hospital opened. Day hospital patients showed an improvement in activities of daily living (ADL) at 6 weeks but not at 5 months; however, they sustained an improvement in mood. The early improvement suggested that day hospital treatment was effective.

Day hospitals are a popular and effective resource for the rehabilitation of selected patients though not necessarily cheaper than institutional care (Hildick-Smith, 1985). They are useful as part of the rehabilitation process after hip fracture – not only as part of the move to earlier discharge but also in providing a 'booster' treatment some time later for those whose recovery is slow. This is particularly important as some patients take a longer time than others to regain their former function (Barnes and Donovan, 1987). Physiotherapy, occupational therapy and chiropody can all be provided in the day hospital, the role of which should be considered therapeutic rather than merely social (Martin and Millard, 1978). Good communication and planning are required to ensure that there are no delays between discharge and the commencement of day hospital treatment. Furthermore, it must be understood that attendance is for a finite period and not merely for social day care. In practice approximately 5% of our elderly orthopaedic patients attend the day hospital following discharge and a further 5% attend during the subsequent 12 months.

Delayed functional recovery

It is recognized that many elderly patients never regain full function after significant musculoskeletal injury. This is particularly the case following hip fracture and Jensen, Tondevold and Sorenson (1979) found that 76% of subjects reported poorer functional status 6 months after such an injury. Barnes and Donovan (1987) reported that whilst only 41% were independent 60 days after surgery 83% were able to walk independently at the end of the first year. Ungar and Warne (1986) found that reduction in mobility, pain and fear of falling interfered with many activities of daily living particularly those outside the house. Moreover, they also showed that the fittest and most independent of their sample remained so but those with some degree of disability were likely to become more dependent in a relatively short time. All these authors argued for an intensive initial treatment programme and some form of ongoing assessment and rehabilitation to ensure all patients attained their maximum potential.

The family and general practitioner

Reference has been made earlier in this chapter to the key role that the family plays in the rehabilitation process of elderly orthopaedic patients. We assist the family of 'at-risk' patients during supervised 4-day 'trial' leaves with the provision of social worker and district nurse support. If a patient is found not to be not

coping satisfactorily the geriatric service assumes immediate responsibility for ongoing management which may include the organization of increased support, admission to the assessment and rehabilitation unit, attendance at the day hospital or respite care.

Communication with general practitioners is of special importance. This includes a promptly written discharge letter giving a clear indication of medications and follow-up arrangements. It must also offer prompt help for those patients who do not manage successfully after discharge.

Community and district physiotherapy

Increasing use is being made of community physiotherapy in early home rehabilitation programmes (Ceder, Thorngren and Wallden, 1980; Pryor and Williams, 1989). Where physiotherapy can be provided in the home there is evidence (Sikorski, Davis and Senior, 1985; Pryor and Williams, 1989) that hospital stays can be reduced and patients can return more quickly to prefracture levels of independence. Sadly, most domiciliary teams are understaffed, resulting in the provision of only a limited amount of 'hands on' treatment. In practice the function of the domiciliary therapist is often to give advice to patients and relatives and to alert general practitioners or the local geriatric service to those patients who need further intensive treatment.

Aged persons' homes and sheltered accommodation

The emphasis in modern rehabilitation is on rapid discharge from the ward to home or sheltered accommodation. While this is a desirable objective it must not be achieved at the expense of the patient regaining his or her full potential. The amount of rehabilitation treatment available in aged persons' homes and similar accommodation is variable from district to district and country to country. If a patient is being discharged to a home where rehabilitation opportunities are limited he must be offered day hospital follow-up, domiciliary physiotherapy or periodic hospital review. If the staff of an aged persons' home report a resident who has deteriorated some time after discharge he or she should be re-assessed by the local geriatric physician to determine whether further therapy is required. All too often such patients are referred at a later date with a request that a long-stay hospital bed be provided when a short but intensive further period of rehabilitation is the more appropriate course of action. Orthopaedic review may also be needed if the problem is local pain or loss of function and should not be withheld simply because the person is resident in a home.

Continuing hospital care ('long-term' care)

Sadly for some patients functional rehabilitation is not possible and continuing hospital care is needed. In our orthopaedic–geriatric unit this amounts to approximately 6% of patients admitted with all fractures (Sainsbury *et al.*, 1986). The decision when continuing care is needed requires fine judgement by the entire rehabilitation team, patient and family. On the one hand it must be recognized when further attempts at rehabilitation are futile and on the other it is vital that a decision to transfer a patient to continuing care is not made in the presence of untreated or partially treated medical conditions. Some units have an arbitrary review period at about 6 weeks but it is essential that those with unfulfilled potential at the review are given more time. The team should never regard those patients who need continuing care as 'failures'. Continuing care is a skilled discipline in its own right that depends heavily on the collective commitment and expertise of the staff – particularly nursing staff. The aim should be as full and worthwhile a life within the hospital as the patient's infirmities allow and death must be with dignity and comfort. There is still a place for physiotherapy and occupational therapy in the long stay wards although the emphasis changes to maintenance of existing function. Periodic review is essential as there are a small number of patients who rehabilitate late and who pleasantly surprise one and all by going home from the continuing care wards.

Conclusion

Ideal rehabilitation after fracture – and in particular fracture of the hip – consists of restoring full function and mobility and returning the patient to his or her former residence in the shortest possible time. While this is not always possible much is known about how to provide good care and a number of exciting possibilities for improved management are being investigated. These are particularly in the field of collaborative rehabilitation with orthopaedic surgeons and geriatricians working together to facilitate early discharge and home rehabilitation programmes. This is very timely as the pressure on acute orthopaedic beds is considerable.

References

Barnes, W. and Donovan, K. (1987) Functional outcomes after hip fracture. *Phys. Ther.*, **67**, 1675–1679

Boyd, R.V., Wallace, W.A., Compton, E.H., Hawthorne, J. and Worlock, P.H. (1983) The Nottingham orthogeriatric unit after 1000 admissions. *Injury*, **15**, 193–196

Brocklehurst, J.C. and Tucker, J.S. (1980) *Progress in Geriatric Day Care*, King Edward's Hospital Fund, London

Ceder, L., Thorngren, K. and Wallden, B. (1980) Prognostic indicators and early home rehabilitation in elderly patients with hip fracture. *Clin. Orthopaed.*, **152**, 173–184

Devas, M.B. (1977) *Geriatric Orthopaedics*, Academic Press, London.

Fordham, R., Thompson, R., Holmes, J. and Hodkinson, C. (1986) A cost benefit study of geriatric-orthopaedic management of patients with fractured neck of femur, University of York Centre for Health Economics, Discussion Paper No. 14

Gilchrist, W.J., Newman, R.J., Hamblen, D.L. and Williams, B.D. (1988) Prospective randomised study of an orthopaedic–geriatric inpatient service. *Br. Med. J.*, **297**, 1116–1118

Hempsall, V.J., Robertson, D.R.C., Campbell, M.J. and Briggs, M.S.J. (1990) Orthopaedic geriatric care – is it effective? *J. Roy. Coll. Phys.*, **24**, 47–50

Hildick-Smith, M. (1985) Geriatric rehabilitation in day hospitals. *Int. Rehab. Med.*, **7**, 120–124

Irvine, R.E. (1982) A geriatric orthopaedic unit. In *Establishing a Geriatric Service* (ed. D. Coakley), Croom Helm, London

Irvine, R.E. (1985) Rehabilitation in geriatric orthopaedics. *Int. Rehab. Med.*, **7**, 115–120

Jensen, J.S., Tondevold, E. and Sorenson, P.H. (1979) Social rehabilitation following hip fractures. *Acta Orthop. Scand.*, **50**, 777–785

Kauffman, T.L., Albright, L. and Wagner, C. (1987) Rehabilitation outcomes after hip fracture in persons 90 years old and older. *Arch. Phys. Med. Rehab.*, **68**, 369–371

Kennie, D.C., Reid, J., Richardson, I.A., Kiamari, A.A. and Kelt, C. (1988) Effectiveness of geriatric rehabilitative care after fractures of the proximal femur in elderly women. *Br. Med. J.*, **297**, 1083–1086

Mair, A. (1972) Report of Subcommittee of the Standing Medical Advisory Committee. Scottish Health Service Council on Medical Rehabilitation, Edinburgh, HMSO

Makai, F. (1990) The tasks and objectives of geriatric orthopaedics. *Acta Chir. Orthop. Traumatol. Cech.*, **57**, 322–327

Martin, A. and Millard, P.H. (1978) Day hospitals for the elderly. Therapeutic or social? Report of a study of the day hospitals taking elderly patients in the South West Thames Region. Geriatric Teaching and Research Unit, St George's Hospital, London

Pryor, G.A. and Williams, D.R.R. (1989) Rehabilitation after hip fractures. Home and hospital management compared. *J. Bone Joint Surg.*, **71**, 471–474

Robbins, J.A. and Donaldson, L.J. (1984) Analysing stages of care in hospital stay for fractured neck of femur. *Lancet*, **ii**, 1028–1029

Sainsbury, R. and Benton, K.G.F. (1981) When a geriatrician can contribute to orthopaedics. *Geriat. Med.*, **11**, 64–65

Sainsbury, R., Gillespie, W.J., Armour, P.C. and Newman, E.F. (1986) An orthopaedic geriatric rehabilitation unit: the first two years experience. *N.Z. Med. J.*, **99**, 583–585

Sikorski, J.M., Davis, N.J. and Senior, J. (1985) The rapid transit system for patients with fractured necks of the proximal femur. *Br. Med. J.*, **290**, 439–443

Tucker, M.A., Davison, J.G. and Ogle, S.J. (1984) Day hospital rehabilitation – effectiveness and cost in the elderly: a randomised controlled trial. *Br. Med. J.*, **289**, 1209–1212

Ungar, D.M. and Warne, R.W. (1986) Morbidity following successful treatment of proximal femoral fractures. *Aust. Fam. Phys.*, **15**, 1157–1158

Versluysen, M. (1987) Pathogenesis of pressure sores in elderly patients with hip fractures. Report to City and Hackney Health District

Villar, R.N., Allen, S.M. and Barnes, S.J. (1986) Hip fractures in healthy patients: operative delays versus prognosis. *Br. Med. J.*, **293**, 1203–1204

17

Special collaborative rehabilitation schemes following femoral neck fracture

Raymond J. Newman

With a greater proportion of the population living to a much older age than their parents, orthopaedic surgeons are now finding that they are dealing with an increasing number of elderly patients many of whom have sustained femoral neck fractures or other osteoporosis-related injuries (Figure 17.1). The immediate surgical goal is the attainment of a pain-free stable hip and with modern anaesthesia, together with the newer techniques of hemiarthroplasty and internal fixation described in chapter 12, the vast majority of such patients are rendered at least partly mobile within a day or so of their injury. However, once the fracture has been 'fixed and forgotten' it becomes apparent that the overall management problem of that individual still exists and is complicated by a poor mental state, the co-existence of non-surgical illnesses and often isolated and somewhat hostile social circumstances that were precarious even before the injury. Multiple pathology is virtually the rule in the elderly and the older the patient is the more likely it will be that the patient will suffer a greater number of simultaneous illnesses. All those working with the aged, whether they be physicians or surgeons, are familiar with this observation and have to be appropriately prepared. In one prospective study of female patients with femoral neck fracture Campbell (1976) found more than one-third to be suffering from dementia, almost another third to have had strokes or other neurological disease, a quarter to have heart disease, one in six respiratory disease and more than one in 10 to suffer from some form of cancer. In a similar series Thomas and Stevens (1974) found that 82% of

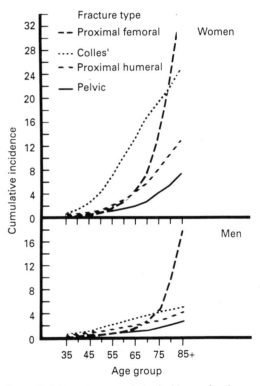

Figure 17.1 Percentage cumulative incidence of various age-related (osteoporotic) fractures over a lifetime for male and female residents of Rochester, Minnesota. (*Source:* Melton and Riggs, 1987; reproduced by permission of the publishers)

their femoral neck fracture patients had significant medical disabilities which contributed to or complicated their injury.

Confusion is common in these individuals and is often multifactorial in its origin with blood loss, dehydration, disorientation and perhaps infection all simultaneously contributing to it. Some patients are apparently lucid on admission but have both mild mental impairment and some sensory deficits such as deafness and poor vision which make a postoperative confusional episode all the more likely.

Although it would perhaps be going too far to agree totally with the medical student who remarked that the orthopaedic unit was 'not so much a surgical unit as a geriatric unit that did operations' there is an uncomfortable truth in this observation. 'Many elderly trauma patients are distinguishable from patients admitted to geriatric assessment units only by the fact that they also have a fracture' (Currie, 1987).

It is therefore not surprising that many of these elderly, frail patients rehabilitate very slowly following their injury and readily come to be regarded as 'bed-blockers' since their prolonged presence prevents the admission of other patients for elective orthopaedic surgery. The waiting list for procedures such as total hip and knee arthroplasty as well as for relatively more minor operations such as bunion surgery is inevitably prolonged. Furthermore, it is not uncommon for the simultaneous admission of several elderly patients with femoral neck fractures to result in the 'boarding out' of some convalescent orthopaedic patients into beds of other acute specialties so leading to secondary delaying effects.

The Department of Health and Social Security report (1981) into the waiting time for orthopaedic outpatient appointments and inpatient treatment was aware of these facts and stated that elderly patients (those aged 65 years or more) occupied 44% of available orthopaedic beds and of those almost one-fifth were being treated for femoral neck fractures. It is clear from reading the report that unless more effective and efficient rehabilitation techniques are introduced to shorten the length of stay of such patients and to increase the throughput of orthopaedic units the current hospital system will rapidly become overburdened.

The desired objective of post-trauma rehabilitation is the concerted effort to maximize the patient's physical, mental and social potential and so facilitate the achievement of his or her maximum functional potential. Contrary to popular belief it is a dynamic, interventional process, goal orientated and time limited, undertaken by doctors in cooperation with other health care workers. In the case of the elderly, and especially those with hip fracture, it must be completed in the shortest possible time so facilitating the best residential placement to occur as quickly as possible. Several factors interact in this process including medical, surgical, nursing and paramedical as well as those of the social services. These considerations have been discussed individually in other chapters of this book making it a salient fact that surgery is only a single instant in the rehabilitation process of elderly patients, especially those with hip fracture.

It is a curious fact highlighted by the DHSS report (1981) that, although so much contemporary trauma and elective orthopaedic surgery is performed on the elderly, the training of orthopaedic surgeons and nurses rarely includes specific experience in those skills necessary to combat the physical, mental and social disabilities which manifest themselves in the elderly traumatized individual. This is not the case for geriatricians who, of course, specialize in this very field of care. It has therefore been suggested by some that the quality and speed of the rehabilitation of infirm elderly patients, especially those with femoral neck fractures, can be improved by a combination of the resources of the orthopaedic and geriatric medicine departments together with those of physiotherapy, occupational therapy and the social services.

Several types of such collaborative rehabilitation schemes have been developed for which beneficial claims have been made and this chapter will describe five different and as yet only partially evaluated organizational models.

Orthopaedic–geriatric collaboration ('orthogeriatrics')

Though currently topical the concept of formal orthopaedic–geriatric collaboration is far from new. Devas established his combined unit in Hastings in 1962 and presented the results of his initial experience in 1963 (Irvine and Devas, 1964). Clark and Wainwright founded their department along similar lines in 1961 and notified their results 5 years later (Clark and Wainwright, 1966). Subsequently, several descriptions of the Hastings scheme appeared incorporating results of rehabilitation which were particularly impressive for their era (Devas and Irvine, 1969; Devas, 1977; Irvine, 1983, 1985). Undoubtedly, these exciting observations have led to the current widespread introduction of collaborative rehabilitation projects for elderly patients with hip fractures. For example, a recent circular to all 289 geriatric departments in the United Kingdom revealed that 43 out of 214 respondents (20%) provided a special orthopaedic unit or service for aged patients with hip fractures (Brocklehurst and Andrews, 1985). This comprised 12% of inland departments compared with 40% of otherwise similar departments in coastal areas (presumably prime sites of retirement).

Both the Duthie working party (DHSS, 1981) and a recent report of the Royal College of Physicians (1989) described the Hastings system in some detail and suggested it to be a valuable rehabilitation model, worthy of development as one possible solution to the increasing demands placed upon orthopaedic services by the large numbers of elderly hip fracture patients currently being treated. Inevitably the method of working of individual 'orthogeriatric' units ('OGUs') – sometimes referred to as 'geriatric–orthopaedic' rehabilitation units (GORUs) – varies according to local circumstances but the following three considerations are common to the planning, organizational and operational policies of most schemes.

1. A clearly identified and appropriately equipped ward or group of beds with independent nursing and physiotherapy staff which may or may not be on the same site as the acute orthopaedic ward.

2. Selection of patients for rehabilitation on the orthogeriatric unit is made either by a geriatrician or an orthopaedic surgeon but the day-to-day administration and medical supervision of the patients on the unit is principally performed by a geriatrician. The selection process for admission and transfer to the unit is completed as soon as possible following injury and certainly within the first week.

3. The triage procedure for the selection of patients is usually into three groups. Those thought not to require specialized rehabilitation facilities are discharged home directly from the acute orthopaedic ward. Similarly, arrangements are made for appropriate long-term care for those patients such as the deeply demented who have little chance of successful rehabilitation. The remaining patients are transferred to the OGU where

the length of stay is regarded as finite. Those patients who are not capable of being discharged within this time (usually 6–8 weeks) are transferred elsewhere in order that the perceived benefits of the scheme can be offered to the maximum number of patients.

In some centres medical advice from a geriatrician is routinely provided before the injured patient is taken to theatre but in most cases only severe medical conditions such as cardiac failure and unstable diabetes are treated at this stage. In general, most medical conditions are better investigated and treated after the fracture has been dealt with surgically.

Once on the orthogeriatric unit patients may stay under the overall care of the orthopaedic surgical staff or the geriatric medical staff but in some units the responsibility is formally shared. No matter what the arrangement, a combined ward round is performed at least weekly by a geriatrician and orthopaedic surgeon together with a senior ward nurse. Physiotherapists, occupational therapists and social workers participate in the ward round or in the case conference that follows. In this way all problems whether they be medical, surgical, social or functional can be considered, fully assessed and dealt with expeditiously by an identified member of the team. Plans for discharge can be made with the appropriate community personnel with the assistance of a liaison nurse.

The orthopaedic–geriatric unit is appropriately equipped for realistic rehabilitation of the elderly injured patient. Some units have additional nurses and therapists over and above those normally found on an orthopaedic ward and this inevitably incurs additional expenses.

This general approach has become widely accepted and Table 17.1 lists the principal publications which describe and at least partly audit the throughput of patients in such units. Though several reports claim to show a benefit of this form of rehabilitation for the elderly patient with hip fracture adverse comment has subsequently been passed regarding patient selection. Control groups have often been retrospective or totally omitted and few workers have formally investigated the value of collaborative orthogeriatric care in a statistically acceptable manner (Gilchrist *et al.*, 1985). This was highlighted in a report of the Royal College of Physicians (1989) which stated 'confirmation or refutation of the

Table 17.1 Principal publications in collaborative care rehabilitation of elderly, traumatized patients

Author	Year	Place	Design	Comments
Devas	1964	Hastings	First description of formal orthopaedic geriatric rehabilitation unit.	
Clark and Wainwright	1966	Stoke-on-Trent	Second description of formal orthopaedic–geriatric rehabilitation unit.	
Devas and Irvine	1969	Hastings	Third description of formal orthopaedic–geriatric rehabilitation unit.	
Cedar et al.	1980	Lund, Sweden	Early postoperative mobilization with weight bearing.	Reduced length of hospital stay.
Lefroy	1980	Perth, Australia	Orthogeriatric unit, uncontrolled study.	Report of outcome with no comparison or reference group.
DHSS	1981	London	DHSS Working Party report on Orthopaedic Services.	The problems of the elderly patient with a femoral neck fracture identified and necessity of orthopaedic–geriatric collaboration stressed.
Ceder and Thorngren	1982	Lund, Sweden	Early mobilization in hospital and early rehabilitation at home in cooperation with social services.	75% of hip fracture patients (mean age 75 years) at home within 2–3 weeks.
Boyd et al.[1]	1982	Nottingham	Comparison of results obtained before and after the establishment of an OGU.	27% reduction in mean length of stay.
Taggart	1983	Belfast	Experience of OGU, uncontrolled	Higher proportion of those patients transferred to OGU went home. Probably this and all other apparently beneficial results were due to the method of patient selection.
Smith	1984	Edinburgh	Geriatrician performed weekly round in orthopaedic wards.	A greater proportion of patients discharged earlier, especially noticeable in the more elderly.
Burley et al.	1984	Edinburgh	Comparison of OGU v. routine care.	No real differences seen in this uncontrolled study of an OGU in its first year.
Sikorski et al.	1985	Queensland, Australia	'Rapid transit system'. Immediate surgery and mobilization without sedation.	90% of patients discharged home within 5 days with appropriate support. Dependent upon large infrastructure of home care assistants.
Desai et al.	1985	West Bromwich	Typical, uncontrolled 'before and after' report.	30% reduction in mean length of stay.
Fordham et al.	1986	Huddersfield	Orthogeriatric unit v. routine care, prospective study.	No difference seen in length of hospital stay. Joint management found to be more expensive than routine orthopaedic care.

Sainsbury *et al.*	1986	Christchurch, New Zealand	Comparison of results obtained before and after the establishment of an OGU.	OGU resulted in shorter mean length of stay.
Murphy *et al.*	1987	London	Comparison of results obtained before and after the establishment of an OGU.	46% reduction in bed-days.
Blacklock and Woodhouse	1988	Newcastle-upon-Tyne	Nurse liaison officer between orthopaedics and geriatrics.	Significant reduction in length of stay and increased patient throughput.
Pryor *et al.*[2]	1988	Peterborough	'Hospital-at-home' within 5 days with appropriate nursing and GP support.	Only 50% of hip fracture patients were suitable for 'hospital-at-home'. System shown to be cost effective in spite of large infrastructure of home care assistants required.
Gilchrist *et al.*	1988	Glasgow	OGU *v.* routine care, prospective study.	No difference in mortality, mean length of stay or placement. No additional cost implications.
Whitaker and Currie	1988	Edinburgh	OGU *v.* routine orthopaedic care, prospective.	Proportion of patients discharged from each group at 6 weeks was the same in spite of OGU patients being shown to be older and more dependent on admission.
Kennie *et al.*	1988	Stirling	OGU *v.* routine orthopaedic care, prospective.	Patients treated in OGU showed greater independence and more satisfactory place of discharge in spite of reduced length of hospitalization. However, study biased.[3]
Harrington *et al.*	1988	London	Geriatric–orthopaedic liaison service.	Liaison service provides an alternative to OGUs but without financial implications.
Reid and Kennie	1989	Stirling	One year follow-up of patients treated on OGU *v.* routine care.	Patients treated in OGU showed higher rate of survival and improved level of independence.[3]
Royal College of Physicians	1989	London	Management strategy for femoral neck fractures.	Recommended close working relationship between orthopaedic surgeons and geriatricians and establishment of specific rehabilitation units.
Hempsall *et al.*	1990	E. Dorset	OGU *v.* routine orthopaedic care, prospective.	Reduced mean length of stay in OGU without difference in independence between the two groups. No difference between the groups at 6 months.

[1] This is a preliminary report of this unit. For definitive report see Boyd *et al.* (1983)
[2] For original description of this scheme see, Mowat and Morgan (1982)
[3] Simpson and Whitaker, 1988; Smith (1988)

value of orthogeriatric units and other management schemes must be carried out by well designed, controlled studies'.

To date few such trials have been performed and these have resulted in conflicting conclusions. Kennie *et al.* (1988) reported that rehabilitation of elderly patients with hip fracture in an OGU setting reduced the mean length of hospital stay from 41 to 24 days. However, there were notable differences between the intervention and control groups with respect to age and mental status at entry to the study which may have accounted for at least some of the apparent improvement in outcome (Simpson and Whitaker, 1988; Smith, 1988).

Gilchrist *et al.* (1988) were one of the first groups to perform a prospective, randomized and suitably controlled study in patients with hip fracture. They reported no difference in the mean length of stay, the mortality or placement at discharge. This investigation included 222 patients but even so was only large enough to detect a 50% change in any chosen outcome indicator with an 80% power and smaller changes could not be excluded (Simpson and Whitaker, 1988). An earlier trial by the Centre for the Health Economics in York (Fordham *et al.*, 1986) was prospective and controlled but limited by the small sample size. Though it showed no savings in bed days utilized (as a general indicator of fixed costs) it did demonstrate a significant increase in some variable costs such as the time spent by physiotherapists, occupational therapists, social workers, etc. The latter made combined orthogeriatric unit management in total £93 per patient more expensive than routine orthopaedic care at 1985 prices, i.e. an increase of 3.6%.

Several publications have reported that the mean length of hospital stay has been reduced following the introduction of a combined orthogeriatric form of rehabilitation (Table 17.1) and this is probably the single most important factor generating enthusiasm for this type of service. Such claims must be rigorously evaluated by controlled trials since it is known that the mean duration of hospital stay for hip fracture patients has been steadily falling since the mid-1960s, i.e. well before the introduction of collaborative care (Greatorex, 1986). Furthermore, length of stay is not necessarily a good performance indicator (Barer and Morrant, 1990) and by itself may be no more than a reflection of the 'aggressiveness' of a particular rehabilitation

unit and its willingness to discharge patients home. This has been amply shown by Fitzgerald *et al.* (1987) who analysed the changing patterns of hip fracture care before and after implementation of a prospective payment system in the United States. This was an attempt by the Federal Government to reduce medical expenditure by the introduction of a fixed price, prospective payment system for particular diagnostic groups. They showed that the implentation of this system was associated with a reduction in the mean length of hospitalization from 16 to 10 days and the mean number of physiotherapy sessions also decreased. Concomitantly, the proportion of patients discharged to a nursing home increased from 21% to 48% as did the proportion receiving nursing home care 6 months following discharge (13–39%).

Consequently, any analysis of the effectiveness of an orthogeriatric unit which shows a reduction in inpatient stay must be accompanied by an equivalent analysis demonstrating that the patients' level of independence and their ability to perform activities of daily living were not detrimentally affected by it. One such trial was performed by Hempsall *et al.* (1990) in East Dorset. They showed by multiple regression analysis that the mean length of stay was more than 9 days shorter in patients treated by a combined orthogeriatric service and this was not associated with a significant difference in outcome 6 months postoperatively in terms of mortality, function, dependency or social status.

The presence of a geriatric physician on the orthopaedic wards must be expected to lead to a greater diagnostic accuracy of medical disorders. Gilchrist *et al.* (1988) reported that 71% of patients in their orthopaedic–geriatric unit were found to have new medical disorders compared with only 55% in the control group. Similarly, whereas only 5% of patients rehabilitated in the orthogeriatric unit were found at review to have been discharged without appropriate treatment for some of their disease processes, the figure was 30% for patients treated on the routine orthopaedic wards. (These conditions were, in order of frequency, vitamin B_{12} deficiency, anaemias, 'biochemical osteomalacia' and diabetes.) In spite of the otherwise impressive activity of the geriatrician in diagnosing and treating new medical problems the authors could not demonstrate any difference in hospital mortality, 6-month mortality, length of stay or placement. Balanced against this negative finding must be the cost and possible iatrogenic complications of the investigations required to make these diagnoses as well as those of the prescribed medications.

Once the hip fracture patient is discharged from hospital the management problem is not necessarily solved since such patients rarely regain their former mobility and many are dependent on others and the social services. Reid and Kennie (1989) reviewed their hip fracture patients 1 year following discharge from either an orthogeriatric unit or a routine orthopaedic ward. They reported that those who had received combined care demonstrated better independence in the activities of daily living and a better type of residence when compared with those patients who had received routine care. Such observations would have great socio-economic implications had there not been statistical problems associated with the patient selection process (Simpson and Whitaker, 1988; Smith, 1988). Similarly, Campion, Jette and Berkman (1983) failed to demonstrate a significant effect of an 'interdisciplinary geriatric consultation service' in reducing readmissions to hospital within 1 year of discharge.

It seems therefore that close cooperation between orthopaedic and geriatric departments in the provision of collaborative rehabilitation services *may* result in the delivery of care which reduces the mean length of hospital stay.

Transferring patients to designated orthogeriatric units is time consuming and expensive and a liaison service in which a geriatrician advises on selected patients on the orthopaedic wards may be a more effective answer. However, what constitutes the best form of liaison has yet to be decided and whether it needs to be performed at consultant level is certainly questionable. For example, the recent introduction of a nurse-based liaison service between the geriatric and orthopaedic units in Newcastle was shown to significantly reduce the mean length of stay on the orthopaedic unit and increase the throughput of a female orthopaedic ward. Unfortunately this report was retrospective and uncontrolled (Blacklock and Woodhouse, 1988). A similar innovative scheme was described by Harrington, Brennan and Hodkinson (1988) in which the orthopaedic–geriatric liaison was in the form of a regular multidisciplinary ward round based at registrar level. Exact figures were not presented but they stated that as a result of

this liaison the numbers of patients requiring transfer for rehabilitation became 'vanishingly small'. A similar model at senior registrar level was reported by Bendall *et al.* (1985).

Collaborative management schemes certainly improve lines of communication between physician and surgeon and also have educational value for those postgraduate doctors involved. This has been shown both in shared care outpatient clinics (Newman *et al.*, 1987) as well as on the wards (Gilchrist *et al.*, 1988). Orthopaedic surgeons who have been exposed to collaborative ward rounds gradually begin to take a greater interest in the medical and social problems of those patients of theirs not treated on designated orthogeriatric units and their patient management changes. It has been shown that notes from ward rounds and discharge summaries on these patients contain more information on the patient's social and medical problems and drug charts generally list fewer drugs with less potential for toxic interaction.

The rapid transit system

This rehabilitation system for patients with proximal femoral fractures has been popularized by Sikorski and colleagues in Australia (Sikorski, Davis and Senior 1985) but is based upon the original ideas of Ceder of early mobilization in hospital followed by early rehabilitation at home (Ceder, Lindberg and Odberg, 1980; Ceder and Thorngren, 1982; Ceder, Stromqvist and Hansson, 1987). It depends principally on reducing the amount of time spent in hospital to an absolute minimum (90% accepted to the system were discharged to their homes within the first 5 days) since the authors consider that prolonged hospitalization is detrimental to the physical, mental and social well-being of the patient. They state that patients tend to be over-investigated and over-treated while in hospital resulting in the development of iatrogenic disorders. They also lose contact with their social situation which often deteriorates rapidly in their absence.

Following admission only those investigations which are clinically indicated are performed. Narcotic and sedative drugs are not used and general anaesthesia is avoided if at all possible. Surgery is performed expeditiously following the injury and this often involves transferring the patient directly from the emergency department to theatre. The surgery is performed by a surgeon with a high level of expertise and postoperatively non-narcotic analgesics are prescribed together with lateral cutaneous nerve or thigh blocks. No limitations are imposed on the mobility of the patients who are encouraged to walk fully weight-bearing within hours of their surgery. Domestic assessments are made within a day or two by dedicated physiotherapy and occupational therapy staff and patients are discharged home as soon as they are able to move around freely in bed, get in and out of a chair and walk a few paces with aids if necessary. Domestic support is provided by nursing, physiotherapy and occupational therapy staff with appropriate medical involvement.

For the first few days following discharge 'a moderate level of general support' is required and this is reduced rapidly. Daily visits by a district nurse and a physiotherapist occur for the first 5–7 days and thereafter their frequency diminishes until after 2 or 3 weeks the patients require no more than before their injury. Home helps to do the cleaning and shopping are often needed and are provided by family, friends, neighbours or a paid agency.

Such a system results in major economic gains as well as many medical and social advantages but clearly it can only be developed when appropriate local facilities exist and there is a suitable infrastructure for creating adequate home support. In practice, the rapid transit system is only possible if the person originates from an institution providing nursing care or has adequate home support. In my experience in this part of the world this is unusual. It also relies on a high provision of domiciliary physiotherapy and other services, including that of the general practitioner, to a level not universally currently available.

The Peterborough 'hospital-at-home'

This scheme is based on that of the 'Santé Service Bayonne' in France and is similar in some ways to the rapid transit system advocated by Sikorski, Davis and Senior (1985). The scheme essentially treats the elderly hip fracture patient as a special case and all such patients are managed by a single team spanning the hospital and the community. The aims are rapid and effective surgery, immediate planning for rehabilitation and early discharge made possible by the hospital-at-home (HAH) service (Mowat and Morgan, 1982). This provides intensive home nursing in addition to the conventional community nursing service. A nurse of whatever grade required can be placed in a patient's home for up to 24 h per day and in addition appropriate physiotherapy and occupational therapy support is arranged. The service is designed to provide short-term care up to 30 days. The only criterion for admission to the hospital-at-home service is that otherwise the patient would be admitted to or remain in hospital.

The Peterborough hospital-at-home is not restricted to hip fracture patients and also caters for patients with terminal care problems and for medical conditions that are incapacitating but can be managed at home by the general practitioner.

The results of this scheme (Mowat and Morgan, 1982; Pryor *et al.*, 1988; Pryor and Williams, 1989; Meeds and Pryor, 1990) suggest that at least half of all hip fracture patients are suitable for early discharge and home rehabilitation providing a hospital-at-home system can be arranged for them. The average inpatient stay for such patients was approximately 8 days with a further 9 days in the hospital-at-home making a total of 17 days' care. Equivalent patients treated as inpatients in hospital stayed an average of 24 days. Furthermore, the early discharge group ceased to require nursing support on average 7 days earlier than the comparison group. Moreover, a nurse was required on average only 20% of the time that a patient was in the hospital-at-home scheme.

Despite the necessity for special funding for travel and overtime for some members of the group, the cost of home nursing proved less than anticipated and certainly less than the cost of nursing patients in hospital. The estimated saving in inpatient days led to a net saving of approximately £75 000 in the first year in the treatment of hip fracture patients by the Peterborough Health District.

It is logical to rehabilitate elderly patients with hip fractures in the environment in which they will have to live and the Peterborough hospital-at-home service has proved cost-effective in doing this. However, only half of all patients sustaining hip fractures are capable of rehabilitation in their own homes.

Essex community orthopaedic project

The group is comprised of a dedicated orthopaedic nurse, an occupational therapist, a physiotherapist and a social worker and is responsible for the immediate assessment of the patient's home and domestic circumstances. It also monitors the rehabilitation process in the ward and the continuing rehabilitation at home and plans an early discharge with the general practitioner who maintains responsibility for the patient while at home. Like Sikorski, Davis and Senior (1985) this group emphasizes that an early postoperative discharge is the principal aim but states that a low mental test score on admission is a strong indication of the patient's unsuitability for early home discharge (Royal College of Physicians, 1989).

South Glamorgan care for elderly hospital discharge service

The hospital discharge service aims to promote a two-tier statutory and voluntary support system for disadvantaged frail elderly patients just after discharge from hospital. The particular features of the scheme include an extremely close liaison between hospital and community services in discharge planning as well as the establishment of a major network of home care assistants who are mostly volunteers but with full-time supervisors. There is a full-time hospital discharge coordinator, a hospital liaison nurse to identify patients requiring the home settlement service, a volunteer organizer to recruit, train and support other volunteers who provide the home support for patients after discharge. These 'settlement aides' provide intensive support for elderly patients in the period shortly after hospital discharge.

A review of this scheme after 2 years has suggested that there is considerable satisfaction among patients but whether such schemes can be adopted elsewhere as an adjunct to existing statutory services remains to be seen.

Conclusion

Despite the plethora of different rehabilitation schemes for the management of elderly patients

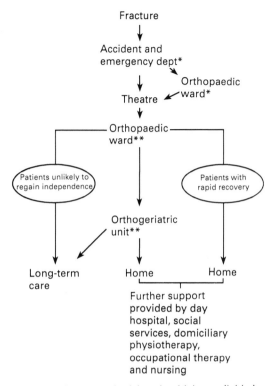

*Advice from a geriatrician should be available in these units.

**In practice these two may be situated on the same ward or in different wards or even on different sites.

Figure 17.2 A model operating policy for the collaborative management of elderly patients with skeletal injury (principally hip fracture). (Modified after Royal College of Physicians, 1989)

with hip fractures which are now available only a minority of such patients are being exposed to them. It appears that a positive attitude to treatment, an emphasis on a team approach, careful planning of a timely discharge from hospital and close liaison between the hospital and community services lead to both increased efficiency in the use of resources and to a better quality of life for these frail patients.

However, most of the schemes described above are labour intensive with an increased number of physiotherapists, occupational therapists and nurses above the norms found in routine orthopaedic rehabilitation wards; the costs of such services requires scrutiny. Some orthogeriatric units such as the one in Glasgow have been established in ways in which additional resource implications do not occur (Gilchrist *et al.*, 1988) but in many centres this is not the case and the expenses are significant (Fordham *et al.*, 1986). Claims that some of these techniques are cost effective have been made (Mowat and Morgan, 1982) but clearly before such schemes proliferate further evaluations require to be performed in statistically suitable manners to be sure that such schemes are truly cost effective.

Currently no one scheme seems to be superior and geriatricians and orthopaedic surgeons will have to decide what is best for them depending on their local resources. The evidence for early discharge along the lines advocated in Sweden, Australia and Peterborough by Ceder, Sikorski and Pryor respectively seems impressive and in view of the increasing demands being placed upon orthopaedic resources by the 'epidemic' of patients with hip fractures more attention will have to be directed to the implementation of such early discharge schemes. However, in order to make these discharges possible reliable supporting organizations such as the 'hospital-at-home' need to be available. It may be that in those situations when early discharge is inappropriate the best form of rehabilitation would be in the form of a combined orthogeriatric programme with care shared between orthopaedic surgeons and geriatricians (Figure 17.2).

Though it is admirable to discharge patients at the soonest possible opportunity, it must be emphasised that the patient must be safe to go home. Adequate medication together with all necessary information must be supplied and appropriate social services support arranged. Furthermore, the patient must feel 'satisfied' at the time of discharge. In this respect, a recent finding of the Royal College of Nursing must be considered – namely, 30% of surgical patients considered their hospital stay to have been too short (Rowlands, 1991).

It is to be hoped that in the future suitable resources will be provided for the implementation of one recommendation in particular of the Duthie Working Party on orthopaedic services (DHSS, 1981). This stated that 'combined orthopaedic–geriatric admission and progressive care units should be encouraged to explore innovative methods of shortening the hospital stay of the elderly orthopaedic patient'.

References

Barer, D. and Morrant, J. (1990) Acute hospital medical care for the elderly – is there a valid performance indicator? *Hlth Trends*, **22**, 3–8

Bendall, R., Vickers, Rh., Whitelaw, M.N. and Millard, P.H. (1985) Hospital care for fractured neck of femur. *Lancet*, **i**, 113–114

Blacklock, C. and Woodhouse, K.W. (1988) Orthogeriatric liaison. *Lancet*, **i**, 999

Boyd, R.V., Compton, E., Hawthorne, J. and Kemm, J.R. (1982) Orthogeriatric rehabilitation ward in Nottingham: a preliminary report. *Br. Med. J.*, **285**, 937–938

Boyd, R.V., Hawthorne, J., Wallace, W.A., Worlock, P.M. and Compton, E.H. (1983) The Nottingham orthogeriatric unit after 1000 admissions. *Injury*, **15**, 193–196

Brocklehurst, J.C. and Andrews, K. (1985) Geriatric medicine – the style of practice. *Age Ageing*, **14**, 1–7

Burley, L.E., Scorgie, R.E., Currie, C.T., Smith, R.G. and Williamson, J. (1984) The joint geriatric orthopaedic service in South Edinburgh: November 1979 – October 1980. *Hlth Bull.*, **42**, 133–140

Campbell, A.J. (1976) Femoral neck fractures in elderly women; a prospective study. *Age Ageing*, **5**, 102–109

Campion, E.W., Jette, A. and Berkman, B. (1983) An interdisciplinary geriatric consultation service: a controlled trial. *J. Am. Geriat. Soc.*, **31**, 792–796

Ceder, L., Lindberg, L. and Odberg, E. (1980) Differentiated care of hip fracture in the elderly. Mean hospital days and results of rehabilitation. *Acta Orthop. Scand.*, **51**, 157–162

Ceder, L., Stromqvist, B. and Hansson, L.I. (1987) Effects of strategy changes in the treatment of femoral neck fractures during a 17-year period. *Clin. Orthop.*, **218**, 53–57

Ceder, L. and Thorngren, K.G. (1982) Rehabilitation after hip repair. *Lancet*, **ii**, 1097–1098

Clark, A.N.G. and Wainwright, D. (1966) The management of the fractured neck of femur in the elderly female: a joint approach of orthopaedic surgery and geriatric medicine. *Geront. Clin.*, **8**, 321–326

Currie, C.T. (1987) Rehabilitating the elderly orthopaedic patient. *Geriat. Med.*, **17**, 42–47

Department of Health and Social Security (1981) Report of a Working Party. *Orthopaedic Services: Waiting time for out-patient appointments and in-patient treatment.* (Chairman Prof. R. B. Duthie) HMSO, London

Desai, H.N., Shakeel, M.H. and El Safty, M.E. (1985) Combined orthopaedic–geriatric care. *Lancet*, **i**, 349–350

Devas, M.B. (1964) Fractures in the elderly. *Geront. Clin.*, **6**, 347–359

Devas, M.B. (1977) *Geriatric Orthopaedics*, Academic Press, London

Devas, M.B. and Irvine, R.E. (1969) The geriatric orthopaedic unit. A method of achieving return to independence in the elderly patient. *Br. J. Geriat. Prac.*, **6**, 19–25

Fitzgerald, J.F., Fagan, L.F., Tierney, W. and Dittus, R.S. (1987) Changing patterns of hip fracture care before and after implementation of the prospective payment system. *J. Am. Med. Ass.*, **258**, 218–221

Fordham, R., Thompson, R., Holmes, J. and Hodkinson, C. (1986) A cost-benefit study of geriatric-orthopaedic management. Centre for Health Economics, University of York, discussion paper 14

Gilchrist, W.J., Newman, R.J., Hamblen, D.L. and Williams, B.O. (1985) Combined orthopaedic-geriatric care. *Lancet*, **i**, 349

Gilchrist, W.J., Newman, R.J., Hamblen, D.L. and Williams, B.O. (1988) Prospective randomised study of an orthopaedic geriatric in-patient service. *Br. Med. J.*, **297**, 1116–1118

Greatorex, I.F. (1986) Femoral neck fractures – improving efficiency in the care of elderly people. *Commun. Med.*, **8**, 185–190

Harrington, M.G., Brennan, M. and Hodkinson, H.M. (1988) The first year of a geriatric-orthopaedic liaison service: an alternative to 'orthogeriatric' units? *Age Ageing*, **17**, 129–133

Hempsall, V.J., Robertson, D.R.C., Campbell, M.J. and Briggs, R.S. (1990) Orthopaedic geriatric care – Is it effective? A prospective population-based comparison of outcome in fractured neck of femur. *J. Roy. Coll. Phys. Lond.*, **24**, 47–50

Irvine, R.E. (1983) Geriatric orthopaedics at Hastings: the collaborative management of elderly women with fractured neck of femur. *Adv. Ger. Med.*, **3**, 130–136

Irvine, R.E. (1985) Rehabilitation in geriatric orthopaedics. *Int. Rehabil. Med.*, **7**, 115–120

Irvine, R.E. and Devas, M.B. (1964) Fractured neck of femur in elderly women. In *Age with a future*. Proceedings of the Sixth International Congress of Gerontology, Copenhagen 1963 (ed. P. F. Hansen), Munksgaard Copenhagen, pp. 276–281

Kennie, D.C., Reid, J., Richardson, I.R., Kiaman, A.A. and Kett, C. (1988) Effectiveness of geriatric rehabilitative care after fractures of the proximal femur in elderly women: a randomised clinical trial. *Br. Med. J.*, **297**, 1083–1086

Lefroy, R.B. (1980) Treatment of patients with fractured neck of the femur in a combined unit. *Med. J. Aust.*, **2**, 669–670

Meeds, B. and Pryor, G.A. (1990) Early home rehabilitation for the elderly patient with hip fracture. The Peterborough hip fracture scheme. *Physiotherapy*, **76**, 75–77

Melton, L.J. III and Riggs, B.L. (1987) Epidemiology of age-related fractures. In *The Osteoporotic Syndrome. Detection, Prevention and Treatment* (ed. L.V. Avioli), 2nd edn, Grune and Stratton, London

Mowat, I.G. and Morgan, R.T.T. (1982) Peterborough hospital at home scheme. *Br. Med. J.*, **284**, 641–643

Murphy, P.J., Rai, G.S., Lowy, M. and Bielawska, C. (1987) The beneficial effects of joint orthopaedic-geriatric rehabilitation. *Age Ageing*, **16**, 273–278

Newman, R.J., Belch, J., Kelly, I.G. and Sturrock, R.D. (1987) Are combined orthopaedic and rheumatology clinics worthwhile? *Br. Med. J.*, **294**, 1392–1393

Pryor, G.A., Myles, J.W., Williams, D.R.R. and Anand, J.K. (1988) Team management of the elderly patient with hip fracture. *Lancet*, **i**, 401–403

Pryor, G.A. and Williams, D.R.R. (1989) Rehabilitation after hip fracture. Home and hospital management compared. *J. Bone Joint Surg.*, **71B**, 471–474

Reid, J. and Kennie, D.C. (1989) Geriatric rehabilitative care after fractures of the proximal femur: one year follow up of a randomised clinical trial. *Br. Med. J.*, **299**, 25–26

Rowlands, B. (1991) The human toll of rapid discharge. *Hosp. Doctor*, **C11**(42), 23

Royal College of Physicians of London (1989) Fractured neck of femur. Prevention and management. Report

Sainsbury, R., Gillespie, W.J., Armour, P.C. and Newman, E.F. (1986) An orthopaedic geriatric rehabilitation unit: the first two years experience. *N.Z. Med. J.*, **99**, 583–585

Sikorski, J.M., Davis, N.J. and Senior, J. (1985) The rapid transit system for patients with fractures of proximal femur. *Br. Med. J.*, **290**, 439–443

Simpson, R.J. and Whitaker, NHG. (1988) Hope for broken hips? *Br. Med. J.*, 1543–1544

Smith, D.L. (1984) The elderly in the convalescent orthopaedic trauma ward: can the geriatrician help? *Hlth Bull.*, **42**, 36–44

Smith, N. (1988) Effectiveness of geriatric rehabilitative care. *Br. Med. J.*, **297**, 1609

Taggart, H. (1983) Geriatric orthopaedic rehabilitation in Belfast. In *Advanced Geriatric Medicine 3* (eds F.I. Caird and J.G Evans), Pitman, London, pp. 144–150

Thomas, T.G. and Stevens, R.S. (1974) Social effects of fracture neck of femur. *Br. Med. J.*, **3**, 456–458

Whitaker, J.J. and Currie, C.T. (1988) An evaluation of the role of geriatric orthopaedic rehabilitation units in Edinburgh. *Hth Bull.*, **46**, 273–276

18

Aids and appliances

Graham P. Mulley

After hip fracture, patients aged 65–74 years spend an average of 30 days in hospital while those over 75 return home after a mean hospital stay of 43 days (Greatorex, 1986). Attention to aids, appliances and the environment can improve the quality of care in hospital and might reduce its duration. We must therefore be aware of those gadgets which facilitate the taking of a full and accurate history (hearing aids and amplified communicators), aids which improve the patient's self-esteem and wellbeing (dentures, spectacles with clean lenses and clothing) and items which improve safety (good lighting, alarms and appropriate floor surfaces). We must also be familiar with equipment which reduces the chances of the patient developing decubitus ulcers as well as the indications for mobility aids. We should also be aware of those aids which allow independent living (feeding, kitchen and dressing aids). If we are to avoid unwittingly doing physical or psychological harm to our patients and inhibiting their successful recovery we must also be vigilant about items which disable or cause distress. Examples of this are chairs which are too high or too low, bedpans, hard trolleys, conspicuous, large volume catheter drainage bags and inadequate or inappropriate footwear.

The prescription of aids and appliances must not be restricted solely to those elderly patients rehabilitating following trauma. They must also be considered for those undergoing elective surgery such as hip and knee arthroplasty and are particularly indicated for the polyarthritic patient and those with neurological disease (Mulley, 1991).

Accessory aids

Older people often have relatively low expectations of their health and tolerate declining vision and hearing, wrongly believing that these are inevitable concomitants of ageing and that nothing can be done to overcome these impediments.

Visual aids

Visual problems are common in hip fracture patients (Stott and Gray, 1980). In a survey of 384 such patients Brocklehurst *et al.* (1978) found that 39% were unable to read small print with either eye, 21% give a history of partial sightedness and 12% had homonymous hemianopia. Impaired vision may therefore have contributed to the fall that caused the fracture. Curiously, those with poor sight fell not by tripping, but by losing balance (Brocklehurst *et al.*, 1978) and of subjects in homes for the aged, blind people were less likely to fall than those whose sight was good (Marulec, Librach and Schadel, 1970).

More than one-third of old people in hospital require attention to their spectacles (Young and George, 1987); simple repairs, cleaning the lenses and ensuring that the spectacles are not too loose can make an enormous difference to a patient's safety and wellbeing.

A medical assessment of an aged person should include examination of the eyes and determination of visual acuity. If vision is impaired, a diagnosis must be sought. If the sight cannot be corrected, then visual aids should be considered. The simple items are often the best: ensuring that illumination is good and providing magnifiers and large-print books (Hillman, 1988). On the pre-discharge home visit, consideration might be given to large numerals on clocks and the telephone, writing aids (to help with addressing envelopes, signing cheques and writing letters), and indicators which give an audible signal when a cup is full (Dudley, 1990).

Hearing aids

Sixty per cent of people over the age of 70 have some degree of hearing loss (Herbst and Humphrey, 1981) and in two-thirds of cases the hearing impairment is socially important. A quarter will have total occlusion of the auditory meatus with wax and in some of these syringing the ear following softening of the wax will restore hearing to a grateful patient (Nassar, 1980).

Taking a history from a deaf old person can be exasperating for the busy doctor, unpleasant for the patient and embarrassing for people within earshot. If every ward had a communicator which amplified the doctor's voice, everyone would benefit. Patients or relatives should be asked about hearing aids on admission. If they have not brought the aid into hospital the family should be asked to fetch it as soon as possible. As part of the general examination the hearing aid should be adequately assessed. Is there a battery in place? Is the battery flat? (to check the battery, switch the aid on and turn up the volume: a feedback squeal will be heard). Does the mould fit properly? Is the mould blocked with wax? Is the flexible tube which carries amplified sound to the ear kinked or blocked with condensation (Corrado, 1988)? If there are problems which cannot be easily rectified on the ward, referral to the audiology clinic is essential.

Dentures

In a survey of edentulous patients attending a dental school, three-quarters of the subjects said that they never wanted to be seen without their dentures. A further 22% avoided being seen without them. Only 4% did not seem to mind being in public without their false teeth. More than two-thirds preferred to clean their dentures when they were alone (Berg, Inglebretsen and Johnson, 1984).

Being without dentures has a dramatic effect on facial appearance; it diminishes self-image and reduces the capacity to enjoy food. We must therefore ensure that patients' dentures are given a high priority by everyone on the rehabilitation team. Dentures should be documented in the medical notes. Nurses should have a care plan for cleaning dentures since in many cases, they are in a poor state of hygiene (Gelbier and Hopes, 1979).

Clothing

We feel comfortable in our own clothes. Clothing expresses our personality and helps give us identity. Unfortunately many institutions favour conformity resulting in the frequent occurrence of patients' clothing being removed on admission. These patients are often dressed in standard nightware – even in the daytime. They may also be issued with back-fastening operating theatre gowns the tapes of which easily become detached immodestly exposing the patients' buttocks when they stand and walk. The undermining of the individual's status is further extended by placing a plastic band around the wrist proclaiming the person's number, name and age.

Let us ensure that our patients are not denied the basic right to be properly dressed in their own clothes. It will help strengthen their sense of individuality and make it more likely that they will be treated as individuals.

Footwear

Patients should be encouraged to wear their own shoes whenever possible since wearing slippers does not facilitate a good gait pattern. Inspection of shoes sometimes provides useful diagnostic clues, e.g. the greater wear of the lateral aspect of the sole and heel in the hemiplegic patient with foot inversion, the uriniferous aroma of the shoes of old people who may be embarrassed to admit to urinary incontinence and the shoes that have been cut away to accommodate feet made oedematous by sitting or sleeping in an easy chair or by heart failure.

Examination of the feet of aged patients often reveals deformities or abnormalities which could be helped by special footwear or eased by chiropody (Williamson *et al.*, 1964). Footwear can not only accommodate deformed feet and relieve pain it can also compensate for leg length inequality (White, 1988). For example, after intertrochanteric hip fracture the affected limb may be up to 2 cm shorter than the other. In this situation the heel can be raised. In those cases with greater degrees of shortening both the heel and sole should be raised but with more raise in the heel tapering towards the toe.

If the patient's foot has become swollen as a result of deep venous thrombosis extra-depth footwear or Drewshoes made from plastazote should be considered. In cases of foot deformity or pressure sores part of this material can be easily cut away so preventing further pressure yet allowing the patient to stand on his feet as soon as possible. Patients who have difficulty with laces will benefit from the use of Velcro fasteners.

Aids to prevent pressure sores

Pressure sores are painful and because they can take months to heal, prolong rehabilitation. Their treatment necessitates much nursing time and skill and therefore everyone on the orthopaedic team should take a keen interest in their prevention and management. Inappropriate aids can contribute to the development of sores whereas low pressure surfaces can help prevent them and are thus of the utmost importance (Young, 1990a).

The incidence of sores in patients with hip fractures varies according to the hospital and patient selection. Of 239 consecutively treated patients with intertrochanteric fractures, 5.3% developed sacral sores and 2.6% had heel sores (Cleveland *et al.*, 1959). In a different study of 50 elderly females admitted to a geriatric–orthopaedic unit, 20 had sores involving the sacral and/or heel areas. In 13 patients, the sores were superficial but were deep in the remainder (Campbell, 1976). In a similar study of 293 patients admitted to a London hospital for elective hip surgery or for treatment of hip fracture, 32% developed sores (Versluysen, 1985). They were most common in elderly women with hip fractures and the sacrum, buttocks and heels were the most frequent sites. Sadly, half the patients had more than one sore. Although 17% of sores were present on admission, 58% developed in the first 2 weeks in hospital.

Why do these sores occur and how can they be prevented? Most are the result of long periods of immobilization on high pressure surfaces on trolleys in accident and emergency departments, wards and operating theatres (Versluysen, 1986). They are therefore partly the responsibility of the doctor who must ensure that time spent on hard surfaces is kept to a minimum and that the hospital has a policy for providing appropriate surfaces for trolleys and beds as well as suitable cushions (King's Fund Centre, 1989). Versluysen (1986) argued that all elderly patients should be treated on low pressure support systems from the time of entry to hospital until mobility had been fully restored.

Equipment is no substitute for good nursing care and can sometimes lead to a false sense of security (Kostuik and Ferrie, 1985). However, low pressure surfaces are a crucial part of pressure sore prevention and management. Standard hospital mattresses are not ideal since they may be covered with a plastic surface. This creates a moist microenvironment which predisposes to the development of superficial sores.

Hospital mattresses are subject to much wear and tear and the inner foam may become wet and soiled. Regular checks to ensure that the mattress is comfortable and springy are recommended as well as a policy for replacing worn out ones (King's Fund Centre, 1989).

Low pressure mattresses may be filled with air or water. Alternating pressure air mattresses ('Ripple mattresses') have been recommended by some as routine for all patients with femoral neck fracture in the acute phase of their illness (Editorial, 1990). Compared with conventional hospital mattresses, large-cell ripple mattresses appear to be effective in preventing and healing sores of heels and trunk (Bliss, McLaren and Exton-Smith, 1967). Small-cell ripple mattresses are less effective in the prevention of pressure sores (Bliss, 1978). Unfortunately, there are problems with ripple mattresses; they may puncture or leak, the air tubes become kinked or detached and the pump and materials are not always reliable (Stapleton, 1986). Staff may be unaware when faults develop, and often do not notice the lights which warn of mechanical faults. Selector switches may be set wrongly and hospital engineers who service the motors and mattresses may have received little training (Bliss, McLaren and Exton-Smith, 1967; Bliss, 1978). These factors may contribute to a patient developing a large sore after only a few hours on a faulty ripple mattress.

Water beds or mattresses may also have a role in pressure sore prophylaxis (Siegal, Vistres and

Laub, 1973) as may low-pressure foam mattresses (Scales *et al.*, 1982). Sheepskins should also be considered – not only are they soft to touch, they are compressible and thus distribute pressure evenly. Their frictional properties provide low resistance to shear and their low porosity under load maintains a low humidity interface. Natural sheepskins are preferred to polyester fabric simulations which are very poor absorbers of water vapour (Denne, 1979).

Although there is a general consensus that low pressure mattresses are effective in preventing pressure sores there are few scientific data to support the claims of manufacturers. In a survey of 48 items of pressure-relieving equipment, Young (1990b) found that there was no published evidence of efficacy in 50%. Anecdotal support was provided in 10 cases, but only two well designed randomized trials had taken place. At present therefore only general recommendations can be made and it is not yet possible to give firm guidelines on which low pressure mattresses to provide for which patients with specific conditions.

Aids for urinary incontinence

Eight per cent of people aged over 75 years living at home have troublesome urinary problems (McGrowther *et al.*, 1986) and following hip fracture surgery about 40% of patients develop urinary retention or incontinence (Campbell, 1976). Some of these will subsequently require in-dwelling catheters. The decision to use urinary catheters must not be taken lightly since it has been estimated that 80% of hospital-acquired infections are related to them. Similarly, one in eight of those who develop bacteraemia from the catheterized urinary tract will die (Waghorn, Griffiths and Kelly, 1988). In addition to the described morbidity, catheterization is associated with significant embarrassment and loss of self-esteem (Belfield, 1988). These psychological problems can be worsened if the patient is supplied not with a discreet drainage bag worn on the thigh or lower leg but rather with a large drainage bag conspicuously placed next to the bed or chair or attached to the walking frame. Such obvious bags advertise that the unfortunate sufferer is incontinent; this can only harm his or her dignity.

External drainage appliances (urinary sheath devices) are a more acceptable alternative for some men. They must be carefully applied and reviewed since they may traumatize the penis or become detached. If the leg bag is secured with straps, skin abrasions may sometimes occur (Smith, 1988).

For those men who are unable to use penile sheaths and for women who are incontinent, pads should be presented. Contemporary ones are highly absorbent, keep the skin dry, and prevent clothing and sheets from becoming wet (Smith, 1988).

The ward environment

Ward design and furnishings should enable those who are temporarily or permanently disabled to do as much as possible for themselves. Unfortunately, the reality often falls short of this ideal. Shiny vinyl floors make patients afraid to walk lest they slip and fall. Equipment and chairs may block the access to the toilet especially at night. Many patients who have high-seat chairs at home are not provided with them when they are in acute wards and therefore require nursing assistance to stand up and sit down (Sklaroff and Atkinson, 1987). Indeed, rather than fostering self-care, the system conspires to render patients unnecessarily dependent. For example, some disabled patients who can wash, bathe, toilet and transfer themselves independently at home may be offered unnecessary assistance with these activities in hospital so promoting reliance on others. Ideally, we need to develop a change in perspective, to ensure the provision of an enabling environment and by the thoughtful use of basic equipment create a milieu which is conducive to successful rehabilitation.

Devas (1976) said it was a poor sort of medicine that left a hip fracture patient lying in bed having to use a bedpan when it is known that the best positions for defaecation are squatting or sitting in a supported position. The use of a bedpan does not allow for ease of comfort and not surprisingly, their use involves much more energy expenditure than a commode (Benton, Brown and Rusk, 1950). They make defaecation difficult, dangerous and undignified and cause irritation and resentment. Commodes are preferred if patients are unable to get to the toilet independently but otherwise the use of the lavatory should be encouraged. It is important to ensure that the lavatory is clearly identified with

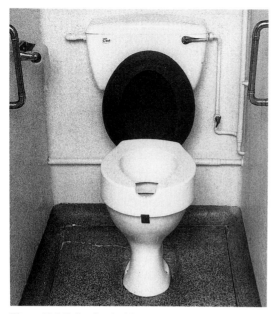

Figure 18.1 Toilet fitted with a secured raised seat and grab-rails on each side

large lettering and a light so that the door is visible at night. The seat should be sufficiently high to allow the patient to use it unaided (Figure 18.1). Grab-rails and toilet frames may be helpful (Penn, 1988) and toilet paper should be provided on both sides. It should preferably be of the type that allows individual sheets to be pulled from a box since hemiplegic patients or those with an arm in a cast may have difficulty tearing off a sheet of serrated paper. The door should open outwards in case the patient falls and requires assistance.

In recent years there has been a quiet revolution in ward equipment. Beds and tables are now of adjustable heights and toilets are designed for access by patients in wheelchairs or using walking frames (Bennett, 1982; Clarke-Williams, 1983). Patients have their own lockers and wardrobes. Chairs are stable and comfortable and thought is being given to the height and angle of the seat, the shape of the backrest, the optimum height and length of the armrests and the material used for covering the chair (Ellis, 1988). However, there is scope for further progress. Hoists (Figure 18.2) can help to move a very disabled elderly person and reduce the risk of backstrain in nurses and other caregivers (Waters, 1988). It is said that one in six nurses in the United Kingdom suffers back pain each year as a result of handling patients (Health Services

Advisory Committee, 1985). Yet many nurses caring for the elderly rarely or never use hoists. This is usually because of inadequate instruction and one in three nurses is unaware of basic safety factors in hoist operation (Connolly *et al.*, 1990).

Hospital wheelchairs are often in a neglected and dangerous condition (Crewe, 1982; Young *et al.*, 1985) with flat tyres, ineffective brakes hard or torn seats and defective footplates. The proposal that a named person on each unit should maintain an inventory of aids and encourage their effective and safe deployment is one that should be seriously considered (Health Services Advisory Committee, 1985).

Mobility aids

The main objective of orthopaedic rehabilitation is to restore the patient's ability to walk and undertake activities of daily living as soon as possible so that he or she can become independent and return to pre-fracture levels of function (Devas, 1976; Karumo, 1977; Jensen, Tondevold and Sorensen, 1979). In practice however many patients who fracture their hips do not regain their former mobility and at 6 months, only one in three survivors is fully mobile (Evans, Prudham and Wandless, 1979). A survey of 360 patients showed that only 51% returned to pre-injury mobility and one-fifth were non-ambulatory at 1 year (Miller, 1978). While 79% of those with subcapital fractures regained pre-fracture mobility indoors, only 50% resumed their previous level of outdoor mobility and stair-climbing (Jette *et al.*, 1987). Similarly, a quarter of hip fracture patients seen at 1 year were more dependent than they had been before the accident (Thomas and Stevens, 1974). Whether these figures would improve with the timely and optimum provision of mobility aids has never been evaluated. Nonetheless, an awareness of these enabling items, the provision of which has been shown to be more cost-effective than providing other forms of help to patients with locomotor disabilities (Hart *et al.*, 1990), should improve the doctor's effectiveness in rehabilitating elderly orthopaedic patients.

Most elderly people who have fractured their hips are frail and usually require some form of mobility aids (Andrews, 1987). These impart confidence and stability and may thus prevent or

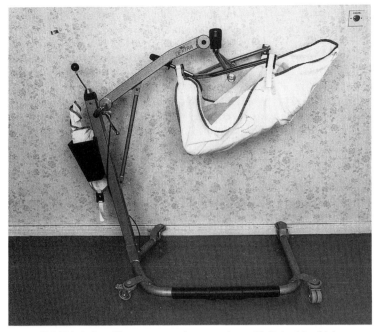

Figure 18.2 This hoist will move even a heavy patient with little risk of injury to the nurse or attendant

postpone further injuries (Braatz and Pino, 1972). They also diminish static forces on painful weight-bearing joints thereby reducing discomfort (Mulley, 1988).

Some mobility aids are inappropriate for the elderly and on all occasions care must be taken to choose the correct aid and ensure that it does not harm the patient. Skill is required in determining whom to wean off mobility aids and at what stage since some individuals become unnecessarily reliant on them and fail to achieve their full rehabilitative potential.

Following hip fracture gait retraining used to begin with the patient walking between parallel bars (Braatz and Pino, 1972; Andrews, 1987). However, this is now only recommended for the extremely timid patient as it tends to instill a false sense of security in an unrealistic situation. More appropriate is the carefully supervised used of a walking frame which is obviously more stable than crutches (Fisher and Jackson, 1988). The first frame is said to have been designed by a 12-year-old boy for his aunt who had fractured her hip (Dobrin, 1980). The basic design has remained unchanged but many varieties are now available and specialist assessment by a physiotherapist is recommended (Mulley, 1990; Hall, Clarke and Harrison, 1990). Simple frames prevent the normal pattern of heterolateral limb movement resulting in a halting gait without truncal rotation. Wheeled frames which are pushed along give a less abnormal gait pattern and allow a faster speed of walking with less energy expenditure (Hamzeh, Bowker and Sayegh, 1988). Though more efficient they do not run well over carpets (Mayfield, 1984) and obviously cannot be used in the vicinity of steps. Furthermore, they are feared by unsteady patients. Care should be taken with wheeled frames by Parkinsonian patients since those with a festinant gait may have difficulty in stopping.

Careful assessment of the patient's physical capability is necessary before crutches are prescribed since energy expenditure when using them can rise by over 60% when compared with the average for normal level walking. Patients with cardiac and chronic chest conditions might therefore be unsuitable for this type of walking aid and in general older patients should be considered for walking frames rather than crutches. It is a frequent observation that many patients aged 60 years and over find the use of axillary, elbow and gutter crutches difficult for non-weight bearing or partial weight bearing purposes – particularly when this has to be sustained for prolonged periods or distances (Ceder *et al.*, 1979; Potter and Wallace, 1990).

Other patients who have particular problems using crutches include those with strokes and poor vision. The use of crutches entails a transfer of weight through the upper limbs and some patients may be unable to tolerate this when muscle power is reduced or when joints are affected by instability or arthritis (Nichols and Mowat, 1972).

The particular problems which are associated with the use of crutches include brachial plexus compression in the axilla, bruising of the antero-lateral chest, blistering or soreness of the hands, carpal tunnel syndrome and, of course, fatigue.

With successful rehabilitation many patients progress in time from frames and crutches to sticks. Those with poor balance (perhaps because of neurological or ocular problems) may welcome the extra support given by a quadropod but tripods are not recommended because of their instability (Nichols and Mowat, 1972).   Rehabilitationists must acquaint themselves with at least some of the basic features of walking sticks (Mulley, 1988). The stick may be made of wood (favoured by many older people being light, cheap and having a welcome traditional feel) or aluminium (which is more robust and usually is adjustable in length). The optimum length of the stick (from the top of the handle to the bottom of the rubber ferrule) should be the same as the vertical distance from the wrist crease to the ground, 15 cm lateral to the shoe heel with the patient standing in everyday footwear with the elbow flexed to 15 degrees. The handle may be curved or straight, the latter being more physiological. Patients with arthritic hands may benefit if the diameter of the handle is appropriately expanded by using foam rubber. Alternatively, a Fischer stick with a wide, moulded handle may be prescribed. The shaft should not be splintered nor too pliable. All sticks should have a secure broad rubber tip, which prevents slipping and reduces the risk of falls.

Sophisticated analysis of the biomechanics of gait indicates that on purely theoretical grounds the most effective way of holding a stick in order to reduce the forces across the hip is in the opposite hand but a reduction in the forces across the hip, knee, ankle or foot can also be procured by holding the stick in the ipsilateral hand (Whittle, 1991). However, this type of stick use results in a lateral lurching gait which is generally considered by physiotherapists to be undesirable. For this reason therapists generally instruct their patients to use the stick in the contralateral hand no matter which joint is to be relieved (Hollis, 1976) since this results in a more normal gait pattern and facilitates a more stable and widely based stance. Certainly patients who have undergone total hip arthroplasty achieve a greater mean stride length with a more normal cadence when the stick is held in the contralateral hand (Edwards, 1986). However, controversy exists on this point even among bioengineers (Paul, 1991) and this is reflected in the fact that sometimes it is observed that a subject uses a stick in the opposite hand to that in which he has been instructed. In some cases this is a mistake on the part of the patient but in others it is a reflection that the observer has failed to fully appreciate all the other subtle compensations of gait and posture which the subject has adopted (Whittle, 1991).

Most patients continue to use mobility aids for many months after their hip fracture. Evans, Prudham and Wandless (1979) found that half the survivors complained of pain in the injured hip 6 months after their fall. At 1 year, half are still fearful of further falls and this limits their range of mobility and is an important factor in the continued use of walking aids (Ungar and Warne, 1986). At 1 year only 20% of hip fracture patients walk without an aid (Ceder *et al.*, 1979; Ungar and Warne, 1986) and this proportion is higher in those discharged to residential and nursing homes.

Ensuring that patients are provided with the appropriate mobility aid and use it correctly is not merely of academic interest. In a survey of patients in a nursing home whose fall resulted in serious injury, the commonest external factor in the genesis of the fall was the inappropriate or incorrect use of a walking aid, usually a frame or stick (Tinetti, 1987).

Aids used in the home

In a survey of more than 1000 people over the age of 75 years living at home in a typical English market town, Clark *et al.* (1984) found that most were able to complete basic activities of daily living without any assistance. However, many required aids to enable them to maintain their independence: one-third used toilet aids (including commodes) and only 43% of women over 85 years could get to and from the toilet without using aids; one-quarter were using bath

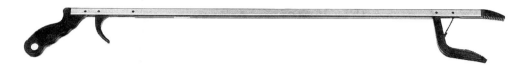

Figure 18.3 A 'helping hand' pick-up stick. These often incorporate a magnet in their tip to facilitate picking up small metallic objects

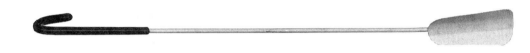

Figure 18.4 A long-handled shoe-horn

aids and one-fifth made use of mobility aids. Many healthy old people therefore use aids for personal hygiene, toileting and mobility. Dressing difficulties are also widespread with approximately half the attenders at a rheumatology clinic experiencing some problem in this regard. Similarly, in a survey of people aged over 75 years living at home, 5.5% required help with dressing and 2% used an aid. These figures of course are higher in those individuals living in residential and nursing homes (Mitchell, 1991).

As might be expected those in whom the arthritic process is so advanced as to be waiting for or who have already undergone total hip replacement have a greater need for aids and equipment. In an Oxford survey, 87% of such patients were using aids prior to admission for surgery with nearly two-thirds using aids for walking, toilet and bathing purposes. One-half benefited from dressing aids including stocking aids, reachers ('helping hands') (Figure 18.3), elasticated shoe laces and long-handled shoe-horns (Figure 18.4). Seventy-four per cent possessed walking aids of which 94% were using them. Three months after operation the need for aids and appliances was generally reduced but

64% were still helped by them. This proportion became progressively smaller with time and when they were reviewed 9 months following surgery only 50% of the group possessed walking aids of which only 71% were still using them. These were overall figures regarding usage of appliances and a more detailed analysis showed a significant difference between the practice of the rheumatoid patients and those with osteoarthrosis. In general, patients with rheumatoid disease possessed and utilized more aids than patients with osteoarthrosis and their overall use of equipment did not materially change with surgery, e.g. at 9 months 50% of rheumatoid patients continued to use toilet aids. In contrast, those patients with unilateral osteoarthrosis made the least use of the prescribed appliances (Haworth and Hopkins, 1980).

A patient returning home after a fracture will be frightened of further injury. The main concern therefore is safety and on the pre-discharge home visit particular attention should be paid to what can be done to reduce the risk of subsequent falls. Other considerations are the need to maintain and improve mobility, to encourage maximum independence in daily living activities, and to be able to contact others should another crisis occur.

In a study of 40 previously independently mobile patients over the age of 65 years who were discharged from an American rehabilitation hospital after treatment for hip fracture, the commonest aid provided was a walking frame (Rosenblatt, Campion and Mason, 1986). Most patients needed bathing equipment and bath aids such as long-handled sponges. About half of the patients received a raised toilet seat and a similar proportion were supplied with a commode. Home visits with a therapist usually result in a number of safety recommendations being made. These include removal of or tacking down of loose rugs, altering the height of chairs and toilets as well as ensuring that the telephone is accessible and that important telephone numbers are conveniently placed next to it. Unfortunately, 20% of people over 85 years have difficulties using the telephone (Hunt, 1978) and after an accident at home many aged people are unable to reach it or use the dial. It is therefore prudent to consider provision of an emergency alarm for an elderly person who is returning home to live alone after a fracture (Davies, 1990). Most alarms consist of a triggering device (a pendant, bracelet or clothes clip) which activates an alarm unit. This then automatically dials a contact point (usually a switchboard manned 24 h per day) or a sequence of pre-arranged numbers of relatives and other carers. Alarms can be bought or rented and they give reassurance to both the aged patient and the family.

There appear to be few studies of the problems encountered by old people who have sustained fractures other than those of the hip and how they might be helped by the provision of aids. One could presume that people whose arm was in a sling or cast because of a fracture would benefit from appropriate feeding aids (Connolly and Wilson, 1990a). Furthermore, the use of non-slip mats minimize the risk of a plate moving across the table, steep-sided plates or plastic plate guards prevent food being pushed off the plate, and a combination knife and fork allows one to eat 'one-handed'. Simple kitchen aids should also be considered, e.g. tap-turners, kettle and teapot tippers and spiked boards which allow food to be stabilized while cutting or peeling (Connolly and Wilson, 1990b). Similarly, a person who has sustained a vertebral compression fracture may have difficulty standing in the kitchen for long periods and a perching stool may afford ease. Trolleys make the task of carrying easier and also facilitate mobility. Many disabled elderly people make use of long-handled shoe-horns (White and Mulley, 1989; Hart *et al.*, 1990) and aids for reaching (North Tyneside Social Services, 1982).

Provision of equipment must be prompt and for this to occur, careful planning before discharge is essential. This is best done by a multidisciplinary case conference during which nurses, therapists and others can determine what equipment is likely to be needed and ensure that provision is smoothly coordinated and speedily provided.

Conclusion

Conventional medical training equips us to treat illnesses with drugs and surgery but unfortunately, few of us have been made fully aware of the importance of aids and appliances which can do so much to improve our patients' wellbeing, facilitate therapy and confer independence. Unless we take an interest in simple items of equipment, our patients may be denied the opportunity to achieve their full capabilities. The account of a retired orthopaedic surgeon describing his personal experience of rehabilitation following an intertrochanteric fracture is salutary (Farrow, 1977). He reported that it was not until his initial home visit that he was fully dressed following his trauma and operation. His poor balance and reduced hip flexion prevented him performing peri-anal toilet and he experienced difficulties putting on socks and shoes as well as lifting the affected leg over the edge of the bath-tub. He also had problems coping with crutches.

The frustration and unhappiness these experiences must have produced could have been mitigated or avoided by the imaginative and prompt provision of appropriate clothing and enabling equipment.

Successful rehabilitation involves paying close attention to little details. The provision of basic aids and appliances which help restore patients to mobility and independence and to maintain their self-esteem is an integral part of the rehabilitation process. This vital aspect of care should therefore be fully considered at all times by all members of the orthopaedic-geriatric rehabilitation team.

References

Andrews, K. (1987) *Rehabilitation of the older adult*. Edward Arnold, London

Belfield, P.W. (1988) Urinary catheters. *Br. Med. J.*, **296**, 836–837

Bennett, G.C.J. (1982) After hip fracture repair. *Lancet*, **ii**, 561–562

Benton, J.G., Brown, H. and Rusk, H.A. (1950) Energy expended by patients on the bedpan and bedside commode. *J. Am. Med. Ass.*, **144**, 1442–1447

Berg, E., Inglebretsen, R. and Johnson, T.B. (1984) Some attitudes towards edentulousness, complete dentures and co-operation with the dentist. *Acta Odontol. Scand.*, **42**, 334–338

Bliss, M.R., McLaren, R. and Exton-Smith, A.N. (1967) Preventing pressure sores in hospital: controlled trial of a large-celled ripple mattress. *Br. Med. J.*, **1**, 394–397

Bliss, M.R. (1978) The use of Ripple beds. *Age Ageing*, **7**, 25–27

Braatz, J.H. and Pino, A.E. (1972) Therapy and rehabilitation for psychogeriatric patients. *Geriatrics*, **27**, 101–106

Brocklehurst, J.C., Exton-Smith, A.N., Lempert-Barber, S.M., Hunt, L.P. and Palmer, M.K. (1978) Fracture of the femur in old age. A two-centre study of associated clinical factors and the cause of the fall. *Age Ageing*, **7**, 7–15

Campbell, A.J. (1976) Femoral neck fractures in elderly women: a prospective study. *Age Ageing*, **5**, 102–109

Ceder, L., Ekelund, L., Inerot, S., Lindberg, L., Odberg, E. and Sjolin, C. (1979) Rehabilitation after hip fracture in the elderly. *Acta Orthop. Scand.*, **50**, 681–688

Clark, M., Clark, S., Odell, A. and Jagger, C. (1984) The elderly at home: health and social status. *Hlth Trends*, **16**, 3–7

Clarke-Williams, M.J. (1983) Ward furniture and equipment. *Care of the Long-Stay Elderly Patient* (ed. M. J. Denham), Croom Helm, London, pp. 71–89

Cleveland, M., Bosworth, D.M., Thompson, F.R., Wilson, H.J. and Ishizvka, T. (1959) A ten-year analysis of intertrochanteric fractures of the femur. *J. Bone Joint Surg.*, **41A**, 1399–1408

Connolly, M.J., Wilkinson, E., Flanagan, S. and Mulley, G.P. (1990) Nurses' attitudes to and use of patient hoists in hospital. *Clin. Rehab.*, **4**, 13–17

Connolly, M.J. and Wilson, A.S. (1990a) Feeding aids. *Br. Med. J.*, **301**, 378–379

Connolly, M.J. and Wilson, A.S. (1990b) Kitchen aids. *Br. Med. J.*, **301**, 114–115

Corrado, O.J. (1988) Hearing aids. *Br. Med. J.*, **296**, 33–35

Crewe, R. (1982) Patient transportation in Wessex. *Care, Sci. Pract.*, **1**, 18–21

Davies, K. (1990) Emergency alarms. *Br. Med. J.*, **300**, 1713–1715

Denne, W.A. (1979) An objective assessment of the sheepskins used for decubitus sore prophylaxis. *Rheumatol. Rehab.*, **18**, 23–29

Devas, M.B. (1976) Geriatric orthopaedics. *Ann. Roy. Coll. Surg. Engl.*, **58**, 16–21

Dobrin, L. (1980) Origin and evolution of the Walkerette. *Mount Sinai J. Med.*, **47**, 172–174

Dudley, N.J. (1990) Aids for visual impairment. *Br. Med. J.*, **301**, 1151–1153

Editorial (1990) Preventing pressure sores. *Lancet*, **ii**, 1311–1312

Edwards, B.G. (1986) Contralateral and ipsilateral cane usage by patients with total knee or hip replacement. *Arch. Phys. Med. Rehab.*, **67**, 734–740

Ellis, M. (1988) Choosing easy chairs for the disabled. *Br. Med. J.*, **296**, 701–702

Evans, J.G., Prudham, D. and Wandless, I. (1979) A prospective study of fractured promimal femur: incidence and outcome. *Publ. Hlth*, **93**, 235–241

Farrow, R. (1977) Rehabilitation of intertrochanteric fractures at home: an insight. *Practitioner*, **219**, 246–250

Fisher, J. and Jackson, M. (1988) Walking aids. *Rehabilitation of the Physically Disabled Adult* (eds C.J. Goodwill and M.A. Chamberlain), Croom Helm, London, pp. 775–786

Gelbier, S. and Hopes, I. (1979) The dental needs of day-patients and in-patients at a London hospital. *Publ. Hlth*, **93**, 350–357

Greatorex, I.F. (1986) Femoral neck fractures – improving efficiency in the care of elderly people. *Commun. Med.*, **8**, 185–190

Hall, J., Clarke, A.K. and Harrison, R. (1990) Guidelines for prescription of walking frames. *Physiotherapy*, **76**, 118–120

Hamzeh, M.A., Bowker, P. and Sayegh, A. (1988) The energy costs of ambulation using two types of walking frame. *Clin. Rehab.*, **2**, 119–123

Hart, D., Bowling, A., Ellis, M. and Silman, A. (1990) Locomotor disability in very elderly people: value of a programme for screening and provision of aids for daily living. *Br. Med. J.*, **301**, 216–220

Haworth, R.J. and Hopkins, J. (1980) Use of aids following total hip replacement. *Occup. Ther.*, **43**, 398–400

Health Services Advisory Committee (1985) *The Lifting of Patients in the Health Services*, HMSO, London

Herbst, K.G. and Humphrey, C. (1981) Prevalence of hearing impairment in the elderly living at home. *J. Roy. Coll. Gen. Pract.*, **31**, 155–160

Hillman, J.S. (1988) Aids for low vision in the elderly. *Br. Med. J.*, **296**, 102–103

Hollis, M. (1976) Re-education of walking. In *Practical Exercise Therapy*, Blackwell Scientific, Oxford, p. 112

Hunt, A. (1978) *The elderly at home. A study on people aged sixty five and over in the community in England in 1976*, Office of Population Censuses and Surveys, HMSO, London

Jensen, J.S., Tondevold, E. and Sorensen, P.H. (1979) Social rehabilitation following hip fractures. *Acta Orthop. Scand.*, **50**, 777–785

Jette, A.M., Harris, B.A., Cleary, P.D. and Campion, E.W. (1987) Functional recovery after hip fracture. *Arch. Phys. Med. Rehab.*, **68**, 735–739

Karumo, I. (1977) Recovery and rehabilitation of elderly subjects with femoral neck fractures. *Ann. Chir. Gynaecol.*, **66**, 170–176

King's Fund Centre for Health Services Development (1989) *The prevention and management of pressure sores in health districts.* A document produced by the Pressure Sore Study Group. King's Fund, London

Kostuik, J.P. and Ferrie, G. (1985) Pressure sores in elderly patients. *J. Bone Joint Surg.*, **67B**, 1–2

McGrowther, C.W., Castleden, C.M., Duffin, H. and Clarke, M. (1986) Provision of services for incontinent elderly people at home. *J. Epidem. Commun. Hlth*, **40**, 134–138

Marulec, I., Librach, G. and Schadel, M. (1970) Epidemiological study of accidents among residents of homes for the elderly. *J. Geront.*, **25**, 342–346

Mayfield, W. (1984) *A survey of walking frame issue and use,* University of Technology, Institute for Consumer Ergonomics, Loughborough

Miller, C.W. (1978) Survival and ambulation following hip fracture. *J. Bone Joint Surg.*, **60A**, 930–933

Mitchell, S.C.M. (1991) Dressing aids. *Br. Med. J.*, **302**, 167–169

Mulley, G.P. (1988) Walking sticks. *Br. Med. J.*, **296**, 475–476

Mulley, G.P. (1990) Walking frames. *Br. Med. J.*, **300**, 925–927

Mulley, G.P. (1991) *More everyday aids and appliances.* A compendium of articles published by the British Medical Journal, London

Nassar, A. (1980) Hearing impairment in the elderly. *Br. Med. J.*, **281**, 1354

Nichols, P.J.R. and Mowat, A. G. (1972) *Splints, walking aids and appliances for the arthritic patient,* Reports on Rheumatic Diseases, No. 48. Arthritis and Rheumatism Council London

North Tyneside Social Services (1982) *The handicapped in the Community. A study of people living in North Tyneside in 1980.* North Tyneside Social Services, Newcastle

Paul, J.P. (1991) Personal communication

Penn, N.D. (1988) Toilet aids. *Br. Med. J.*, **296**, 918–919

Potter, B.E. and Wallace, W.A. (1990) Crutches. *Br. Med. J.*, **301**, 1037–1039

Rosenblatt, D.E., Campion, E.W. and Mason, M. (1986) Rehabilitation home visits. *J. Am. Geriat. Soc.*, **34**, 441–447

Scales, J., Lowthian, P.T., Poole, A.G. and Ludman, W.R. (1982) 'Vaperm' patient support system: a new general purpose mattress. *Lancet*, **ii**, 1150–1152

Siegal, R.J., Vistres, L.M. and Laub, D.R. (1973) The use of water beds for the prevention of pressure sores. *Plastic Reconstr. Surg.*, **51**, 31–37

Sklaroff, S.A. and Atkinson, F.I. (1987) Disabled patients in acute hospital wards. *Clin. Rehab.*, **1**, 127–131

Smith, N. (1988) Aids for urinary incontinence. *Br. Med. J.*, **296**, 772–773

Stapleton, M. (1986) Preventing pressure sores: an evaluation of three products. *Geriat. Nurs.*, March/April, 23–25

Stott, S. and Gray, D.H. (1980) A prospective study of hip fracture patients. *N.Z. Med. J.*, **91**, 165–169

Thomas, T.G. and Stevens, R.S. (1974) Social effects of fractures of the neck of the femur. *Br. Med. J.*, **3**, 456–458

Tinetti, M.E. (1987) Factors associated with serious injury during falls by ambulatory nursing home residents. *J. Am. Geriat. Soc.*, **35**, 644–648

Ungar, D.M. and Warne, R.W. (1986) Morbidity following successful treatment of proximal femoral fractures. *Aust. Fam. Phys.*, **15**, 1157–1159

Versluysen, M. (1985) Pressure sores in elderly patients: the epidemiology related to hip operations. *J. Bone Joint Surg.*, **67B**, 10–13

Versluysen, M. (1986) How elderly patients with femoral fracture develop pressure sores in hospital. *Br. Med. J.*, **292**, 1311–1313

Waghorn, D.J., Griffiths, G.L. and Kelly, T.W.J. (1988) Urinary catheters. *Br. Med. J.*, **296**, 1128

Waters, K. (1988) Hoists. *Br. Med. J.*, **296**, 1114–1117

White, E.G. (1988) Special footwear. *Br. Med. J.*, **296**, 548–550

White, E.G. and Mulley, G.P. (1989) Footwear worn by the over 80s. *Clin. Rehab.*, **3**, 23–25

Whittle M.W. (1991) *Gait Analysis: An Introduction*, Butterworth–Heinemann, Oxford

Williamson, J., Stokoe, I.H., Gray, S., Fisher, M., Smith, A., McGhee, A. and Stephenson, E. (1964) Old people at home: their unreported needs. *Lancet*, **i**, 1117–1120

Young, J.B. and George, J. (1987) When assessing elderly people, don't forget their spectacles. *Geriat. Med.*, **17**, 12–13

Young, J.B., Belfield, P.W., Mascie-Taylor, B.H. and Mulley, G.P. (1985) The neglected hospital wheelchair. *Br. Med. J.*, **291**, 1388–1389

Young, J.B. (1990a) Pressure sores: do mattresses work? *Lancet*, **i**, 182–183

Young, J.B. (1990b) Aids to prevent pressure sores. *Br. Med. J.*, **300**, 1002–1004

19

Medicolegal aspects of care of the elderly

Diana Brahams

Introduction

Elderly patients, like any others, must be treated with skill and care when these can be ascertained, in accordance with their wishes. They must not have medical treatment imposed upon them; treatment given to a lucid adult without his consent or contrary to his stated wishes will be unlawful and a battery/trespass to the person.

Aged patients must therefore be treated with the ordinary respect due to any autonomous individual and their freely given consent, when they have the capacity to give it, must be obtained.

These patients are a vulnerable group, medically and socially, and care must be taken to ensure that their consent is freely given. They should not be intimidated, hurried or coerced into having treatment that they do not really wish to undergo. A need for orthopaedic surgery will often arise as a result of an accident which renders the person distressed, confused and in pain and probably fearful of what may be next. As with any other patient in such circumstances there may be a partner or other family member left at home who requires care and about whose welfare the patient may be concerned. Furthermore, consciously or subconsciously, the elderly patient who has been rushed into hospital after an accident is also likely to suffer a loss of confidence coupled with the anxiety that he or she may not regain sufficient fitness to resume his preferred independent life-style. Similarly, he may worry that he may not be perceived fit enough by well-wishers and family who consider him to be now too frail and vulnerable. In such circumstances, the future may seem to hold little promise and much pain for the elderly patient.

All these factors when added to the patient's pre-existing anxieties and medical and social problems, are likely to affect the patient's judgment and his capability to make logical and reasoned decisions with regard to his treatment. From this, it will be easily appreciated that the patient becomes very vulnerable to pressure (subtle and obvious) from both the medical staff and his family. This should always be borne in mind when consent is sought.

Sometimes the patient may have been rendered unconcious or so confused and upset that he cannot give a reasoned and proper consent to medical treatment – indeed he may have been demented or otherwise impaired well before the need for treatment arose. What then is the legal position? In brief, the law requires the doctor to act in what he considers (on reasonable grounds) to be the patient's best interests. Sometimes, however, the best option will not be clear or may carry significant risks and the doctor will be well advised to take a second opinion and/or to consult with members of the patient's family, carers and other medical or social services personnel.

The patient's family may be able to advise as to what the patient might have wanted but cannot give a valid legal consent on his behalf.

Although the issue of capacity to consent is particularly important with regard to the elderly patient, it is only one of many medicolegal matters which may arise in the course of medical care as with any other patient. Accordingly, some of the key underlying legal principles which apply in this context are considered below as well as the problems which may arise with consent. (See also the recommendations and guidance provided in the Report of the Royal College of Psychiatrists (1989) which is considered at the end of this chapter.)

General principles of law and the doctor's duty of care

The test of competence

The law imposes on the doctor *a duty of care* towards his patient, old and young alike, but the standard or quality of the care he is under a duty to provide will be judged by the courts by reference to medical standards prevailing at the time the treatment was given. A doctor must act with reasonable skill and care and with reasonable competence and in accordance with a practice thought proper by a responsible body of medical opinion, which need not necessarily be a majority view. Thus, a doctor whose practice conformed with one thought proper by a responsible body of medical opinion at the time it was given, will not be found negligent in law. However, if a doctor falls below this standard of practice, he will then be found guilty of professional negligence which should never be confused with neglect.

A doctor may be very caring and attentive and yet incompetent and thus negligent. However, if he is to be able to recover compensation by way of an award of damages, the patient must prove on the balance of probabilities that the doctor's negligence complained of caused him injury and damage. Fortunately, not every negligent medical treatment causes the patient injury; it may be reversed in time or the injury may be minor and transient.

Conversely, many adverse treatment outcomes are not caused by incompetent medical treatment but by the patient's underlying medical condition or extraneous factors. However, a failure to warn of the possibility of such a risk materializing may raise the idea in the patient's mind that it was unexpected and the suspicion that this outcome *should not have happened and that it may due to negligence*. Failure to respond to reasonable enquiries and offer a proper explanation is likely to fuel any suspicions of negligence, incompetence and worst of all, a 'cover-up' by doctors and nursing staff.

Thus a failure to comply with a practice thought proper by a responsible medical opinion will amount to negligence in law, and if it can be shown to have caused injury, will be actionable in damages. This is the test which applies across the board to all kinds of medical treatment and care, from counselling, to operative, to drug prescription and to discharge home. The legal test of a doctor's competence or lack of it was laid down in 1957 by Mr Justice McNair in the case of *Bolam v Friern Hospital Management Committee* [1957] 1 WLR 582, who said: 'A doctor is not guilty of negligence if he has acted in accordance with a practice accepted as proper by a responsible body of medical men skilled in that particualar art ... Putting it the other way round, a doctor is not negligent if he is acting in accordance with such a practice, merely because there is a body of opinion that takes a contrary view ...'

From this it can be seen that the test laid down by the law in *Bolam* provides for doctors' professional treatment to be judged by their 'responsible' medical peers and has since been endorsed many times over. It also calls for a doctor to be judged in accordance with his specialty and post. Thus, a general practitioner should be judged by the standards to be expected of reasonably competent general practitioners generally (irrespective of their date of qualification or personal experience in the field) and a hospital doctor similarly, *Wilsher v Essex Area Health Authority* [1987] QB 730. In that case, the plaintiff was a child who was born very prematurely suffering from various problems including oxygen deficiency. His prognosis was poor. The unit was staffed by two consultants, a senior registrar, several junior doctors and trained nurses. Unfortunately, a junior and inexperienced doctor mistakenly placed a catheter into a vein rather than an artery but then very properly asked a senior registrar to check what he had done. The registrar failed to notice the mistake, and when replacing the catheter some hours later, made exactly the same error himself. In both instances the monitor failed to record accurately the oxygen tension in the plaintiff's arterial blood with the consequence that the plaintiff was given excessive quantities of oxygen.

Subsequently, the baby was found to be almost blind. He sued in negligence claiming that this was caused by the excess of oxygen delivered to him in the unit and the trial judge awarded damages. The Court of Appeal dismissed the appeal but ultimately it was allowed by the House of Lords on the issue of causation

– namely, it was not established that the excess oxygen caused his blindness since there were a number of other possible causes. However, the Court of Appeal's decision included some guidance on the standard of care which was to be expected from doctors holding different hospital posts in a specialist unit and this aspect of the case was not disapproved by the House of Lords.

The Vice-Chancellor, Sir Nicolas Browne-Wilkinson said that the Court had been told that it was not the practice to formulate claims on the basis that a health authority which failed to provide doctors of adequate skill and experience should be directly liable in negligence. However, he saw no reason why this should not be done. Further, the Court found that the lack of experience of any individual doctor (who may be new to the post) did not and should not provide an answer to a claim in negligence (on the basis that given the individual doctor's training and experience more could not reasonably be expected). The doctor was bound in law to meet normal standards of competence in accordance with the post he held.

Errors of judgment

An error of professional medical judgment will not necessarily be negligent; it may or may not be depending on all the circumstances and the application of the *Bolam* test (and see the House of Lords decision in *Whitehouse v Jordan* [1981] 1 All ER 267). In that case a baby was born with brain damage after a trial by forceps followed by an emergency caesarean section. The trial judge found the obstetrician negligent, but this decision was overturned on appeal.

Different schools of thought regarding treatment

Readers will remember that a doctor has only to comply with a practice thought proper by a responsible body of medical opinion, not all medical peers or even a majority of them. In a medical negligence action there are likely to be different schools of medical opinion fielded by the opposing parties, so it is not enough for the plaintiff to find expert medical opinion which supports his claim if there is a responsible body of opinion which supports the case made by the defendant. In such a case the Court in coming to its decision is not entitled to 'prefer' one body of expert evidence or school of thought to another,

see *Maynard v West Midlands Regional Health Authority* [1985] 1 All ER 635. In that case, the trial judge purported to apply the *Bolam* test but the Court of Appeal and later the House of Lords stated that in practice he had found the school of expert medical opinion offered by the plaintiff more to his liking than the other offered by the defendant doctors. (See also *Hughes v Waltham Forest Health Authority*, [1991] 2 Med L R 155).

The doctor owes his patient a duty of care whether or not he is to be paid fees for his treatment under a contract providing a relationship is entered into. A doctor has an ethical obligation but not a legal one to stop and help at the scene of an accident or at a social event, etc. Once he does so he must act with skill and care though if there are special or adverse circumstances and few resources available, this would be taken into account and there are very few instances known of negligence claims brought against doctors acting as 'good samaritans'.

'Informed' consent in the UK

The *Bolam* test of the reasonably competent practitioner in the relevant field applies also in the field of 'informed consent' and indeed the *Bolam* test was specifically endorsed by the House of Lords in the case of *Sidaway v Governors of Bethlem Royal Hospital and Others* [1985] AC 871 as extending to all kinds of treatment with no distinction in law made between 'therapeutic' and 'non-therapeutic', elective or essential, etc. The Court accepted that how much information should be disclosed in an individual case is a matter for the doctor's clinical judgment, but at the same time the Court made it clear that a patient needed to be given sufficient information in order to come to an 'informed' decision.

Since the decision in *Sidaway* two Court of Appeal decisions have made it clear that the law in the UK does not require the doctor to provide a blanket disclosure of all information known to him or his department and/or of every risk however statistically improbable or minor to be spelled out, and/or every possible alternative treatment to be discussed and raised. (See *Blyth v Bloomsbury Health Authority* [1987] PMILL vol 3 no 2).

The plaintiff in the *Sidaway* case had complained about non-disclosure of a 1–2% risk of paralysis before agreeing to an operation on her cervical spine for the relief of long-standing pain. She had not raised any questions of her own, but this aspect was considered by the House of Lords, who said they should be answered as truthfully and as fully as would be required by the plaintiff. The House of Lords also indicated that really serious risks which were not remote should always be disclosed but only gave two examples, a 10% risk of a stroke and 4% risk of death which were extracted from two American cases.

The House of Lords by a majority of 4:1 expressly rejected the North American so-called 'prudent patient' test, i.e. disclosure by the doctor of information which a prudent patient in the position of the individual patient concerned looked at objectively, would want to know. The prudent patient test requires the disclosure of all 'material' risks.

In fact, in the *Sidaway* case Lord Scarman, the sole proponent of the 'prudent patient' test there, held that a 1–2% risk of paralysis was not such a risk, though it was clearly one which *subjectively* the patient in the case, Mrs Amy Sidaway, definitely did want to know about. She had earlier satisfied the trial judge that had she been informed that such a risk of paralysis existed she would never have undergone the treatment – generally a necessary requisite for a successful claim in negligence based on a failure to disclose a risk which occurred. However, other injuries, such as shock and depression, which might have been decreased or avoided by an appropriate warning, may also form the basis for a claim in damages.

In practice, however, statistically significant risks are not the only ones which a doctor may be advised to disclose as doctors have discovered to their costs in claims for damages arising out of a failure to warn of future fertility when carrying out sterilization operations, see *Thake v Maurice* [1986] 1 All ER 497 (but compare *Eyre v Measday* [1986] 1 All ER 488). Litigation in this field, with its concomitant claims for the upkeep of the unwanted baby, has undoubtedly affected current medical practice, encouraging fuller disclosures of possible risks and failures. This fuller disclosure accords generally with what is sought by today's average patients, who by and large (but not uniformly) are eager for more information than earlier generations. The desire for more information by patients at large, which is fanned by well-publicized legal cases

and medicolegal coverage on television, radio and in the press, is being reflected in the content of the current consent forms offered for sterilization and related procedures.

It is also highly significant that the UK Department of Health's management document *Patient Consent to Examination or Treatment, A Guide to Consent for Examination or Treatment* (1990) seems to be keen to promote practices as standard which go well beyond the low watermark currently practised by some 'responsible' medical practitioners and the endorsement of these practices and the minimum bare requirements laid down by the House of Lords in the decision of *Sidaway* and the interpretation given to the *Sidaway* judgments by the Court of Appeal in *Blyth* and other cases. If the Department's new documents and consent forms are indeed to be uniformly adopted and are to form the background for all NHS contracts and medical treatment, practitioners who do not conform with these recommendations as a minimum may find themselves no longer acting in accordance with a practice thought proper by 'responsible' medical opinion.

At the time of issue in September 1990, the advice went beyond what the law required on the basis of the *Bolam* test and the House of Lords guidance given in *Sidaway*. It seems to me to mark a positive step in the right direction of a fuller disclosure of options and risks and a response to modern patient demands. Some would take a different view (Heneghan, 1991). The new advice does not seem to me to banish the doctor's clinical discretion on how much detailed information must be provided in each case, but to provide broad general norms for guidance on how 'well-informed' (as opposed to mere 'informed') consent is to be achieved. It suggests that 'where treatment carries substantial risks the patient must be advised of this by a doctor so that consent may be well-informed'.

The disclosure by the doctor of alternative treatment options though, alas, not necessarily required unless all responsible medical opinion would support it, is also promoted by the new documents in fairly circumscribed terms – note the inclusion of the word 'reasonably' and 'may': '... where a choice of treatment might reasonably be offered the health professional may always advise the patient of his/her recommendations together with reasons for selecting a particular course of action'. The advice considers that sufficient information must normally be given to ensure that the patient understands the nature, consequences and substantial risks, and can thus take a decision on the basis of that information'.

If the patient refuses treatment on the grounds that he regards the risks to outweigh the benefits as he perceives them, that is his right, and it should be honoured. However, it is the doctor's clinical responsibility to present the medical picture in a sensible and balanced way which does not discourage the patient from undergoing treatment which is indicated and likely to be of benefit. Risks and percentages of risks should be explained in terms which are readily understandable by the patient. However, at the end of the day, it must never be forgotten that though a risk may be statistically small, say 1 in 200, when it actually materializes, it is a 100% disaster for that individual not a 0.5% disaster.

Consequences of treatment given without 'informed consent'

Where a patient has consented to the treatment but was not told of certain risks which unluckily materialized, he/she is not entitled to claim that his/her consent was vitiated from the start and to sue the doctor in battery. This was made quite clear by Mr Justice Bristow in the case of *Chatterton v Gerson* [1981] QB 432. Any claim must be framed in negligence and prove on the balance of probabilities that the doctor in failing to warn of the risk that materialized was negligent and fell below the standard to be expected of a reasonably competent doctor in his field.

Mr Justice Bristow explained that 'What the court has to do in each case is to look at all the circumstances and say, "Was there a real consent?" I think justice requires that in order to vitiate the reality of consent there must be a greater failure of communication between doctor and patient than that involved in a breach of duty if the claim is based on negligence. When the claim is based on trespass to the person, once it is shown that the consent is unreal, then what the plaintiff would have decided if she had been given the information which would have prevented vitiation of the reality of her consent is irrelevant. In my judgment once the patient is informed in broad terms of the nature of the procedure which is intended, and gives her consent, that consent is real, and the cause of the

action on which to base a claim for failure to go into risks and implications is negligence, not trespass. Of course if information is withheld in bad faith, the consent will be vitiated by fraud.'

Thus, in a claim for negligent non-disclosure of risks, the patient has not only to prove negligence but also as in any other case, causation, namely, that had he or she been appropriately informed he/she would have refused the treatment. However, there may be circumstances where even if it can be proved that consent would have been given the failure to warn caused actionable shock and distress to the patient (which was one of the heads of damage in *Malette v Shulman*, the case of the Jehovah's witness who was given an unauthorized blood transfusion and which is considered below).

An unsuccessful repeat operation on the cervical spine of a woman performed in 1981 resulted in immediate tetraplegia. The surgeon recognized that there was a substantial risk of total paralysis (up to 25%) from the operation even when competently done, but that on the other hand, if the condition remained untreated, total paralysis would supervene within 9 months. He did not advise the patient of these factors before seeking her consent for the operation. In an action brought for negligence, Mr Justice Hutchinson sitting in the High Court found that even if she had been warned the patient would have elected to have the operation (which with the benefit of hindsight she denied). However, the judge nonetheless awarded compensation to the plaintiff for shock and depression consequent on discovering without prior warning that she had been rendered tetraplegic.

In the UK the legal concept of 'informed consent' is more circumscribed than in North America. That said, it must not be forgotten that it is the right of a lucid adult to decide what shall be done to his/her body. Medical treatment which is imposed without consent or against the will of the patient in such a case will amount to a battery (or in layman's terms, an assault) and/or a trespass on the person which will be actionable in law. This may occur by mistake, for example, if there is confusion over the identity of the patient or which part of his anatomy is to be operated on. Thus, a consent to an operation on the right hip will not validate an operation performed on the left one and the patient would be entitled to sue in battery and presumably also in negligence.

Similarly, consent given for specific treatment does not extend to any further treatment which is not essential to preserve the life of the patient but which the surgeon thinks might be conveniently carried out at the same time (see *Marshall v Curry* [1933] 3 DLR 260).

When an unconscious patient is admitted to a hospital as an emergency, treatment which is necessary to preserve life and health should be performed; the patient's consent will be deemed unless there are clear indications to the contrary such as in the case of a Jehovah's witness who carries a 'No transfusion!' card or the patient concerned has clearly left prior instructions to cover the eventuality. In a recent Canadian case, a casualty surgeon disregarded a Jehovah's witness's card and transfused her (saving her life) after a serious car accident. She sued him for battery and was awarded damages (but not her costs) (see the Canadian case of *Malette v Shulman et al* [1988] 47 DLR (4TH) 18 and see also Brahams, 1990).

In Britain it is uncertain whether more than nominal damages would have been awarded in these circumstances. However, where refusal was ignored and the outcome was unsuccessful, there could be substantial liability in damages, as where the patient contracted AIDS. In such a case, though the courts in Britain might be reluctant to support such a claim, the doctor could nonetheless conceivably find himself liable in damages for all that ensued, whether reasonably foreseeable or not, which could include long-term private care, loss of earnings and pain and suffering (see the remarks of Bristow J in *Chatterton v Gerson* above and the Canadian case of *Allen v Mount Sinai Hospital* below).

Where the procedure is elective and not an emergency, and the patient refuses to allow a blood transfusion, the doctor may decline to undertake treatment if he regards this as imposing an unreasonable fetter on his clinical and management options. He may, however, accept the conditions, but in such a case he should warn the patient of the potential dangers to her life and limb to which she is likely to be exposed. He should also ensure that her wishes and his warning of the consequences are witnessed and evidenced.

Where a patient does impose a restriction on treatment, such as not receiving a particular drug or not using a particular vein, for example in her right arm, this must be respected. Treatment given against the patient's expressed views will be a battery and the adverse consequences which flow will be actionable in damages. In the Canadian case of *Allen v Mount Sinai Hospital et al* [1980] 109 DLR (3d) 634, the plaintiff entered the defendant hospital for a minor procedure. She met the anaesthetist outside the operating theatre and said to him, 'Please don't touch my left arm, you'll have nothing but trouble there'. The doctor's response was, 'We know what we are doing'.

The plaintiff was then taken into the theatre where the doctor injected sodium pentothal and the other required drugs into her left arm. He had no trouble finding a vein. However a short time afterwards he noticed that the needle had slipped out of the vein causing part of the solution to leak into the interstitial tissues of the limb.

Although normally this would cause the patient to have no more than a sore arm for a day or two, the plaintiff suffered a very severe reaction. She successfully sued the doctor in battery and negligence for damages. The court held that although the doctor had not been negligent in allowing the needle to slip out, the administration of an anaesthetic is a surgical operation which will be a battery unless the patient consents to it. The plaintiff had not consented – indeed she had expressly instructed the doctor not to start the operation in her left arm yet he had done so. It was a battery. Because his responsibility was founded in battery, he was liable for all the consequences which flowed therefrom, whether they were foreseeable or not. Even had nothing gone wrong he would have been liable for nominal damages.

Research and clinical trials

Where the doctor proposes to include the patient in a clinical trial, he should ideally first obtain his consent to do so and if the treatment is new and relatively untested, he should say so and the patient should not feel under pressure to agree. It should also be made clear that he can withdraw at any time. The law as stated in *Sidaway* and applied since does not seem to require doctors to set out all the alternative options in and outside the trial, which may be randomized, provided the treatment on offer is regarded as a proper one and as good as any others available and is appropriate for that patient and in his best interests. This selection of treatment for a patient without a discussion of all alternatives with him accords with what actually occurs in UK hospitals where patients tend not to ask probing questions. The randomization of patients in a clinical trial which compares existing treatments is not a fundamentally very different process but remains a relatively low watermark on compulsory disclosure. Where the treatment is new or relatively untested, for example on elderly patients who may respond differently from young healthy volunteers, this should normally be disclosed.

In the case of *R v Mental Health Act Commission ex parte W*, W was a 27-year old compulsive paedophile who had repeatedly offended. He sought the help of a psychiatrist who initially treated him with high doses of the anti-androgen, cyproterone acetate, but despite increasing dosages, this failed to curb W's sexual urges. The psychiatrist then suggested an experimental regime with goserelin which was manufactured for the treatment of prostatic cancer. He explained how it worked and gave W the data sheet. W was enthusiastic. He had two monthly injections which curbed his sexual urges and a third monthly injection was given. In the meantime the Mental Health Act Commission had been contacted by the psychiatrist, interviewed W and refused their consent to further treatment which they said fell within s57 of the Mental Health Act 1983.

At a hearing the Divisional Court found the treatment fell outside the Mental Health Act and that the Commission had wrongly concluded that W had not given a real consent. Dealing with the question of information with regard to new and experimental treatments, Lord Justice Stuart-Smith (who gave the judgment of the Divisional Court) did not base his decision on *Sidaway*, though he did expressly consider and apply the decision in *Chatterton v Gerson* (neither case was concerned with experimental treatment) which he said was equally appropriate in a public law setting. In response to the argument that it was not, said: 'I confess I do not follow this distinction. He submits that whether or not a patient consents is a matter for the subjective judgment of the Commissioners and they can apply any test which in their discretion they think fit. I cannot accept this. No doubt consent has to be an informed consent in that he knew the nature and likely effect of the treatment. There can be no doubt that the applicant knew this. So too in this case where

the treatment was not routinely used for control of sexual urges and was not sold for this purpose, it was important that the applicant should realize that the use on him was a novel one and the full implications with use on young men had not been studied, since trials had only been involved with animals and older men.'

The incompetent adult patient and medical treatment

For some time it was realized that there was an apparent lacuna in the law dealing with incompetent adults with regard to medical treatment for physical (as opposed to mental) ailments. Where treatment for a mental condition is necessary and consent is not possible or in some cases not forthcoming, treatment may be given under the relevant provisions in the Mental Health Act 1983 or, in very limited circumstances, under the common law where the patient and/or the public are put at risk.

In practice, however, relatives are usually consulted and necessary treatment given on an *ad hoc* commonsense basis, but in truth the relatives giving the 'consent' cannot validly do so in law. The problems arising from a lack of capacity to consent for ethically controversial treatments, such as the sterilization of a mentally handicapped adult woman, surfaced as doctors became concerned about their legal position and applications were made to the court. This concern was heightened further when the House of Lords ruled in *In re B* [1987] 2 All ER 206, that parents on their own could not consent to the sterilization of a mentally handicapped girl below the age of 18 years and before the operation could be performed she had to be made a ward of court so that the court could decide whether the treatment was in truth in her best interests.

In 1989, the House of Lords finally clarified the position in the case of *F v West Berkshire Health Authority* [1989] 2 All ER 545 (see also Brahams, 1989).

Giving the leading judgment, Lord Brandon said that the common law allowed a doctor to treat adults who were incapable of consenting provided the procedure (operation or other treatment) was in the best interests of the patient. The law would regard a treatment as being in the patient's best interests only if it was performed to save life or to ensure improvement or prevent deterioration in physical or mental health. Sick, mentally incapable patients who cannot make decisions on their own behalf will need to rely on others, including doctors, to see their needs are met.

A mentally disabled adult who cannot consent to treatment will, accidents and emergencies apart, usually be in the care of guardians and referred to doctors for treatment or reside in a mental hospital. It would be up to doctors to use 'their best endeavours' to do what was in the best interests of the patient. The lawfulness of such treatment would depend not only on any approval or sanction of the court but on whether the operation or other treatment was in the patient's best interests. The standard that would be applied by the court would be that of the reasonably competent doctor practising in the speciality (as laid down in the *Bolam* test) in deciding medical negligence claims.

Sometimes elderly patients may be depressed and confused by the idea of hospital treatment, but not necessarily lack capacity to decide in relatively simple terms whether or not they want to undergo treatment. They will frequently want to rely on the doctor's advice but should not be coerced into agreement if they are fundamentally unwilling.

It may be difficult on occasion for doctors to assess capacity and whether a patient's mental state is preventing the patient from coming to an 'informed' choice. This problem has recently been considered by the Royal College of Psychiatrists. As its Report (1989) recognizes, the scope of the problem is wide-ranging and there is particular concern about the plight of the demented elderly – some 5% of the population aged over 67 years suffer from dementia, i.e. 375 000 patients. Of these, about 20% are in institutions. The other major group are those adults who suffer from mental handicap, many of whom also reside in institutions of one sort or another. As the Report indicates, 'Issues of how, and how far, to treat patients who cannot give their consent, and whether and how far to restrain them when their behaviour may endanger themselves or others are commonplace. They pervade areas of the health and social services where the Mental Health Act Commission cannot reach, e.g. general and geriatric wards in general hospitals and residential homes. It would be quite arbitrary to suggest

legislation applicable only to those who happened to be in psychiatric wards, when so many very similar incompetent patients presenting identical dilemmas are elsewhere. For example, only 11 000 of the demented elderly are in psychiatric wards, leaving 64 000 in other institutions.'

In its report, the Working Group considered the problems of lack of capacity to consent. It accepted as it had to, that 'When people lacked capacity to take medical treatment decisions, others have to take them on their behalf or they would be deprived of the care they needed and to which they were entitled. In many cases it would not only be lawful for doctors to give treatment, but their common law duty.' (See *In Re F (Mental Patient: Sterilisation) [1990] 2AC 1, HL(F)* and Brahams (1989).

The Working Group began 'with the premise that no one can legally consent to the treatment of a non-volitional patient. Nevertheless, doctors are unlikely to leave such patients to suffer the effects of untreated mental or physical disorder but are likely to continue to treat where appropriate.

There is clearly a distinction between patients who accept treatment, even if they cannot comprehend its nature or purpose, and those who resist it. In the latter case, the first question is: 'Is this treatment essential?' For conditions like diabetes requiring hypoglycaemic agents, and pernicious anaemia needing vitamin B_{12} injections, it evidently is. Second, 'what can be achieved by persuasion?' The answer is, very often, a great deal, in a setting with the right ambience and where staff have established a caring, sympathetic, trustworthy relationship and the approach is not a confrontation. Third, if treatment is needed and persuasion fails: 'is subterfuge justified?' (e.g. secreting medication in food or drink). Occasionally, where the desired objective is thus attained without a battle, it is, and the practice is probably widespread. Finally, 'how far is coercion ever justified?' At this stage, if the treatment is for mental disorder, patients' needs will be best met and their rights best be protected by being placed on an appropriate section of the Mental Health Act. This does not apply, however, to treatment of physical disorder. Here coercion can only be considered if there is danger to life or the risk of serious disability without prompt intervention (e.g. to arrest haemorrhage or to internally fix a fractured bone.

What to do in practice

The report of the Royal College of Psychiatrists (1989) made some helpful suggestions including the following categories of people who might be consulted about matters of treatment. The greater the degree of difficulty the greater should be the degree of consultation.

1. Relatives: but they may not agree with each other and their interests may sometimes be at odds with those of the patient.

2. The general practitioner and/or the community social worker: especially when either or both has a good previous knowledge of the patient.

3. Hospital administrators or Health Authority members: lay people who might reasonably be involved.

4. The local ethical committee: might be persuaded to extend its interest to treatment decisions but would be too unwieldly except for occasional controversial matters which should probably go to court.

5. The consultant making the final decision after consultation with the multidisciplinary team and others, as appropriate, including, perhaps another consultant psychiatrist.

6. Exceptionally, the courts but only appropriate for highly controversial treatments.

Some illustrative practical problems

Below is a 'hierarchy' of treatment situations considered in the report of the Royal College of Psychiatrists.

1. A patient has an infection and needs an antibiotic:
   The doctor should decide which antibiotic and prescribe it. If he decides not to treat the patient however, because the patient's quality of life is so poor that to continue seems inhumane, this decision should be shared with the patient's relatives and the multidisciplinary team.

2. A hospitalized severely mentally handicapped patient's restlessness, wandering, destructiveness and aggression constitute a danger to himself and/or others:
   This is a decision for the multidisciplinary team (including the clinical psychologist), with a big say from the nurses who have to live with the problem most of the time. It may be that the use of a tranquillizer seems the least restrictive alternative when such methods as distraction, occupation, behavioural modification techniques and eliminating a treatable underlying cause (such as faecal impaction or toothache) have not succeeded. It is then up to the doctor to choose the drug and the dosage regimen. If this behaviour is not transitory, but likely to continue, the patient should probably be on Section 3 of the Mental Health Act.

3. A patient needs surgery for a painful condition: acute abdominal:
   The doctor will consult with the senior available surgeon, inform the next of kin, and the operation will be performed. This is regarded as urgently necessary treatment.

4. An elderly paranoid schizophrenic patient on Section 3, refuses an antibiotic for delusional reasons:
   The patient's need for treatment and the irrationality of his refusal will be discussed with any relatives and the multidisciplinary team, and the best strategy for giving the treatment, not excluding subterfuge (even though this may to some extent validate the patient's paranoia!) devised. Coercion will only be justified for life-saving treatment. (The counsel of perfection – to cure the patient's paranoia first – is usually impractical in this situation.)

5. A demented patient has a dense cataract, is partially blind and the ophthalmic surgeon believes that her sight will be much improved by enucleation of the cataract and a lens implant:
   The consultant will explain the situation to the relatives and ward staff and arrange surgery as under (3).

6. A demented patient has cancer of the bowel:
   If the prognosis of surgical treatment is fairly good, (3) applies. If not, palliative surgery may still be justified, to give the patient a more comfortable end. The patient's quality of life after a colostomy may not warrant surgery, or the disease may be too extensive for surgery, in which case that best terminal care will be arranged.

7. A demented patient needs an amputation for gangrene of the foot:

Unless death is very near, the case for amputation to improve the quality of the remaining life could be strong, even though there is no hope that the patient will be able to use crutches, let alone an artificial limb. The support of the family especially and also of the ward team would be sought. If the patient had previously expressed the view, though, that he would rather die than lose a leg, that view, if substantiated, should be respected.

8. Now patient (4) has a fractured femur and will not permit surgery on delusional grounds:

   The consultant consults the senior available orthopaedic surgeon, who advises that without surgery the patient will never walk again. The matter is discussed with the family and the ward staff team, who probably accept that the balance of risk favours surgery, which then goes ahead, as under (3). The operation would be urgently needed to prevent serious irreversible disability but not to prevent loss of life. If, however, there is strong dissent from the family or, possibly, from within the team, another orthopaedic opinion should be sought. If there is still dissent, this is a case when the consultant should consider the options under 'What to do in Practice' (above). How far to go through the options and the final decision itself (which should be capable of justification to a court) would be matters for the consultant's judgment in the particular circumstances and with the background of this guidance. Clearly, the surgeon also would be sharing the burdens and risks of

the case. This is a case where an outside opinion, lay or legal, or a court might be welcomed. As it is, there is likely to be a good deal of variation from one place to another as to whether the patient's femur is operated on.

While the best interests of the patient are clear, as is the duty of care on the doctor, these may conflict with the lack of consent from the patient and the dissent of others. It is unclear what view a court might take.

Conclusion

Surgeons and physicians have to manage the care of elderly individuals by taking into account all of the basic principles of autonomy and best interests, the general guidance available and most particularly, the welfare of the individual person. The doctor must always act with care, competence and compassion and in the best interests of his patient whose views he must always respect if the patient is capable of holding them and making them known.

References

Brahams, D. (1989) Sterilisation of mentally handicapped woman approved by House of Lords. *Lancet*, **i**, 1089

Brahams, D. (1990) Religious beliefs and parental duty. *Lancet*, **336**, 107–108

Heneghan C. (1991) Consent to medical treatment. *Lancet*, **335**, 421

Royal College of Psychiatrists (1989) Consent of non-volitional patients and *de facto* detention of informal patients. Council Report CR6

Appendix

Sources of useful information and organizations specializing in the care of the elderly

Throughout the world there are many organizations which will provide assistance, advice and appliances to ease the lives of elderly patients suffering from orthopaedic and related complaints. The facilities that they provide will also be useful for the spouses, family and carers of such individuals.

Below is a list of such organizations to be found in the United Kingdom but sister organizations and equivalent associations can be found throughout the world.

1. Organizations

Age Concern Bernard Sunley House, 60 Pitcairn Road, Mitcham, Surrey CR4 3LL

Alzheimer's Disease Society Bank Buildings, Fulham Broadway, London SW6 1EP

Arthritis Care 6 Grosvenor Crescent, London SW1X 7ER

Arthritis and Rheumatism Council Copeman House, St Mary's Court, St Mary's Gate, Chesterfield, Derbyshire, S41 7TD

Association of Disabled Professionals The Stables, 73 Pound Road, Banstead, Surrey SM7 2HU

Back Pain Association Grundy House, 31–33 Park Road, Teddington, Middlesex TW11 0AB

British Association for the Hard of Hearing 7–11 Armstrong Road, London W3 7JL

Carers National Association 29 Chilworth Mews, London W2 2RG

Chest, Heart and Stroke Association CHSA House, Whitecross Street, London EC1Y 8JJ

Community Health Group for Ethnic Minorities 28 Churchfield Road, London W3 6EB

Crossroads Care Attendant Scheme 94 Coton Road, Rugby, Warwickshire CV21 4LN and 24 George Square, Glasgow G2 1EG

Help the Aged 32 Dover Street, London W1A 2AP

Jewish Welfare Board 315–317 Ballards Lane, London N12 8LP

National Ankylosing Spondylitis Society 6 Grosvenor Crescent, London SW1X 7ER

National Association for the Relief of Paget's Disease 413 Middleton Road, Middleton, Manchester M24 4QZ

National Council for Carers and their Elderly Dependants 29 Chilworth Mews, London W2 3RG

National Osteoporosis Society PO Box 10, Radstock, Bath BA3 3YB

Parkinson's Disease Society 36 Portland Place, London W1N 3DG

The Royal British Legion 48 Pall Mall, London SW1Y 5JY

St John's Ambulance Brigade 1 Grosvenor Crescent, London SW1X 7EF

2. Appliances and equipment

The Disabled Living Foundation, 380–384 Harrow Road, London W9 2HU, produces publications on many aids of daily living and gives advice and information on all aspects of disability and handicap. Much of its computerized database is accessible by external users via both packet switched (PSS) and direct dial ordinary telephone lines (PSTN).

Disabled Living Centres are to be found in many parts of the UK. They exhibit a large selection of aids for the disabled and provide information for disabled people and their families as well as for health care professionals. As a rule, they do not provide disability aids but they do advise where suitable aids can be obtained.

Rehabilitation Engineering Movement Advisory Panels (REMAP), 25 Mortimer Street, London W1N 8AB, offers solutions to problems which have not been overcome by standard items of equipment. It arranges for engineers to design, make or adapt equipment to meet the special needs of disabled people.

Mary Marlborough Lodge, Nuffield Orthopaedic Centre, Headington, Oxford OX3 7LD, produces a series of authoritative guides on aids and equipment. Titles include 'Wheelchairs', 'Hoists and Walking Aids', 'Personal Care' and 'Clothing and Dressing'.

3.   Housing

Royal Association for Disability and Rehabilitation (RADAR), 25 Mortimer Street, London W1N 8AB, offers guidelines on all aspects of housing for disabled people.

4.   Motoring

The Motability Scheme enables those who receive the mobility allowance to use this to lease cars (which can be adapted if necessary). Details are available from Motability, Boundary House, 91–93 Charterhouse Street, London EC1M 6BT.

The Orange Badge Parking Scheme allows those who are seriously disabled to park in restricted areas and use meters without charge. These badges can be obtained from local authorities.

5.   Financial help and general advice for the disabled

The Department of Social Security produces a range of explanatory leaflets. Titles include:

'Which benefit?' – a particularly useful guide
'Attendance allowance'
'Mobility allowance'
'Aids for the disabled'
'Help with mobility – getting around'
'Long-term sick and disabled – cash help for people at home'
These can be obtained free of charge from DSS Leaflets, PO Box 21, Stanmore, Middlesex HA7 1AY.

6.   Travel, holidays and leisure

The British Red Cross Society, 9 Grosvenor Crescent, London, SW1X 7EJ, provides helpful advice to disabled people wishing to travel within the United Kingdom. They can provide escorts to travel with disabled people, and provide private ambulance and car transport. Contact the local branch, whose address will be in the telephone directory.

The Automobile Association Hotel and Information Services Department, Fanum House, Basingstoke, Hampshire RG21 2EA, produces the 'AA Guide for the Disabled', which gives details of amenities in restaurants and accommodation in Great Britain.

Arthritis Care, 6 Grosvenor Crescent, London SW1X 7ER, has specially adapted holiday centres in England and Scotland.

A range of leaflets on holidays for the disabled is obtainable from Holiday Care Service, 2 Old Bank Chambers, Station Road, Horley, Surrey RH6 9HW.

RADAR produces access guides to many British towns and cities. Their 'Directory for Disabled People' published by Woodhead-Faulkner (Publishers Ltd) is an invaluable guide to holidays, leisure and numerous other aspects of coping with disability.

7.   Sex

The Association to Aid the Sexual and Personal Relationships of the Disabled (SPOD), 286 Camden Road, London N7 0BJ, advises on sexual problems encountered by disabled people.

The Arthritis and Rheumatism Council, 41 Eagle Street, London WC1R 4AR, produces a helpful booklet entitled 'Marriage, Sex and Arthritis'.

Index